VOLUME **5**

Reducing Risks and Complications of Interventional Pain Procedures

VOLUME

5 Reducing Risks and Complications of Interventional Pain Procedures

Volume Editors
Matthew T. Ranson, MD, MS

Assistant Director and Staff Physician
Center for Pain Relief
St. Francis Hospital
Charleston, West Virginia

Jason E. Pope, MD

Napa Pain Institute
Napa, California
Assistant Professor of Clinical Anesthesiology
Division of Multispecialty Anesthesiology
Vanderbilt University Medical Center
Nashville, Tennessee

Series Editor
Timothy R. Deer, MD, DABPM, FIPP

President and CEO
The Center for Pain Relief
Clinical Professor of Anesthesiology
West Virginia University School of Medicine
Charleston, West Virginia

ELSEVIER
SAUNDERS

1600 John F. Kennedy Blvd.
Ste 1800
Philadelphia, PA 19103-2899

REDUCING RISKS AND COMPLICATIONS OF INTERVENTIONAL PAIN
PROCEDURES
(Volume 5: A Volume in the Interventional and Neuromodulatory Techniques
for Pain Management Series by Timothy Deer)   ISBN: 978-1-4377-2220-8

International Standard Book Number: 978-1-4377-2220-8

Content Strategist: Pamela Hetherington
Content Development Specialist: Lora Sickora
Publishing Services Manager: Jeff Patterson
Project Manager: Megan Isenberg
Design Direction: Lou Forgione

Printed in China

Last digit is the print number: 9 8 7 6 5 4 3 2 1

Working together to grow
libraries in developing countries

www.elsevier.com | www.bookaid.org | www.sabre.org

ELSEVIER   BOOK AID International   Sabre Foundation

For Missy for all your love and support.

For Morgan, Taylor, Reed, and Bailie for your inspiration.

To some of those who have taught me a great deal:
John Rowlingson, Ken Alò, Richard North, K. Dean Willis, Eric Grigsby, Giancarlo Barolat, Sam Hassenbusch, Elliot Krames, Peter Staats, Nagy Mekhail, Robert Levy, Sudhir Diwan, David Caraway, Kris Kumar, Joshua Prager, Gabor Racz, and Jim Rathmell.

To my team:
Christopher Kim, Richard Bowman, Matthew Ranson, Brian Yee, Doug Stewart, Wilfrido Tolentino, Jeff Peterson, Venus Welcome, Linda Harless, and Michelle Miller.

To my good friends for their support:
Paul, Kelly, Salim, and Jason.

Timothy R. Deer

I would like to thank my family and partners for their patience and support throughout the course of this work.

Matthew T. Ranson

For Emily for all of her love, prayers, patience, and unyielding support.
For Vivienne for her inspiration.
For my family for keeping me focused.
To my father for his wisdom.

For those whose mentorship has shaped my career:
Timothy Deer, Nagy Mekhail, Eric Grigsby, Leo Kapural, Michael Stanton-Hicks, David Kloth, Salim Hayek, Joshua Prager, David Caraway, and Michael Richardson.

To my friends for all of their support:
Mike, Keith, Sean, and Eric.

Jason E. Pope

Contributors

Pari Azari, MD
Adjunct Professor, Duke University Medical Center, Department of Anesthesiology, Division of Pain Management, Durham, North Carolina
Chapter 12: Complications Associated with Head and Neck Blocks, Upper Extremity Blocks, Lower Extremity Blocks, and Differential Diagnostic Blocks

Jonathan D. Carlson, MD
Clinical Assistant Professor, Midwestern Medical School, Glendale, Arizona
Chapter 7: Complications Related to Radiofrequency Procedures for the Treatment of Chronic Pain

Collin F. M. Clarke, MD, FRCPC
Department of Anesthesiology and Perioperative Medicine, The University of Western Ontario, London, Ontario, Canada
Chapter 12: Complications Associated with Head and Neck Blocks, Upper Extremity Blocks, Lower Extremity Blocks, and Differential Diagnostic Blocks

Eric G. Cornidez, MD
Interventional Pain Specialist, The Pain Center of Arizona; Fellow, Pain Medicine, Department of Anesthesiology, Mayo Clinic Arizona, Scottsdale, Arizona
Chapter 18: Complications of Intraarticular Joint Injections and Musculoskeletal Injections

Justin S. Field, MD
Orthopedic Spine Surgeon, Desert Institute for Spine Care, Phoenix, Arizona
Chapter 8: Complications of Lumbar Spine Fusion Surgery

Patrick W. Hogan, DO
Interventional Pain Medicine Specialist, Clinical Assistant Professor, Midwestern Medical School, Glendale, Arizona
Chapter 7: Complications Related to Radiofrequency Procedures for the Treatment of Chronic Pain

Billy K. Huh, MD, PhD
Professor, Department of Anesthesiology, Pain Division, Duke University Medical Center, Durham, North Carolina
Chapter 12: Complications Associated with Head and Neck Blocks, Upper Extremity Blocks, Lower Extremity Blocks, and Differential Diagnostic Blocks

Iain H. Kalfas, MD, FACS
Cleveland Clinic, Department of Neurosurgery, Cleveland, Ohio
Chapter 9: Complications of Nucleus Replacement and Motion-Sparing Technologies

Chang Po Kuo, MD
Department of Anesthesiology and Pain Medicine, Trigeneral Hospital, Taipei, Taiwan
Chapter 12: Complications Associated with Head and Neck Blocks, Upper Extremity Blocks, Lower Extremity Blocks, and Differential Diagnostic Blocks

Paul J. Lynch, MD
Co-founder, Arizona Pain Specialists, Scottsdale, Arizona
Chapter 2: Complications of Peripheral Nerve Stimulation: Open Technique, Percutaneous Technique, and Peripheral Nerve Field Stimulation
Chapter 6: Complications of Therapeutic Minimally Invasive Intradiscal Procedures
Chapter 17: Complications of Percutaneous Vertebral Augmentation: Vertebroplasty and Kyphoplasty

Christi Makas, DO
Chapter 6: Complications of Therapeutic Minimally Invasive Intradiscal Procedures

Tory L. McJunkin, MD, DABA
Co-founder, Arizona Pain Specialists, Scottsdale, Arizona
Chapter 2: Complications of Peripheral Nerve Stimulation: Open Technique, Percutaneous Technique, and Peripheral Nerve Field Stimulation
Chapter 6: Complications of Therapeutic Minimally Invasive Intradiscal Procedures
Chapter 17: Complications of Percutaneous Vertebral Augmentation: Vertebroplasty and Kyphoplasty

Parag G. Patil, MD, PhD
Assistant Professor, Department of Neurosurgery, University of Michigan Health System, Ann Arbor, Michigan
Chapter 4: Avoidance, Recognition, and Treatment of Complications in Cranial Neuromodulation for Pain

Tristan C. Pico, MD
Interventional Pain Medicine Physician, Arizona Pain Specialists, Chandler, Arizona
Chapter 11: Radiation Safety and Complications of Fluoroscopy, Ultrasonography, and Computed Tomography

Jason E. Pope, MD

Napa Pain Institute, Napa, California; Assistant Professor of Clinical Anesthesiology, Division of Multispecialty Anesthesiology, Vanderbilt University Medical Center, Nashville, Tennessee

Chapter 1: Complications of Spinal Cord Stimulation
Chapter 3: Complications of Cranial Nerve Stimulation
Chapter 14: Complications of Facet Joint Injections and Medial Branch Blocks
Chapter 15: Complications of Radiofrequency Rhizotomy for Facet Syndrome
Chapter 16: Complications of Sacroiliac Joint Injection and Lateral Branch Blocks, Including Water-Cooled Rhizotomy

Matthew T. Ranson, MD, MS

Assistant Director, Staff Physician, Center for Pain Relief, St. Francis Hospital, Charleston, West Virginia

Chapter 5: Complications of Intrathecal Drug Delivery Systems
Chapter 13: Complications of Epidural Injections

Elizabeth Srejic, MS

Louisiana Pain Specialists, New Orleans, Louisiana

Chapter 2: Complications of Peripheral Nerve Stimulation: Open Technique, Percutaneous Technique, and Peripheral Nerve Field Stimulation
Chapter 17: Complications of Percutaneous Vertebral Augmentation: Vertebroplasty and Kyphoplasty

William C. Thompson IV, MD

Interventional Pain Medicine Physician, Valley Pain Consultants, Phoenix, Arizona

Chapter 10: Complications of Spinal Injections and Surgery for Disc Herniation

Preface

I am honored to write this foreword for *Interventional and Neuro-modulatory Techniques for Pain Management Series Volume 5: Reducing Risks and Complications of Interventional Pain Procedures.* While interventional pain management as a specialty has evolved rapidly over the last three decades, so has the technical complexity of the interventions performed. As such, the interventional specialist must be ever cognizant of the potential complications associated with these evolving techniques. In this volume, Deer and colleagues have produced a sentinel collection of practical clinical strategies to which the interventional practitioner can adhere. In doing so, they will not only reduce risks and complication rates but also improve their diagnostic and therapeutic outcomes. While several resources have touched on these topics, none has provided such a comprehensive review of such a varied number of modalities within our armamentarium. The value of this concise outline of best practices, assimilated with the clinical pearls and experience of recognized leaders in the field, cannot be measured or overstated. As such, it is and will remain a fundamental reference for interventional pain medicine for years to come.

Kenneth M. Alò, MD
Clinical Member, The Methodist Hospital Research Institute
President, Houston Texas Pain Management
Houston, Texas
Director, Neurocardiology Section,
Department of Cardiology and Vascular Medicine,
Monterrey Technical University
Monterrey, Mexico

Acknowledgments

I would like to acknowledge Jeff Peterson for his hard work on making this project a reality, and Michelle Miller for her diligence to detail on this and all projects that cross her desk.

I would like to acknowledge Lora Sickora, Pamela Hetherington, and Megan Isenberg for determination, attention to detail, and desire for excellence in bringing this project to fruition.

Timothy R. Deer

Contents

I Neurostimulation

1 Complications of Spinal Cord Stimulation

Jason E. Pope

CHAPTER OVERVIEW

Chapter Synopsis: Implantation of spinal stimulators for relief of neuropathic and ischemic pain has grown tremendously in recent years. As the technique becomes more prevalent, its associated complications should be considered. Appropriate subspecialty training and proper attention to patient selection can reduce the risk of complications. Roughly one-third of patients who receive spinal stimulation experience complications, most of which require a revision in device placement. Despite the need for revision, most patients still rate the procedure a success. The risk of complications arising drops dramatically 1 year after implantation. Problems arise mainly from technical limitations of the device, notably lead migration or fracture. Biologic complications have become far less common as the implantation technique has matured. The most common side effects are pain over the device and surface infections. Rarely, more severe consequences can arise, including deep infection, epidural abscess, seroma or hematoma, dural puncture, and immune reactions.

Important Points:

- Appropriate Accreditation Council for Graduate Medical Education mentored subspecialty training in interventional pain management is vital to ensure patient-centered care.
- Accurate and expertly placed needles in appropriately selected patients are essential to ensure accurate diagnosis and successful treatment.
- Complications associated with spinal cord stimulation (SCS) rarely impact patient morbidity or mortality.
- Approximately 30% to 40% of patients undergoing SCS will have a complication, and nearly 80% of them require a revision.
- Despite this, 85% of patients undergoing revision surgery are satisfied with the results.
- About 11% of patients who have a spinal cord stimulator have a complication requiring explant.
- Biologic complications commonly occur within 3 months of implant, although infections can rarely present much later. Technical complications typically occur within 2 years of implant.
- Common biologic complications include infection, pain over the device, seroma, and dural puncture.
- Common technical complications include lead migration and lead fracture and (less commonly) battery malfunction.
- Devastating infectious and technical complications, although rare, have been reported and deserve special attention.

Introduction

Neurosurgical treatments for pain have historically fallen under the headings of anatomic, ablative, or augmentative, and before the gate control theory was proposed by Melzack and Wall,[1] little attention was directed toward augmentative therapies. Spinal cord stimulation (SCS) has become one of the most useful interventional therapies to treat neuropathic and ischemic pain since its introduction as an intrathecal device by Shealy et al[2] in 1967.

Current estimates suggest that more than 27,000 spinal cord stimulator implants were performed in 2007 alone in the United States,[3] and this number will likely increase as SCS is used earlier in treatment algorithms for neuropathic pain,[4] supported by cost effectiveness and successful outcomes.[5]

One can appreciate that increased use of the technique also increases the incidence and prevalence of associated complications, which range from the mundane to the devastating. Recent reviews place the overall incidence of complications associated with spinal cord stimulation to be approximately between 14% and 43%.[6] Cameron[7] performed an extensive review of the literature extending over 3679 patients, concluding an overall mean complication rate with SCS of 36%. Moreover, Kumar et al[8] reported that complications requiring revisions were approximately 25% to 33% and

approximately 85% of reoperation patients were satisfied with the results.[9] Furthermore, Rosenow et al[10] retrospectively determined that in 289 patients who underwent spinal cord stimulator implants, 46% required revision, and of those, almost half required more than one.

It should be noted, however, that the innate nature and limitations of current SCS technology requires vigilance and, as a consequence of changes in impedance and battery life, either reprogramming or surgical revision. It is far from a "just set it and forget it" device, and although adjustments need to be made, the incidence of complications dramatically decreases after the first 12 months.

As with any treatment plan, complication avoidance begins with patient selection. Patients with local infection near the injection site, coagulopathy, allergy to injectate, or comorbidities or conditions that prevent fluoroscopic needle guidance or consent should be avoided. Patient selection regarding psychometric testing deserves special mention. It is well established that concurrent psychiatric illness reduces interventional treatment success rates[11] and that approximately 20% to 45% of pain patients have accompanying psychopathology.[12] Therefore it is essential that appropriate measures be taken to diagnose, treat, or exclude unsuitable

Table 1-1: Reported Complications of Spinal Cord Stimulation

Complication	Frequency
Overall	14%–43%[6,17]
Complication requiring revision	25%–33%,[8] 23%[17]
Complication requiring explant	11%[17]

Table 1-2: Technical Complications Reported for Spinal Cord Stimulation

Complication	Frequency
Lead migration (loss of stimulation) requiring revision	11%,[21] 13.2%[22]
Lead integrity violation requiring revision	6%,[21] 9%[22]
Loose connection	0.4%[7]
Hardware malfunction, equipment failure	2.9%,[7] 6.5%[17]
Battery failure	1.6%[7]
Central nervous system electrical injury from aberrant stimulator activation	Case report[25]
Misplacement of epidural lead	Case report[24]

candidates. Instruments described to aid in identifying the presence of clinically significant psychopathology include the Symptom Checklist 90 (SCL-90-R) and the Minnesota Multiphasic Personality Inventory (MMPI-2). Poor treatment outcome was identified in patients with presurgical somatization, depression, anxiety, and poor coping.[13]

It is also crucial to appropriately use the spinal cord stimulator for the appropriate indications (neuropathic pain states and ischemic pain), as approved by the Food and Drug Administration. Disease states that yield themselves to successful treatment with SCS include postherpetic neuralgia, intercostal neuralgia, postlaminectomy pain, complex regional pain syndrome, phantom limb pain, angina, painful peripheral neuropathy, focal peripheral neuropathies, ischemic limb pain, and radiculitis and radiculopathy.[14]

A clear understanding of spinal anatomy, utilization of image guidance, and proper surgical technique are vital to ensure both quality treatment and reduced patient morbidity and mortality.[15] Furthermore, it should be understood that appropriate training within Accreditation Council for Graduate Medical Education accredited programs and mentorship is pivotal to ensure treatment success and limit iatrogenic morbidity; interventional hobbyists and weekend crusaders only serve to undermine the accessibility of this valuable therapy to patients.

Spinal cord stimulator complications can be broadly divided into those that are technical or those that are biologic or surgical in nature. The consequences of these complications can range from the mundane to the devastating. Most complications of SCS do not impact patient mortality,[7] unlike that for intrathecal drug delivery, as recently reported by Coffey et al.[16] Although the range of various complications varies from 0% to 81% across studies,[17] the frequencies of the complications in the tables in this chapter are presented as the means. Refer to **Table 1-1** for reported rates of complications, revisions, and explants associated with SCS.

Selected Complications

Technical Complications

Innately, the restrictions current technology places on the spinal cord stimulator device plays a role in the associated complications. Advances in system technology have largely reduced many early complications related to device failure, including loss of stimulation. Van Buyten et al[18] described such a relationship, commenting in a 5-year prospective study of 84 patients with 85 spinal cord stimulator systems, with overall 54% of patients reporting greater than 50% pain relief at 5 years. Satisfaction and employment of the patient programmer were at least 95% after stimulator therapy began (**Table 1-2**).

Furthermore, stimulation, regardless of the choice of the numerous mechanisms proposed,[14] depends on the integrity and characteristics of the "circuit created." Spinal cord stimulator contact to target structure length varies with patient position, as described by Abejon and Feler,[19] and predictively, so too do the circuit created and the resultant therapeutic stimulation. Recumbence reduced impedance and energy requirement (measured in thoracic and cervical implanted leads), and therefore stimulation was perceived to be "stronger," although the difference was not statistically significant. Clinical implications longitudinally require further study.

Lead Migration   The most common complication of SCS is lead migration[7,14,17,20] and loss of therapeutic stimulation. Cameron et al[7] reported that 27.2% of spinal cord stimulator cases were technical in nature, and of those, 87% were related to the lead. Estimates place migration incidence to be between 11% and 13%, with a greater propensity for migration in the cervical spine,[8] likely related to greater mobility, compared with the lumbar spine.

Understandably, migration occurs when directional forces and tensile load on the electrode exceed the stabilizing forces of the anchor. These forces depend on lead-spanning mobile areas, trajectory into the epidural space, anchor orientation, the type of tissue the anchor is sutured to, suture technique, and the site of battery placement. It has been suggested that percutaneous electrodes are more prone to migration than their laminectomy counterparts and that battery location in the abdomen may be associated with less lead migration than in the gluteal region, however work by Henderson and Kumar suggest otherwise. Those studies have suggested that the closer the implanted pulse generator (IPG) is to the lead insertion site, the lower the risk of lead movement. IPG placement choices include the buttocks, midflank, abdominal wall, or infraclavicular regions.[7] Rosenow et al,[10] however, in a study of 289 patients, reported that migration was slightly higher in the surgical laminectomy lead.

Mitigating migration involves reducing iatrogenic cofounders. These include the angle of spinal cord lead entry into the epidural space, stress loops, battery site choice, and anchor or suturing technique. Bedder and Bedder[15] detail basic surgical technique and nomenclature that will not be further discussed here. Kumar et al[8] suggest that proper anchoring and placement of the tip of the anchor into the supraspinal ligament might reduce anchor failure. Strain relief loops of approximately 1 inch in diameter, both near the anchor and at the generator site, may reduce tensile load (**Fig. 1-1**).

Sometimes extensions are needed to allow placement of the battery in a desirable location from the paraspinal access. Extensions are also used when the implanted percutaneous trial method is used; when a trial is deemed successful, the extension portion

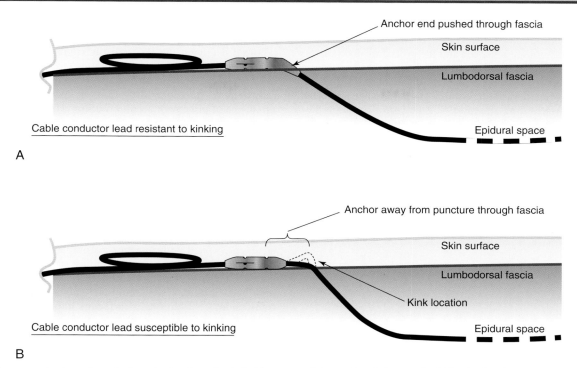

Anchor end pushed through fascia

Skin surface

Lumbodorsal fascia

Cable conductor lead resistant to kinking

Epidural space

A

Anchor away from puncture through fascia

Skin surface

Lumbodorsal fascia

Kink location

Cable conductor lead susceptible to kinking

Epidural space

B

Fig. 1-1   Proper anchoring of a spinal cord stimulator lead. **A,** The nose of the anchor is invested within the fascia, minimizing lead migration and lead kinking. **B,** The nose of the anchor is superficial to the fascia, creating a potential nidus for migration and kinking. (Modified from Kumar K, Buchser E, Linderoth B, et al: Avoiding complications from spinal cord stimulation: practical management recommendations an international panel of experts, *Neuromodulation* 10:24-33, 2007.)

can be removed distally from the externalized extension to the IPG location and a new extension can be tunneled to the subcutaneous IPG location, while maintaining the neuroaxial segment.

Lead Fracture   Lead fracture occurs approximately 5% to 9%,[21-23] with contradictory reports regarding fracture rates with percutaneous versus laminectomy leads. Kumar et al[23] described percutaneous lead fracture more often than laminectomy leads; in contradiction, Rosenow et al[10] reported more lead fracture with laminectomy. Clearly, lead fracture depends on lead tensile strength, the friction coefficient of the internal wires composing the lead, and a vector of force that challenges the lead integrity. Iatrogenic ways to lessen lead fracture are similar to strategies used to reduce lead migration and include appropriate anchoring, using stress loops, placement of the IPD in the abdomen,[8] and avoidance of tunneling around mobile structures (i.e., joints).

Hardware Malfunction and Battery Failure   Exclusive to lead migration of fracture, other hardware complications occur with a frequency of 2.9% and include battery failure (exclusive to predicted nonrechargeable battery depletion) with a frequency 1.6% per Cameron et al.[7] Turner et al[17] described equipment failure rates of 6.5%.

Iatrogenic measures mitigating equipment failure again focus on good surgical skill because of diligent testing of connections and a keen understanding of the limitations of the technology. Each stimulator company's IPG has a different recommendation regarding depth from skin, and every attempt should be made to be compliant. Readers are directed to each company's literature for details.

Misplacement of Epidural Lead   Therapeutic stimulation requires epidural placement of the spinal cord stimulator lead.

Intrathecal and subdural placement have been reported.[24] Troubleshooting of lead placement centers on fluoroscopic guidance and impedance testing. Anterior epidural lead placement is suggested by muscle contraction of adjacent or distal spinal nerves and painful stimulation within the appropriate expected stimulation parameters. Intrathecal lead placement is suggested by very low-impedance testing, and the hallmark of subdural stimulation is segmental, low-amplitude stimulation that is often uncomfortable to the patient. A case report of intramedullary lead placement is described in the next section.

Aberrant Stimulation   Aberrant activation of stimulation rarely occurs, although an infamous case report is often sited. Eisenberg and Waisbrod[25] described a patient who had a cervical spinal cord stimulator that was activated by an antitheft device. Six months after implantation, upon entering a store, the patient felt an electrical shock in the back of his skull and fell unconscious. He awoke in the emergency department with confusion, ataxia, upper extremity intention tremor, weakness, and dysarthric speech. Initial computed tomography (CT) scan and electroencephalogram were normal, although 6 months later, with continued symptoms, follow-up CT demonstrated a left basal ganglia infarct. The authors postulate that the anti-theft device triggered a sudden bolus of current, causing damage that contributed to the injury.

Kumar et al[8] reported that whereas device or technical complications typically occur within 2 years of implant, biologic complications of SCS typically occur within 3 months.

Biologic Complications

Biologic complications typically present themselves within 3 months of implant and usually do not cause significant untoward sequelae. Historically, dorsal column stimulation was performed in the subarachnoid space instead of the epidural space, and more devastating complications were reported, including paraplegia and death. As the technology advanced and the procedure evolved, it is well understood that serious biologic consequences are a rarity and usually do not have a significant impact on patient morbidity and mortality.[7] However, devastating complications have been reported more recently, warranting attention.[8,26-28] The most common biologic complications reported include pain over the device, superficial infection, seroma formation, and dural puncture or leak with frequencies of 5.8%, 5%, 2.5%, and 2%, respectively (**Table 1-3**).[14,17,21,29] Less frequent complications are discussed in turn.

Table 1-3: Reported Biologic Complications of Spinal Cord Stimulation

Complication	Frequency
Infection	5%,[21] 3.4%[22]
Deep infection	0.1%[17]
Contact dermatitis	Case report[46]
Epidural fibrosis	[30]
Aseptic meningitis	Case reports[7]
Allergy	Case report[47]
Gastrointestinal side effects	Case reports[52,53]
Renal failure	Case report[49]
Headache	Case report[45]
Epidural hematoma	0.3%,[8] case report[43]
Subdural hematoma	Case report[26]
Epidural abscess	Case report[27]
Dural puncture or CSF leak	2%,[14] 0.3%[8]
Seroma	2.5%[29]
Pain over device	0.9%[8], 5.8%[17]
Skin erosion	0.2%[8]
Foreign body reaction	Case report[48]
Micturition inhibition or urologic	Case reports[50,51]
Quadriparesis after mechanical spinal cord injury	Case report[28]
Insulin sensitivity	Unpublished Cleveland Clinic Report

Pain Over the Device Pain overlying the spinal cord stimulator device components ranges from 0.9% to 5.8%.[8,17] Pain has been reported overlying the IPG and the epidural entry site (may be related to anchors between the spinous processes). Treatment can involve topical or injection therapy, although anecdotally, it typically requires revision. Mitigation of device site pain includes avoidance of placement around friction-generating sites; ensuring adequate distance from osteal structures; and most importantly, a clear consensus with the patient regarding IPG placement preoperatively.

Infection The risk of infection is always a concern when undergoing surgery and even more so when implanting a foreign body. Infections have been reported years after implantation,[30] and a high index of clinical suspicion is necessary to make the diagnosis because signs and symptoms are often subtle and vague. Risk factors associated with infections of implanted hardware include immunosuppressive therapy (including steroids), diabetes, rheumatoid arthritis, tobacco, alcohol use, malnutrition, obesity, prolonged hospital stay, multiple surgeries, or perioperative transfusion.[15,31] Additional risk factors implicated perioperatively include inappropriate or inadequate timing of preoperative antibiotic therapy, shaving of the operative site (versus clipping), improper surgical site skin preparation, inadequate preoperative hand scrub, and lack of ventilation in the operative suite.[15]

Superficial and Deep Infections Superficial infections are the most common infectious complication associated with SCS, occurring with a frequency of approximately 5%, with coagulase-negative *Staphylococcus* spp., *Staphylococcus aureus*, and *Enterococcus* spp. being commonly implicated in decreasing order of occurrence.[15] Deep infections occur less frequently, and intraspinal infections, including epidural abscesses, are very infrequent and are also caused primarily by *S. aureus*, although gram-negative, anaerobic, mycobacteria, and fungi have been described.[32,33] Torrens et al[31] describe a case of methicillin-resistant *S. aureus* (MRSA) meningitis diagnosed on postoperative day 8 after a superficial infection despite an enteral antibiotic course and removal of the lead (**Fig. 1-2**).

Iatrogenic sources of superficial infections can be reduced by proper patient preparation and operative technique and were reviewed by Bedder and Bedder.[15] Antimicrobial prophylaxis should occur within 30 minutes of skin incision and cover the most commonly implicated organisms. First-generation cephalosporins are frequently used (including cefazolin) to cover gram-positive bacteria. Fourth-generation cephalosporins (cefepime) broaden coverage to gram-negative bacteria while maintaining

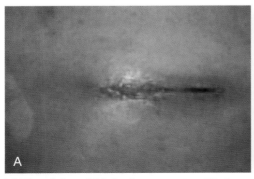 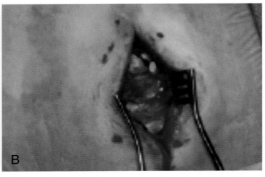

Fig. 1-2 Superficial (**A**) and deep (**B**) infection. (From Deer TR, Stewart CD: Complications of spinal cord stimulation: identification, treatment and prevention, *Pain Med* 9(suppl):S93-S101, 2008.)

gram-positive coverage, providing treatment for *Enterobacter* and *Pseudomonas* spp. Cephalosporins do not cover against enterococci. Clindamycin is an option for patients who require antimicrobial prophylaxis with a severe penicillin allergy. The decision to provide postoperative prophylactic antibiotics continues to be a controversial topic. Many practitioners continue to do so despite only anecdotal evidence.[34] Furthermore, unnecessary antibiotic use increases microbial resistance and health care costs.

Surgical preparation includes optimizing and mitigating patient comorbidities that increase infectious risk, ensuring proper scrub, and promoting a sterile and accessible operative field. Hair removal should be performed immediately before the procedure and should including clipping because shaving increases the chance of infection.[35] Skin preparation is usually accomplished by chlorhexidine gluconate, povidone–iodine, or alcohol-based solutions. Each deserves special mention. Povidone–iodine preparations need to have sufficient time to be thoroughly dry to maximize their antimicrobial effects. Alcohol is extremely bacteriocidal, but its use may be limited by flammability. Chlorhexidine has a longer duration of action and is more bacteriocidal than iodine preparations.[36]

Intraoperative strategies to reduce infection include meticulous sterile technique, layered wound closure to avoid dead space, appropriate hemostasis, avoidance of placing sutures overlying the device, and nonpressured irrigation (the adage "the solution to pollution is dilution" holds true in clean, uncontaminated surgeries).

If infection is suspected, it is usually heralded by erythema, induration, temperature of greater than 101.4°F, purulent discharge, or wound dehiscence, and an infectious disease consult is suggested. Superficial infections around the IPG site remote to epidural entry may be treated with a course of antibiotic therapy with aggressive and daily vigilance. If systemic signs or symptoms are present or suspected or if infection is encroaching on the epidural access site, an infectious disease consultation is mandatory, and all the hardware (IPG and leads) should be removed. If reimplantation is desirable, this should not be considered until the patient is infection free and medically stable for at least 12 weeks.

Skin Erosion
Skin erosions are a consequence of superficial lead placement and are more a consequence of peripheral nerve stimulation. IPG battery erosion or evisceration can be reduced by appropriate IPG placement away from mobile or osteal sites and careful layered closure with avoidance of suture lines over the implanted device.

Epidural Abscess
Epidural abscess occur spontaneously with a reported incidence of 0.2 to 1.2 per 10,000 hospital admissions.[37] Meglio et al[27] reported a case of paraplegia after discovery of an epidural and intradural abscess of a patient with a recently explanted spinal cord stimulator. Early diagnosis is paramount to reduce morbidity and mortality.[38] Progressive clinical phases have been described for epidural infection leading to epidural abscess, described by Van Zundert.[39] Phase I involves backache and local tenderness; phase II is associated with radicular pain, fever, neck stiffness, and rigidity and commonly occurs 2 to 3 days later; phase III presents with sensory, motor, or reflex depression (often 3 to 4 days later); and phase IV is associated with paralysis.[39]

About 80% to 90% of epidural abscesses are correctly diagnosed using MRI with gadolinium contrast.[37] When neurologic deterioration occurs, decompression via laminectomy is warranted and should be used within 36 hours to limit morbidity, although neurologic sequelae can still be significant.[40] Intravenous bacteriocidal antibiotics should be started as early as possible and continued for

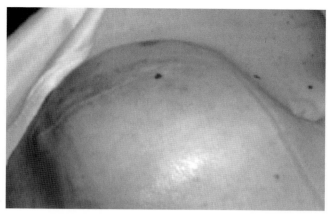

Fig. 1-3 Seroma. (From Deer TR, Stewart CD: Complications of spinal cord stimulation: identification, treatment and prevention, *Pain Med* 9(suppl):S93-S101, 2008.)

4 weeks, with enteral or parenteral therapy continued for at least 8 to 12 weeks.[41] Therapy should be modified according to speciation and an antibiotic resistance profile, if isolation is achievable.

Seroma A seroma is a collection of serosanguineous fluid that may occur secondary to friction forces of two tissue planes and excessive surgical trauma (**Fig. 1-3**).[29] Iatrogenic mitigating factors include limiting aggressive blunt dissection, reducing excessive cautery, achieving careful hemostasis, and performing a layered closure to limit dead space. If a seroma forms, treatment includes abdominal binder and drainage, although care must be taken not to introduce infection.

Neuraxial Hematoma The incidence of epidural hematomas is largely unknown, although it has been estimated to be near one in 150,000 epidurals and one in 222,000 spinal anesthetics.[42] Franzini et al[43] described a large epidural hematoma after implantation of a laminectomy lead with an immediate postoperative presentation of progressive lower extremity weakness. The authors suggested postoperative vigilance in patients with increased risk. Independent risk factors for epidural hematoma after spinal surgery include male gender (4:1) and patients in the fifth or sixth decade of life.

Subdural hematomas have been described as a complication of SCS. Chiravuri et al[26] published a case of a subdural hematoma temporally associated with stimulator placement but complicated by a preoperative fall with associated head trauma.

Although a review of the American Society of Regional Anesthesia 2010 guidelines for neuraxial interventions in patients receiving anticoagulation therapy is beyond the scope of this chapter, it is vital that readers use the guidelines.[42] Treatment is contingent on hematoma evacuation within 8 hours of neurologic deficit.[44]

Quadriparesis Meyer et al[28] report a case describing quadriplegia after inadvertent intramedullary spinal cord stimulator lead placement in a patient under general anesthesia. This unfortunate incident occurred in a 25-year-old woman with chronic regional pain syndrome of the left upper extremity who had an existing stimulator that improved her pain and function but required revision of the IPG for "technical reasons." The patient was placed under general anesthesia for the procedure. Intraoperatively, it was discovered that her percutaneous leads also needed revision. The

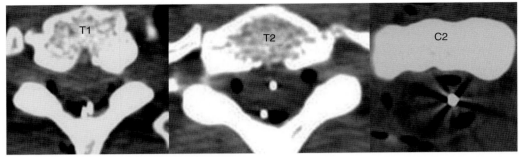

Fig. 1-4 Serial computed tomography images of an intramedullary lead. (From Meyer SC, Swartz K, Johnson JO: Quadriparesis and spinal cord stimulation: case report, *Spine* 2007 (32):E565-E5658.)

existing leads were removed, and new percutaneous leads were introduced via the "standard closed percutaneous technique at T2-3 interspace." Immediately after surgery, the patient had severe neurologic compromise. Postoperative CT demonstrated a lead within the spinal cord at the tip of C2 (**Fig. 1-4**).

The lead was eventually removed via an open procedure, further compromising neurologic function, with persistent worsening function at last follow-up. The authors suggest that revision procedures should be performed in an "open" manner; however, placement of spinal cord stimulator electrodes under general anesthesia should never be performed and is the more prudent learning point.

Dural Puncture Dural puncture, unfortunately, remains a relatively common complication of SCS[30], with estimates centering around 2%. Furthermore, postdural puncture headache (PDPH) after 16- to 18-gauge needle entry is estimated to be as high as 86%.[24] Risk factors include previous surgery at needle entry, calcified ligamentum flavum, and an uncooperative patient.[30] Very commonly, conservative measures fail to treat the headache, and an epidural blood patch is required, with a success rate of approximately 60% to 70%. Very commonly, when accidental dural puncture occurs, a prophylactic blood patch is placed. The volume of autologous blood depends on the puncture site, but often at least 20 mL or patient discomfort guides the necessary amount. The trial can continue with a more cephalad interspace used for epidural needle placement and entry.[30]

Headache Exclusive to PDPH, SCS has been implicated in headache. Ward and Levin[45] described persistent headaches subsequent to placement of a percutaneous cervical spinal cord stimulator at C3 that responded to ergotamine and sumatriptan and resolved with lead repositioning. The authors contend the possibility of migraine (**Fig. 1-5**).

Immunologic Reactions Contact dermatitis, allergy, and foreign body reactions have reported as case reports after SCS.[46-48] McKenna and McCleane[46] reported a patient with a skin reaction overlying the IPG site 1 month after stimulator placement. The authors describe the reaction as an isomorphic response to the expansion of underlying tissues rather than a nickel allergy, however, despite a prior atopy and patch testing suggesting a nickel allergy.

Ochani et al[47] described a case of suspected allergic reaction 6 weeks after cervical and lumbar placement for chronic regional pain syndrome after left sympathectomy for atypical face pain after facial trauma. The patient presented 2 weeks after implantation with a burning sensation adjacent to implanted leads and tenderness overlying the generator pocket. Infectious workup

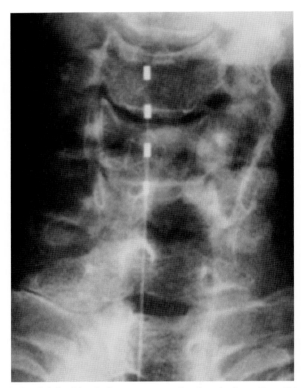

Fig. 1-5 Original lead placement causing headaches. (From Ward TN, Levin M. Case reports: headache caused by spinal cord stimulator in the upper cervical spine, *Headache* 40:689-691, 2000.)

was negative. Two weeks later, then patient again presented with generalized hives and edema, which responded to steroid therapy. Patch dermatologic allergy testing revealed sensitization to platinum, silicone, and polyurethane. The stimulator was removed, resolving the complaints.

Lennarson and Guillen[48] reported a foreign body reaction to the lead after explant, resulting in symptomatic compression of the spinal canal, necessitating multilevel cervical laminectomy, excision of the mass, and fusion. The diagnosis is clouded, however, because a superficial MRSA infection was discovered at the neck incision, although deep culture results were negative. Histiopathic analysis of the mass excised revealed a giant cell reaction (**Fig. 1-6**).

Epidural Fibrosis Epidural fibrosis has also been described as a complication of SCS, although it is inherent to its placement. Scarring begins within 2 weeks of electrode placement and

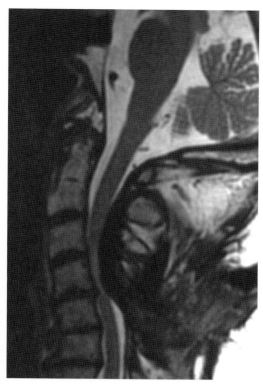

Fig. 1-6   Compressive foreign body reaction. (From Lennarson PJ, Guillen T: Spinal cord compression from a foreign body reaction to spinal cord stimulation: a previously unreported complication, *Spine* 35(25): E1516-E1519, 2010.)

continues throughout the lifetime of the device. The fibrosis may alter the circuit created to produce stimulation, governed by Ohms law, resulting in failed or loss of therapeutic stimulation.[30] This phenomenon was described by Kumar et al[23] as system tolerance despite continued coverage of the painful area and an intact system.

Urologic Complications   Renal failure, micturition inhibition, and other urologic complications have been reported.[49-51] Larkin et al[49] reported a case of renal failure temporally associated with placement of a spinal cord stimulator. The patient was anuric and hypotensive, and serum blood urea nitrogen and creatine were 83 mg/dL and 8.1 mg/dL, respectively. The authors suggested the sympathectomy from the SCS might have compromised renal perfusion.

Loubser et al[51] described a case report of a patient with partial T12–L1 spinal cord injury and subsequent SCS to treat his neuropathic or central pain. The patient required large amplitudes to produce the desired paresthesias, and at these therapeutic amplitudes, urethral sphincter spasm occurred, preventing self-catheterization. Even after the spinal cord system was explanted, the patient continued to have urinary retention and associated infections attributed to the device. The author suggested routine urologic functional testing to be incorporated during the trial period.

More recently, micturition inhibition complicating SCS was reported by Grua and Michelagnoli.[50] The patient had cauda equina syndrome from an angioma at T12. After failing conservative therapy, he underwent percutaneous spinal cord stimulator with cephalad end of the lead left of center at T12. The patient

reported complete resolution of his pain but urge incontinence. Only after 30 days from the interrupted trial, the patient had complete return of bladder function. The stimulation was again initiated with immediate reappearance of the bladder dysfunction. The decision was made to explant. The authors postulated the autonomic effects of stimulation may have imbalanced the signals, altering urinary function.

Gastrointestinal Complications   Sporadic case reports of gastrointestinal complications associated with SCS have been described.[52,53] Thakkar et al[52] described two cases of patients with SCS who experienced symptoms exacerbated by stimulation, namely nausea, diarrhea, worsened gastrointestinal reflux, and flatulence; these were hypothesized to have occurred because of the associated sympathectomy and unopposed parasympathetic gastrointestinal effects.

Kemler et al[53] described a case of relapsing colitis caused by SCS. The patient had a spinal cord stimulator system placed with the lead placed at C4 and the IPG placed left lower abdominal quadrant for upper extremity chronic regional pain syndrome. The patient's ulcerative colitis relapsed and remitted twice with using and discontinuing the device. The authors postulated that there may have been an electromagnetic effect on the colon, aberrancy of the GABAergic system, or an electrical effect on intestinal circulation.

Anecdotal, unpublished reports of insulin sensitivity have been described. At the Cleveland Clinic, a patient with uncontrollable insulin-dependent diabetes had a spinal cord stimulator placed for neuropathic visceral abdominal pain with the stimulator lead distal segment at the cephalad portion of T5. Three days later, after her typical insulin regimen, the patient was found to be hypoglycemic and was admitted to the intensive care unit for stabilization. During her admission, the therapeutic stimulation was ceased, whereupon her insulin insensitivity increased to baseline. Upon resuming the therapeutic stimulation, the patient again became hypoglycemic, suggesting that the reduced resistance could be attributed to the stimulation.

Summary

Spinal cord stimulation is an important tool in the armamentarium of interventional pain physicians. As with any intervention, success is contingent on the appropriately selected patient. Furthermore, because it is a device used for a lifelong therapy against chronic pain, revision (of some nature) is expected. The recapturing of therapeutic stimulation can be achieved with reprogramming, revision, or both and is limited by the current technology. Iatrogenic sources of spinal cord stimulator complications need to be mitigated by meticulous surgical care and attention to detail. This includes keeping a keen eye on the reported side effects. As the mystery surrounding the mechanisms of SCS become more understood, so too can the accompanying side effects.

References

1. Melzack R, Wall PD: Pain mechanisms: a new theory. *Science* 150:971-979, 1965.
2. Shealy CN, Mortimer JT, Reswick JB: Electrical inhibition of pain by stimulation of the dorsal columns: preliminary clinical report. *Anesth Analg* 46(4):489-491, 1967.
3. Prager J: Estimates of annual spinal cord stimulator implant rises in the United States. *Neuromodulation* (13):68-69, 2010.
4. Simpson BA: The role of neurostimulation: the neurosurgical perspective. *J Pain Symptom Manage* 4(suppl):S3-S5, 2006.

5. North RB, Shipley J, Taylor RS: The cost effectiveness of spinal cord stimulation. In *Neuromodulation*, vol II, St. Louis, 2009, Elsevier, pp 355-376.

6. Eldrige JS, Weingarten TN, Rho RH: Management of cerebral spinal fluid leak complicating spinal cord stimulator implantation. *Pain Practice* 6(4):285-288, 2006.

7. Cameron T: Safety and efficacy of SCS for the treatment of chronic pain: a 20-year literature review. *J Neurosurg* 100:254-267, 2004.

8. Kumar K, Buchser E, Linderoth B, et al: Avoiding complications from spinal cord stimulation: practical management recommendations an international panel of experts. *Neuromodulation* 10:24-33, 2007.

9. North RB, Kidd DH, Farrokhi F, Piantadosi SA: Spinal cord stimulation versus repeated lumbosacral spine surgery for chronic pain: a randomized, controlled trial. *Neurosurgery* 56:98-107, 2005.

10. Rosenow JM, Stanton-Hicks M, Rezai AR, Henderson JM: Failure modes of spinal cord stimulation hardware. *J Neurosurg Spine* 5:183-190, 2006.

11. Fishbain D, Goldberg M, Meagher BR, et al: Male and female chronic pain patients characterized by DSMIII psychiatric diagnostic criteria. *Pain* 26:181-197, 1986.

12. Gallagher R: Primary care and pain medicine: a community solution to the public health problem of chronic pain. *Med Clin North Am* 83:555-583, 1999.

13. Celstin J, Edwards RR, Jamison RN: Pretreatment psychosocial variables as predictors of outcomes following lumbar surgery and spinal cord stimulation: a systematic review and literature synthesis. *Pain Med* 10(4):639-653, 2009.

14. Pinzon EG: Spinal cord stimulation. *Pract Pain Med* May/Jun:69-75, 2005.

15. Bedder MD, Bedder HF: Spinal cord stimulation surgical technique for the nonsurgically trained. *Neuromodulation* 12:1-19, 2009.

16. Coffey RJ, Woens ML, Broste SK: Medical practice perspective: identification and mitigation of risk factors for mortality associated with intrathecal opioids for non-cancer pain. *Pain Med* 11:1001-1009, 2010.

17. Turner JA, Loeser JD, Deyo RA, Sanders SB: Spinal cord stimulation for with failed back surgery syndrome or complex regional pain syndrome: a systematic review of effectiveness and complications. *Pain* 108:137-147, 2004.

18. Van Buyten JP: The performance and safety if an implantable spinal cord stimulation system in patients with chronic pain: a 5 year study. *Neuromodulation* 6:79-87, 2003.

19. Abejon D, Feler C: Is impedance a parameter to be taken into account in spinal cord stimulation? *Pain Physician* 10(4):533-554, 2007.

20. Devulder J, Vermeulen H, De Colvenaer L, et al: Spinal cord stimulation in chronic pain: evaluation of results, complications, and technical considerations in sixty-nine patients. *Clin J Pain* 7:21-28, 1991.

21. Sarubbi F, Vasquez J: Spinal epidural abscess associated with the use of temporary epidural catheters: report of two cases and review. *Clin Infect Dis* 25:1155-1158, 1997.

22. Kemler MA, De Vet HCW, Barendse GAM, et al: The effect of spinal cord stimulation in patients with chronic reflex sympathetic dystrophy: two years follow-up of the randomized controlled trial. *Ann Neurol* 55:13-18, 2004.

23. Kumar K, Wilson JR, Taylor RS, Gupta S: Complications of spinal cord stimulation, suggestions to improve outcome, and financial impact. *J Neurosurg Spine* 5:191-203, 2006.

24. Pope JE, Stanton-Hicks M: Accidental subdural spinal cord stimulator lead placement and stimulation. *Neuromodulation* 14(1):30-33, 2010.

25. Eisenberg E, Waisbrod H: Spinal cord stimulator activation by an antitheft device. *J Neurosurg* 87:961-962, 1997.

26. Chiravuri S, Wasserman R, Chawla A, Haider N: Subdural hematoma following spinal cord stimulator implant. *Pain Physician* 11:97-101, 2008.

27. Meglio M, Cioni B, Rossi GF: Spinal cord stimulation in management of chronic pain. A 9-year experience. *J Neurosurg* 70:519-524, 1989.

28. Meyer SC, Swartz K, Johnson JO: Quadriparesis and spinal cord stimulation: case report. *Spine* (32):E565-E5658, 2007.

29. Beer GM, Wallner H: Prevention of seroma after abdominoplasty. *Aesthet Surg J* 30(3):414-417, 2010.

30. Deer TR, Stewart CD: Complications of spinal cord stimulation: identification, treatment and prevention. *Pain Med* 9(suppl):S93-S101, 2008.

31. Torrens K, Stanely PJ, Ragunathan PL, Bush DJ: Risk of infection with electrical spinal cord stimulation. *Lancet* 349:729, 1997.

32. Ergan M, Macro M, Benhamou CL, et al: Septic arthritis of lumbar facet joints: a review of six cases. *Rev Rhum Engl Ed* 64:386-395, 1997.

33. Bruma OJ, Craane H, Kunst MW: Vertebral osteomyelitis and epidural abscess due to mucormycosis, a case report. *Clin Neurol Neurosurg* 81(1):39-44, 1979.

34. McDonald M, Grabsch E, Marshall C, Forbes A: Single versus multiple dose antimicrobial prophylaxis for major surgery: a systematic review. *Aust N Z J Surg* 68:388-396, 1999.

35. Alexander JW, Fischer JE, Boyajian M, et al: The influence of hair-removal methods on wound infections. *Arch Surg* 118:347-352, 1983.

36. Grabsch EA, Mitchell DJ, Hooper J, Turnidge TJ: In-use efficacy of a chlorhexidine in alcohol surgical rub: a comparative study. *ANZ J Surg* 74:769-772, 2004.

37. Alcock E, Regaard A, Browne J: Facet joint injection: a rare form cause of epidural abscess formation. *Pain* 103:209-210, 2003.

38. Mackenzie AR, Laing RBS, Kaar GF, Smith FW: Spinal epidural abscess: the importance of early diagnosis and treatment. *J Neurol Neurosurg Psychiatry* 65:209-212, 1998.

39. Van Zundert A: The epidural abscess: diagnosis and treatment. In *Highlights in regional anaesthesia and pain therapy IX*. Rome, Italy, 2000, ESRA and Cyprint, pp 159-162.

40. Danner RL, Hartman BJ: Update of spinal epidural abscess: 35 cases and review of literature. *Rev Infect Dis* 9:265-274, 1987.

41. Darouiche RO, Hamil RJ, Greenberg, et al: Bacterial spinal epidural abscess: review of 43 cases and literature survey. *Medicine* 71:369-385, 1992.

42. Horlocker TT, Rowlingson JC, Enneking FK, et al: Regional anesthesia in the patient receiving antithrombotic or thrombolytic therapy: American Society of Regional Anesthesia and Pain Medicine Evidence-Based Guidelines (Third Edition). *Reg Anesth Pain Med* 35(1):64-101, 2010.

43. Franzini A, Ferroli P, Marras C, Broggi G: Huge epidural hematoma after surgery for spinal cord stimulation. *Acta Neurochir (Wien)* 147: 565-567, 2005.

44. Vandermeulen EP, Van Aken H, Vermylen J: Anticoagulants and spinal-epidural anesthesia. *Anesth Analg* 79:1165-1177, 1994.

45. Ward TN, Levin M: Case reports: headache caused by spinal cord stimulator in the upper cervical spine. *Headache* 40:689-691, 2000.

46. McKenna KE, McCleane G: Dermatitis induced by a spinal cord stimulator implant. *Contact Dermatitis* 41:279, 1999.

47. Ochani TD, Almirante J, Siddiqui A, Kaplan R: Allergic reaction to spinal cord stimulator. *Clin J Pain* 16:178-180, 2000.

48. Lennarson PJ, Guillen T: Spinal cord compression from a foreign body reaction to spinal cord stimulation: a previously unreported complication. *Spine* 35(25):E1516-E1519, 2010.

49. Larkin TM, Dragovich A, Cohen SP: Acute renal failure during a trial of spinal cord stimulation: theories as to a possible connection. *Pain Physician* 11:681-686, 2008.

50. Grua ML, Michelagnoli G: Rare adverse effect of spinal cord stimulation: micturition inhibition. *Clin J Pain* 26:433-434, 2010.

51. Loubser PG: Adverse effects of epidural spinal cord stimulation on bladder function in a patient with chronic spinal cord injury pain. *J Pain Symptom Manage* 13:251-252, 1985.

52. Thakkar N, Connelly NR, Vieira P: Gastrointestinal symptoms secondary to implanted spinal cord stimulators. *Anesth Analg* 97:547-549, 2003.

53. Kemler MA, Barendse GA, van Kleef M: Relapsing ulcerative colitis associated with spinal cord stimulation. *Gastroenterology* 117:215-217, 1999.

2 Complications of Peripheral Nerve Stimulation: Open Technique, Percutaneous Technique, and Peripheral Nerve Field Stimulation

Tory L. McJunkin, Paul J. Lynch, and Elizabeth Srejic

CHAPTER OVERVIEW

Chapter Synopsis: Peripheral nerve stimulation (PNS) has emerged as an effective treatment for chronic neuropathic pain with the advantages of being cost effective, reversible, nonaddictive, and nonpharmacologic. Several approaches may be used for implantation and stimulation, including an open surgery technique (PNS:OT), a percutaneous implantation technique (PNS:PT), and a nonperineural technique called peripheral nerve field stimulation (PNfS). As the neuromodulatory techniques have evolved, side effects have become uncommon but should be considered as the treatments become more prevalent. Certain areas of implantation, notably the nerves of the brachial plexus, present greater risks than others. Infection ranks as the most common side effect, but technical problems such as lead migration or lead fracture can also arise. The risk of biologic complications is usually immediate; technical complications usually occur within 2 years of implant. Whereas surgical implantation (PNS:OT) of a stimulating electrode requires exploration and nerve visualization, PNS:PT relies on fluoroscopic imaging for guidance. PNfS places a stimulating device in the peripheral subcutaneous area of pain. As with any neurostimulation technique, a thorough patient selection process can increase the chances for success of the procedure and lower associated risks. A psychological assessment may be required in advance of implantation, but screening by response to nerve block is no longer indicated as predictive of success. Risk can be minimized with vigilance by the physician.

Important Points:

- PNS is a neuromodulation technique involving application of an electrical current adjacent to peripheral nerves to treat chronic, intractable, debilitating neuropathic pain conditions that are refractory to less invasive treatments.
- There are three main variants of PNS: PNS performed with an open surgical technique (PNS:OT); PNS executed with a percutaneous technique (PNS:PT), and a subcutaneous; nonperineural technique called peripheral nerve field stimulation (PNfS).
- PNS techniques, which are reversible, cost effective, nonaddictive, and nonpharmacologic, are based on delivery of low-level electric impulses to pain-generating nerves via an implantable system, consisting of a programmable generator connected to electric transmission leads.
- Common neural targets amenable to PNS include cranial nerves, occipital nerves, segmental truncal nerves, and upper and lower extremity plexus and peripheral nerves or areas not accessible or effectively treated by spinal cord or spinal nerve root stimulation.
- The risk of serious problems resulting from PNS therapies appears to be relatively low in clinical practice, especially for PNfS. However, PNS therapy is not without risk, and lead placement along specific target areas may be more challenging technically than in other implantable therapies.
- The most common complication is infection. Other reported complications include peripheral nerve trauma and damage to other tissues, pain over the device, and seroma.
- Technical complications generally involve equipment failure, including lead migration and lead fracture, and less commonly, battery malfunction.
- Devastating infectious and technical complications, although rare, have been reported and deserve special attention.
- Biologic complications commonly occur within 3 months of implant, although infections can rarely present much later. Technical complications typically occur within 2 years of implant.
- Meticulous attention to surgical technique is the best measure against the development of infection, the most common PNS complication. In addition, adequate patient screening, use of high-quality imaging, practitioner expertise, and familiarity with the different types of available hardware are recommended to preclude adverse outcomes.

Introduction

Peripheral nerve stimulation (PNS) is a neuromodulation technique in which an electrical current is applied adjacent to peripheral nerves to diminish pain. For the sake of this chapter, *PNS techniques* will describe stimulation of structures that are anatomically outside of the spinal canal. There are three main variants of PNS: PNS performed with an open surgical technique (PNS:OT); PNS executed with a percutaneous technique (PNS:PT); and a subcutaneous, nonperineural technique called peripheral nerve field stimulation (PNfS). No matter which technique is chosen, PNS is used for chronic, intractable, debilitating neuropathic pain conditions that are refractory to less invasive treatments.

Using PNS:OT, a lead, often a paddle lead, is surgically placed directly adjacent to the target nerve. An example is placement of a paddle lead along the sciatic nerve for a person with neuropathic sciatica. Using PNS:PT, a percutaneous lead is placed through a needle that is usually guided via a nerve stimulator or by ultrasonography. An example is placement of a percutaneous lead through a needle under ultrasound guidance along nerves of the brachial plexus for a painful brachial plexopathy. Using PNfS, which is also called *subcutaneous field stimulation*, a lead is typically placed through a needle into the subcutaneous tissue in the direct area of pain experienced by the patient, remote to named peripheral nerves. An example is a lead placed in the subcutaneous tissues for axial low back pain in a patient with postlaminectomy syndrome.[1]

Neuromodulation has a fascinating history that long predates modern understanding of electricity. The Egyptians used electric stimulation to treat pain as early as 2500 BC, as seen on stone carvings depicting placement of electric catfish on people. In ancient Greece and Rome, torpedo fish were used to deliver electric shocks of as many as 200 volts (which may be sufficient to kill a human adult) to combat pain and common maladies such as headache, gout, and arthritis.

In contemporary times, PNS techniques, which are reversible, cost effective, nonaddictive, and nonpharmacologic, are based on delivery of low-level electric impulses to pain-generating nerves via an implantable system, consisting of a programmable generator connected to electric transmission leads. Over the past decade, they have been used increasingly to treat a wide range of conditions involving pain in peripheral or cranial neural distributions. In particular, they may be an effective treatment for neuropathic pain that is not accessible or effectively treated by spinal cord or spinal nerve root stimulation. Common neural targets amenable to PNS include cranial nerves (e.g., trigeminal peripheral terminal branches), occipital nerves, segmental truncal nerves (e.g., nerve root, intercostal, ilioinguinal, iliohypogastric, genitofemoral), and upper and lower extremity plexus and peripheral nerves (e.g., ulnar, median, radial, lateral femoral cutaneous, sciatic, anterior and posterior tibial nerves).[2]

Another reason PNS therapies have increased in popularity may be their lower incidence of complications. In spite of reported complications including infection, lead migration, and device failure, the risk of serious problems resulting from PNS or PfNS therapies appears to be relatively low in clinical practice. Although there has been no formal comparison of PNS versus spinal cord stimulation (SCS) complications, when compared with intrathecal drug delivery, electrical neuromodulation techniques rarely impact morbidity or mortality significantly.[3]

Notwithstanding the preceding, PNS therapy is not without risk, and lead placement along specific target areas may be more challenging technically than SCS therapy. For example, placement of PNS leads using an open or closed technique to treat nerves of the brachial plexus, which lie in close proximity to the subclavian and axillary vessels, might be associated with comparable or greater risks than SCS lead placement in the cervical epidural space to treat upper extremity neuropathic pain.

Selected Complications

Perhaps one of the most significant advantages of PNS is its relatively low rate of complications (**Table 2-1**). Mobbs et al[4] mention relatively minor complications in their retrospective study (currently the largest in the literature), which examines the role of the implantable PNS device in the chronic pain patient. In 38 patients who received implanted PNS devices, six stimulators were removed after implantation (15%). Two were removed due to infection, representing a 5% infection rate. One of these patients had hemophilia despite factor VIII cover, and an episode of bleeding that was further complicated by infection, necessitating stimulator removal. Despite a positive result during the trial period, one stimulator was removed after one month because of minimal effect post-implantation. This patient subsequently improved again after his workers' compensation issues were resolved. One stimulator was removed at 4 years post-implantation since the patient maintained it was no longer needed. Two stimulators in one patient had an initially positive effect, lasting 3 months, followed by a rapid decline in effect. The patient did not wish to have the stimulators re-trialed or re-implanted. A single lead had to be replaced as it was fractured following a fall from a tree. The stimulator continued to function

Table 2-1: Complications of PNS (OT; PT, fS)	
Complication	**Reported Rate (If Reported)**
Overall revision rate	27%[32]
Requiring explant	15%[4]
Procedural	
Tissue trauma	Theoretical
Allergic reactions	Case reports,[33]* 0.8%[34]
Specific anesthesia-related complications	Anecdotal evidence
Hemorrhage	Theoretical
Peripheral nerve trauma	60%[4]
Organ trauma	Theoretical
Post-Procedural	
Infection	5%,[4] 3%-5%,[17] 4.5%,[18] 1%[35]
Seroma	2.5%[36]
Lead migration	27%-33%,[34,37] 2%[35]
Skin erosion	12.5%,[21] 7%[35]
Pain at generator site	0.9%-5.8%[38,39]*
Excessive bleeding	Theoretical
Sepsis	Theoretical, unpublished case report at the Cleveland Clinic
Battery failure/hardware failure	1.6%,[40]* 2%[35]
Lead migration	33%,[27] 24%[30]

*Extrapolated from spinal cord stimulation devices.

following revision of the lead. During the follow-up period, two battery generators were replaced because of battery failure and a further two generator/lead combinations were repositioned as they were uncomfortable and restricted arm movement. One electrode was relocated during the trial period due to a substantial, uncomfortable motor effect in an adjacent muscle. A further 8 electrodes were resutured during the second operation due to electrode lead migration.

The overall risk of complications associated with PNS therapies appears to be very low. In contrast to SCS, PNS techniques target nerves external to the spinal canal, eradicating potential development of bleeding and infection within the epidural space, catastrophic central neurologic deficit, and emergent spine surgery. However, there exists a risk of a range of procedural, postprocedural, device-related, and infectious complications even when PNS is performed by the most experienced practitioners. Consequently, any physician who undertakes a PNS procedure must be prepared to manage any unexpected sequelae.

Before undertaking a PNS procedure, several factors should be considered, according to a review of surgical procedures pertaining to implantable neuromodulation technology.[5] These factors include the incidence, severity, and time to resolution of complications, as well as the net impact on the patient given that complications may detract from the beneficial effect of the procedure.

One of the cornerstones of iatrogenesis avoidance in PNS is patient selection. This includes restricting PNS eligibility to patients with neuropathic pain who have failed to gain relief from more conservative therapies. Because infection is one of the most common complications of PNS procedures, patients must be free of serious skin and systemic infections and must not be immunocompromised. Furthermore, patients receiving PNS must be able to tolerate weaning from nicotine, steroids, and blood thinners and must be thoroughly prescreened to determine their psychological suitability for undergoing PNS procedures.

Procedural Complications

Common potential procedure-related complications surrounding PNS procedures involve tissue trauma, infection, allergic reactions, and anesthesia-related complications. In general, avoidance of such complications necessitates high-quality fluoroscopic guidance to promote optimal lead placement, as well as meticulous surgical technique to prevent infection from contaminated skin, implanted equipment, and other causes. However, development of complications from PNS procedures is still possible even with extensive preventive measures, use of technologically advanced equipment, and years of practitioner expertise.

Harm caused to tissues during PNS procedures may consist of bleeding, peripheral nerve trauma, and damage to vital structures (e.g., vessels and organs). Because vital internal structures are vulnerable in PNS, the use of high-quality fluoroscopy is indicated; for example, pneumothorax, a potential organ-related complication of PNS device installation in the thoracic region, is best circumvented by high-quality imaging.[6] In deeper tissues, damage to vessels can be evaded by using an open rather than percutaneous technique, which may help to prevent blind injury of vasculature, embolism, and other negative sequelae.

Hemorrhage is a potential adverse outcome in any surgical procedure. In PNS, bleeding can occur in the region of the generator or lead incision, promoting hematoma and wound dehiscence. In some instances, serosanguineous fluid rather than blood may accumulate, leading to seroma. Both of these problems are limited to the area of surgery and do no usually result in life-threatening disorders.

Because the risk of excessive bleeding and seroma development exists, standard precautions against hemorrhage and fluid leakage should be exercised. Specifically, in the preoperative period, patients should discontinue medications likely to promote bleeding, and patients with a history of excessive bleeding should have a coagulation profile performed. During the procedure, the practitioner should focus on careful tissue dissection, containment of bleeding, and thorough inspection of the wound before closure. In addition, expert surgeons recommend irrigation and complete closure of surgical wounds to diffuse any sources of infection and restriction of pocket size to no larger than necessary to inhibit seroma formation.

The use of PNS therapy was commonly used to treat pain after previous nerve damage as described by Mobbs et al[4] in their retrospective study (currently the largest in the literature) of 38 patients implanted with 41 nerve stimulators. The previous nerve damage included blunt and or sharp nerve trauma (in 14 of 38 patients) and inadvertent injection of a nerve (in nine of 38 patients). The incidence of nerve damage from PNS therapy itself is unknown and believed to be rare. To avoid nerve damage, practitioners should maintain excellent knowledge of relevant anatomy and watch for patient neuralgia and radicular pain in the postoperative period. Treatment of suspected nerve injury may include steroid protocol, anticonvulsants, and referral for neurologic consult.

Allergic events in PNS procedures can range from mild topical reactions to full anaphylaxis. Allergic events generally surround the use of preoperative skin preparations, antibiotics, local anesthetics, latex, and sedative medications (e.g., midazolam). Rarely, patients have reported allergic events to the PNS equipment itself, although this seems to be a delayed reaction.

Taking a thorough patient history is beneficial in determining whether the patient is allergic to any of the agents used in PNS therapies. Because the patient may be unaware of any allergies surrounding these products, the physician should remain vigilant for development of allergic sequelae during PNS. For example, local anesthetics are common elicitors of adverse reactions with clinical symptoms such as anaphylaxis with tachycardia; hypotension; and subjective feelings of weakness, heat, or vertigo.[7] Furthermore, during general anesthesia or sedation, anaphylactic response to IV hypnotics and other drugs can occur; cardiovascular collapse and bronchospasm are frequent in immunoglobulin E–dependent reactions.[8] In addition, latex can produce allergic reactions as serious as anaphylaxis.[9]

Although the incidence of allergic or toxic reactions to skin preparations is unusual, practitioners should remain aware that iodine tincture and chlorhexidine can produce adverse outcomes in some patients. It is advisable to take a thorough patient history to avoid cutaneous manifestations, particularly in patients with skin sensitivity or other drug allergies. Iodine is associated with adverse effects ranging from minor skin irritation to anaphylaxis, with symptoms occurring within minutes and up to 8 hours after contact.[10] In addition, the incidence of contact dermatitis to chlorhexidine in atopic patients is approximately 2.5% to 5.4%, and acute hypersensitivity reactions to chlorhexidine are often not recognized and therefore may be underreported.[11]

Skin preparations are a topic of concern not only because of their allergic potential but also because of choice of agent (e.g., iodine tincture vs. chlorhexidine). According to a 2010 study published in the New England Journal of Medicine,[12] preoperative cleansing of the patient's skin with chlorhexidine–alcohol was superior to cleansing with povidone–iodine for preventing surgical site infection (SSI) after clean-contaminated surgery.

Chlorhexidine–alcohol was significantly more protective than povidone–iodine against both superficial incisional infections (4.2% vs. 8.6%; $P = 0.008$) and deep incisional infections (1% vs. 3%, $P = .05$), although it was not effective against organ space infections (4.4% vs. 4.5%). Furthermore, according to Barenfanger et al,[13] in choosing a skin preparation for surgical site antisepsis in PNS, it should be noted that although iodine tincture has been called the "gold standard" in preoperative skin preparation, it does not provide statistically greater utility than chlorhexidine in terms of contamination rates, and chlorhexidine may be safer, less expensive, and preferred by staff members. Furthermore, iodine tincture has the disadvantage of being toxic when used repeatedly, but toxicity or sensitization caused by chlorhexidine is very uncommon. However, Barenfanger et al[13] found that the average contamination rate with chlorhexidine was found to be slightly greater than with iodine (3.13%, or 186 contaminants in 5936 cultures, vs. 2.72%, or 158 contaminants in 5802 cultures).

Numerous randomized, controlled trials in the literature underscore the benefits of giving prophylactic antibiotics to the patient immediately before surgical procedures such as PNS to inhibit development of infection, although the risk of allergic reaction to antibiotics exists. Classen et al[14] prospectively monitored the timing of antibiotic prophylaxis and development of surgical wound infections in 2847 patients undergoing surgical procedures. Among patients who received antibiotics up to 24 hours before surgery, 2 hours before surgery, 3 hours after surgery, and more than 3 hours after surgery, those who received antibiotics 2 hours before surgery had the lowest rates of subsequent surgical wound infections. Furthermore, according to a surgeon's perspective by Nichols,[15] it is generally recommended in elective clean surgical procedures using a foreign body and in clean-contaminated procedures that IV antibiotics should be administered in the operative suite immediately before incision.

Although innumerable clinical trials demonstrate the efficacy of preoperative administration of antibiotics against subsequent infection, physicians should remain mindful of the possibility of unexpected antibiotic allergy in these patients. Although allergic reactions to antibiotics account for only a small proportion of reported adverse drug reactions and estimates of their prevalence vary widely, they are associated with substantial morbidity and mortality and increased health care costs.[16]

Although infectious complications of PNS and PNfS techniques have generally been associated with less morbidity and mortality as compared to spinal cord stimulation, serious infectious complications have been described. In an unpublished case at the Cleveland clinic, a patient underwent PNfS for somatic abdominal pain, placing the lead in transversus abdominal plane using US guidance. Six weeks later the patient presented with an acute abdomen and sepsis secondary to erosion of the leads into the peritoneal cavity, with subsequent death from septic complications.

Post-Procedural Complications

The most common complication after a PNS procedure is infection, which is estimated at the approximate rate of 3% to 5%,[17] and is most likely to occur at the site of implantation. Infection may include wound cellulitis, gross infection at the generator and lead sites, and sepsis. Close adherence to specific guidelines to prevent infection and meticulous attention to sterile technique during the procedure and throughout wound closure are considered to be the best measures against infection.

Signs and symptoms of PNS-related infection may include pain, swelling, rubor, and purulent drainage, as well as fever, nausea, vomiting, and chills. Of particular concern are signs of advanced infection, including elevated white blood cell, C-reactive protein, and sedimentation rate counts. Wound infection can vary from mild cellulitis to dehiscence and frank pus requiring explantation of the system. Cellulitis at the surgical site, the precursor to skin erosion and dehiscence, may occur when the lead, anchor, or generator irritates the skin. Careful screening of patients for skin abnormalities, special attention to wound closure with optimal tissue alignment, and postoperative wound monitoring work in concert to help preclude development of such complications.

Wound infections involving the generator, tunneled area, or lead incision site can occur in up to 4.5% of patients based on reported incidences.[18] To avoid development of wound infections, meticulous surgical technique is necessary to prevent primary contamination of the implanted equipment even from common skin flora. In infected patients, subsequent wound dehiscence with external exposure of any of the implant requires explantation of the total device, although a previously infected area can be successfully reimplanted after successful treatment of the affected area.

To lower the incidence of infection, some experts recommend swabbing of the wound for microbiologic analysis in the stage subsequent to the trial period and before permanent implantation. According to Rudiger et al,[19] swabbing should function as a prerequisite for permanent implantation, with the anchoring site wound opened and inspected for visible signs of infection and swabbed for microbiologic analysis, including sensitivities for positive results. Furthermore, Rudiger et al[19] noted a lowered incidence of infection in patients given a double-layer hydrocolloid dressing and noted that this type of dressing reduced movement and prevented dislocation of temporary leads at the wound exit site. In addition, another study noted silver-impregnated wound covers lowered infection rates in 786 patients implanted with a neurosurgical device, including spinal cord stimulators.[20]

Seroma formation may occur in PNS wound sites, particularly in patients with connective tissue conditions such as lupus, rheumatoid arthritis, and scleroderma. Development of seroma occurs most frequently in the wound circumventing the generator and in serious cases can lead to device explantation. History of seroma formation should alert practitioners to remain particularly mindful of this potential complication.

Although it is recommended that pocket size be minimized to inhibit seroma formation, an excessively small pocket can promote inadequate wound closure as well as pressure on the tissue with gradual skin erosion over the hardware components. For PNS specifically, lead migration can occur at the skin when the leads are placed too superficially. For example, Slavin et al[21] reported one of eight patients who received PNS of trigeminal nerve branches for infraorbital pain developed skin erosion over an electrode requiring removal and eventual reimplantation. Eruption of device components through the skin can be caused by poor tissue health from chronic disease, weight loss, and excessively superficial placement of hardware. Skin erosion can occur at any place along the device whether it is the implanted pulse generator, the electrodes, the leads, or the anchoring devices. It occurs most frequently at the generator site, requiring surgical revision to preclude system failure, which warrants complete removal of the system. If an anchoring method is used to secure the leads, the tissue must be closed in multiple planes to protect the anchor from erosion. Alternatively, some experts choose to use nonabsorbable sutures and secure the lead without creating a formal anchor. This technique is not well studied and is not recommended in most clinical scenarios.

An overly small pocket can also cause pain in the region of the implanted hardware. For example, pain at the generator site is commonly seen in patients with histories of myofascial pain syndromes such as fibromyalgia. The risk of developing pain surrounding the device can be reduced by creating the pocket in a location that receives the least pressure during daily activities. To treat this type of pain, consider topical anesthetics, padding, or surgical revision if necessary.

Another postoperative complication seen in PNS is excessive bleeding. Meticulous control of bleeding throughout the procedure should help to eliminate this risk for most patients. Patients who receive long-term anticoagulation therapy are at greater risk of postoperative hemorrhage, and the risk of excessive bleeding should be considered when returning to the postoperative anticoagulation protocol.

Development of sepsis from PNS, although uncommon, is still a cause for concern, particularly because bacteria tend to thrive on the surface of implanted devices.[22] Recent data indicate that *Escherichia coli* and *Staphylococcus aureus* continue to be the most frequent pathogens isolated in bloodstream infection;[23] growth of these and other bacteria on the biomaterial surface of PNS hardware may multiply and physiologically transform into a "biofilm" community, which bolsters their resistance to antibiotic therapy and host immunity. Because of the hardiness of the resulting biofilm, treating sepsis without removing all foreign bodies and necrotic bone fragments is often ineffective.

Infection

Because infection is considered the most probable and potentially serious complication of PNS therapy, the practitioner should attempt to mitigate the risk of topical and systemic infection in the patient. Beyond screening patients for topical infections, immunocompromised status, and systemic conditions, the most important measure against infection is meticulous surgical technique.

According to Centers for Disease Control and Prevention (CDC) guidelines[24] for prevention of SSIs:

- Whenever possible, identify and treat all infections remote to the surgical site before elective operation and postpone elective operations on patients with remote site infections until the infection has resolved.
- Do not remove hair preoperatively unless the hair at or around the incision site will interfere with the operation.
- If hair is removed, remove it immediately before the operation, preferably with electric clippers.
- Adequately control serum blood glucose levels in all patients with diabetes and particularly avoid hyperglycemia perioperatively.
- Encourage tobacco cessation. At minimum, instruct patients to abstain for at least 30 days before elective operation from smoking cigarettes, cigars, pipes, or any other form of tobacco consumption (e.g., chewing or dipping).
- Do not withhold necessary blood products from surgical patients as a means to prevent SSI.
- Require patients to shower or bathe with an antiseptic agent on at least the night before the operative day.
- Thoroughly wash and clean at and around the incision site to remove gross contamination before performing antiseptic skin preparation.
- Use an appropriate antiseptic agent for skin preparation.
- Apply preoperative antiseptic skin preparation in concentric circles moving toward the periphery. The prepared area must be large enough to extend the incision or create new incisions or drain sites if necessary.
- Keep preoperative hospital stay as short as possible while allowing for adequate preoperative preparation of the patient.

- There is no recommendation to taper or discontinue systemic steroid use (when medically permissible) before elective operation.
- There is no recommendation to enhance nutritional support for surgical patients solely as a means to prevent SSI.
- There is no recommendation to preoperatively apply mupirocin to nares to prevent SSI.
- There is no recommendation to provide measures that enhance wound space oxygenation to prevent SSI.

Furthermore, for optimal asepsis and surgical technique, the CDC recommends that the practitioner:

- Adhere to principles of asepsis when placing devices and administering IV drugs.
- Assemble sterile equipment and solutions immediately before use.
- Handle tissue gently, maintain effective hemostasis, minimize devitalized tissue and foreign bodies (i.e., sutures, charred tissues, necrotic debris), and eradicate dead space at the surgical site.

And for postoperative incision care and surveillance:

- Protect the wound with a sterile dressing for 24 to 48 hours postoperatively for an incision that has been closed primarily.
- Wash hands before and after dressing changes and any contact with the surgical site.
- When an incision dressing must be changed, use sterile technique.
- Educate the patient and family regarding proper incision care, symptoms of SSI, and the need to report such symptoms.
- There is no recommendation to cover an incision closed primarily beyond 48 hours, nor on the appropriate time to shower or bathe with an uncovered incision.
- Assign the surgical wound classification upon completion of an operation. A surgical team member should make the assignment.
- For each patient undergoing an operation chosen for surveillance, record variables shown to be associated with increased SSI risk (e.g., surgical wound class, American Society of Anesthesiologists class, and duration of operation).

An additional means of reducing the number of SSIs is rapid screening and decolonizing of nasal carriers of *S. aureus*, according to a study by Bode et al.[25] A total of 1270 nasal swabs from 1251 patients were positive for *S. aureus*; 917 of these patients were enrolled in an intention-to-treat analysis, and 808 (88.1%) underwent a surgical procedure. All *S. aureus* strains identified on polymerase chain reaction assay were susceptible to methicillin and mupirocin. The rate of *S. aureus* infection was 3.4% (17 of 504 patients) in the mupirocin–chlorhexidine group compared with 7.7% (32 of 413 patients) in the placebo group, and the authors noted that the effect of mupirocin–chlorhexidine treatment was most pronounced for deep SSIs.

Another study suggesting the importance of eradication of *S. aureus* concerned a group of patients with SCS implants.[26] Of the 158 patients who participated in a weeklong trial of SCS, six (4%) developed infections. Of the 68 patients who received the implant after participating in the trial, eight (12%) developed infections. In five of the 14 total infected individuals, the site of infection was cultured. In each case, *S. aureus* was the only isolated pathogen.

As part of an infection management protocol, the practitioner should review signs of infection with the patient and monitor postoperatively. Upon suspicion of infection, a general testing and treatment protocol should be developed (e.g., blood work, computed tomography scan, opening up wound, device explantation). In general, wound exploration is recommended instead of oral antibiotic treatment if SSI is suspected.

If seroma develops, a protocol for optimal timing of drainage should be developed, as well as guidelines on where to drain (e.g., in the office, ambulatory surgery center, hospital). Typically, seroma exploration should be performed in a sterile environment, and the wound should be carefully monitored to avoid introduction of pathogens into the wound site.

Device-Related Complications

Although recent technologic improvements have allowed for improved quality and complexity of stimulators and better lead extensions, PNS therapies still carry a risk of complications pertaining to implanted components, particularly within the first 2 years after implantation of the device.[5]

An important hardware-related complication is loss of paresthesia coverage, which can result from device failure, component breakage or disconnection, development of fibrosis surrounding the lead, increasing tolerance to stimulation, and lead migration. Painful stimulation can also occur from these causes, and positional stimulation can be caused by inadequate contact between lead and tissue in certain positions such as standing or sitting and may resolve over time or require surgical revision. Development of stimulation problems should be addressed with a thorough evaluation of the hardware system, including physical examination, imaging studies, and computer analysis.

Although percutaneous implantation of electrodes should be a relatively straightforward and simple technique, the procedure can still produce undesirable sequelae, leading to low patient satisfaction and overall increase in costs associated with the procedure.[5] Lead migration felt as a change in the stimulation by the patient may be diagnosed by an inability to obtain coverage over the painful area and comparison of imaging studies of current lead position with those taken at baseline. In fact, lead migration is probably the most common problem related to PNS cases and may be responsible for 33% of reoperations, according to a retrospective analysis performed by Ishizuka et al.[27]

Correlates can be drawn to literature of SCS migration and its prevention. Studies in SCS show lead migration in 22% of patients, although the percentage of patients that needed surgical intervention has not been disclosed.[28] In another case, 14.8% of patients required surgical intervention because of SCS lead migration or fracture.[29] And in occipital nerve stimulation, lead migration occurred in 12 of 51 (24%) subjects in a multicenter, randomized, blinded, controlled feasibility study.[30]

To examine how mechanical failures such as lead breakage and migration can undermine the efficacy of implantable technologies, a panel of experienced implanters interpreted a systematic analysis of surgical techniques coupled with extensive in vivo and in vitro biomechanical testing of system components and related them to clinical observations.[31] A computer model based on morphometric data was used to predict movement in a standard SCS system between an anchored lead and pulse generator placed in various locations, and these displacements were then used to determine a realistic range of forces exerted on components of the SCS system. Leads and anchors were subjected to repetitive stresses until failure occurred. In addition, an in vivo sheep model was used to determine system compliances and failure thresholds in a biologically

realistic setting. According to panel consensus, use of a soft Silastic anchor pushed through the fascia to provide a larger bend radius for the lead was associated with a time to failure 65 times longer than an anchored but unsupported lead. In addition, whereas failures of surgical paddle leads occurred when used with an anchor, without an anchor, no failures occurred to 1 million cycles. Based on these findings, the panel recommended a paramedian approach, abdominal pulse generator placement, maximizing bend radius by pushing the anchor through the fascia and anchoring of the extension connector near the lead anchor.

To reduce lead migration risk, patients should be instructed to avoid movement in the immediate postoperative period, including bending, lifting, and vigorous motion. The physician should select ligament or fascia for anchoring purposes, avoiding muscle, which is associated with lead migration because of its high mobility. The anchor should be placed as proximally as possible to where the lead enters the ligament or fascia to avoid room for migration distal to the anchor, and the wound should not be closed if bleeding is ongoing because hematoma can compress the anchor. It should be remembered that the anchor is only one factor in securing the system, and total dependence on the anchor can lead to migration; for example, if possible, the lead should be placed in an area of minimal movement.

Although most PNS complications have revolved around lead migration, improved anchoring techniques and continuing medical education opportunities for implanters should help to decrease the risk of migration.

Although no formal study has been performed specifically for PNS because the hardware is largely the same, surgical guidance to mitigate lead migration may be extrapolated. According to an expert panel, the optimal material for anchoring percutaneous leads for SCS is 0 black braided nylon, if possible.[5] Some practitioners prefer 2.0 silk sutures; however, according to the same panel, these should not be tied too tightly, and thin sutures may cut through the anchor or insulation. Furthermore, the lead should be anchored to deep fascia, and the nose of the Silastic anchor should be pushed through it; if this is not performed properly, a kink in the lead may result, which can be responsible for fracturing of the lead.[5] Another consideration is that a strain relief loop should be used after anchoring the lead and before connection to an extension cable, if used; even though fibrous tubular casing may develop around the loop, the extension cord moves within this fibrous casing, which does not promote extra strain.[5] In addition, generator placement close to the area of stimulation and minigenerators may help to reduce migration problems.

Battery failure is another hardware-related complication in PNS. Battery failure may be directly associated with high energy use; battery conservation may be promoted by use of a cycling mode, low frequencies, and a limited number of active electrodes.[5] Furthermore, a rechargeable system may be optimal when a patient requires continuous high-voltage stimulation that would otherwise shorten battery life of nonrechargeable systems.[5]

A general article published by the New York School of Regional Anesthesia (NYSORA)[41] points out that the use of nerve stimulators does not exclude the possibility of nerve damage[42,43] and recommends caution when stimulation is obtained with currents of less than 0.02 mA. The article further states that stimulation with such low-intensity current is often associated with paresthesia on injection, perhaps suggesting an intraneural placement of the needle. In this scenario, the NYSORA recommends that the practitioner routinely withdraw the needle until the motor response is obtained at a current of 0.2 to 0.5 mA. The NYSORA also states that nerve stimulators used for peripheral nerve blockade can vary greatly in their features, stimulating frequency, maximum voltage output, stimulus duration, and accuracy, and although most modern units it studied performed adequately within a clinically relevant range of currents and impedance loads, some older models may be grossly inaccurate. For that reason, the NYSORA states the recommendations on the current intensity in older books may not be applicable with all nerve stimulators.

Conclusion

PNS appears to be a safe, effective, multimodal means of treating otherwise refractory pain resulting from a variety of etiologies. Although there remains a need for additional large, randomized controlled trials studying PNS techniques, the available data suggest open, percutaneous, and field techniques of PNS have high efficacy in the treatment of neuropathies and carry a relatively low risk of complications. Furthermore, the therapy has advanced significantly in recent years, with advancements such as improved leads, more sophisticated programmable generators, and a wide variety of electrical arrays for achieving neuromodulation.

However, despite the technological advances that have rendered PNS an encouraging therapeutic option for chronic pain, as with any invasive maneuver, PNS carries some degree of risk. It is critical for physicians to identify and reduce the occurrence of probable pitfalls and treat negative outcomes appropriately to reduce permanent complications. Because the primary risk of PNS appears to be infection, meticulous attention to surgical technique is the best measure against the development of complications. In addition, measures such as adequate patient screening and use of high-quality imaging are necessary to avoid adverse outcomes, as are development of practitioner expertise and familiarity with the different types of available hardware.

Provided that adequate cautionary measures are taken and the physician remains vigilant, carefully selected patients are positioned to gain tremendous pain relief and enhanced functionality from PNS therapies.

References

1. Paicius RM, Bernstein CA, Cheryl Lempert-Cohen C: Peripheral nerve field stimulation for the treatment of chronic low back pain: preliminary results of long-term follow-up: a case series. *Neuromodulation* 10(3):279-290, 2007.
2. Stanton-Hicks M: *Neuromodulation*, London, 2009, Elsevier, pp 2:400.
3. Coffey RJ, Woens ML, Broste SK, et al: Medical practice perspective: identification and mitigation of risk factors for mortality associated with intrathecal opioids for non-cancer pain. *Pain Med* 11:1001-1009, 2010.
4. Mobbs RJ, Nair S, Blum P: Peripheral nerve stimulation for the treatment of chronic pain. *J Clin Neurosci* 14(3):216-221; discussion 222-223, 2007.
5. Kumar K, Buchser E, Linderoth B, et al: Avoiding complications from spinal cord stimulation: practical recommendations from an international panel of experts. *Neuromodulation* 10(1):24-33, 2007.
6. Liu SS, Gordon MA, Shaw PM, et al: A prospective clinical registry of ultrasound-guided regional anesthesia for ambulatory shoulder surgery. *Anesth Analg* 111(3):617-623, 2010.
7. Ring J: Anaphylactic reactions to local anesthetics. *Chem Immunol Allergy* 95:190-200, 2010.
8. Moneret-Vautrin DA, Mertes PM: Anaphylaxis to general anesthetics. *Chem Immunol Allergy* 26(8-9):719-723, 2010.
9. Heitz JW, Bader SO: An evidence-based approach to medication preparation for the surgical patient at risk for latex allergy: is it time to stop being stopper poppers? *J Clin Anesth* 22(6):477-483, 2010.
10. Rahimi S, Lazarou G: Late-onset allergic reaction to povidone-iodine resulting in vulvar edema and urinary retention. *Obstet Gynecol* 116(suppl 2):562-564, 2010.
11. Lim KS, Kam PC: Chlorhexidine—pharmacology and clinical applications. *Anaesth Intensive Care* 36(4):502-512, 2008.
12. Darouiche RO, Wall MJ, Jr, Itani KM, et al: Chlorhexidine-alcohol versus povidone-iodine for surgical-site antisepsis. *N Engl J Med* 362(1):18-26, 2010.
13. Barenfanger J, Drake C, Lawhorn J, Verhulst SJ: Comparison of chlorhexidine and tincture of iodine for skin antisepsis in preparation for blood sample collection. *J Clin Microbiol* 42(5):2216-2217, 2004.
14. Classen DC, Evans RS, Pestotnik SL, et al: The timing of prophylactic administration of antibiotics and the risk of surgical-wound infection. *N Engl J Med* 326(5):281-286, 1992.
15. Nichols RL: Preventing surgical site infections: a surgeon's perspective. *Emerg Infect Dis* 7(2):220-224, 2001.
16. Gruchalla RS, Pirmohamed M: Antibiotic allergy. *N Engl J Med* 354(6):601-609, 2006.
17. De Leon-Casasola O: Spinal cord and peripheral nerve stimulation techniques for neuropathic pain. *J Pain Symptom Manage* 38(2 suppl):S28-S38, 2009.
18. Deer T: *Atlas of implantable therapies for pain management*, New York, 2011, Springer.
19. Rudiger J, Thomson S: Infection rate of spinal cord stimulators after a screening trial period. A 53-month third party follow-up. *Neuromodulation* 14(2):136-141, 2011.
20. Turner MS, Flint KJ, Davis KE: Infection rates and use of silver-impregnated wound covers when implanting neurosurgical devices. *AANS Neurosurgeon* 19(3), 2010.
21. Slavin KV: Peripheral nerve stimulation for neuropathic pain. *Neurotherapeutics* 5(1):100-106, 2008.
22. Gallo J, Kolár M, Novotný R, et al: Pathogenesis of prosthesis-related infection. *Biomed Pap Med Fac Univ Palacky Olomouc Czech Repub* 147(1):27-35, 2003.
23. Kern WV: [Bacteraemia and sepsis]. *Dtsch Med Wochenschr* 136(5):182-185, 2011.
24. Mangram AJ, Horan TC, Pearson ML, et al: Guideline for prevention of surgical site infection, 1999. Centers for Disease Control and Prevention (CDC) Hospital Infection Control Practices Advisory Committee. *Am J Infect Control* 27(2):97-132; quiz 133-1334; discussion 96, 1999.
25. Bode LG, Kluytmans JA, Wertheim HF, et al: Preventing surgical-site infections in nasal carriers of Staphylococcus aureus. *N Engl J Med* 362(1):9-17, 2010.
26. Halwani M: LD-30: *Infection spinal cord stimulator placement: a retrospective cohort study*. Infectious Diseases Society of America. Presented Saturday, October 23, 2010; Vancouver, British Columbia.
27. Ishizuka K, Oaklander AL, Chiocca EA: A retrospective analysis of reasons for reoperation following initially successful peripheral nerve stimulation. *J Neurosurg* 106(3):388-390, 2007.
28. North RB, Kidd DH, Zahurak M, et al: Spinal cord stimulation for chronic, intractable pain: Experience over two decades. *Neurosurgery* 32(3):384-394; discussion 394-395, 1993.
29. Ubbink DT, Vermeulen H, Spincemaille GH, et al: Systematic review and meta-analysis of controlled trials assessing spinal cord stimulation for inoperable critical leg ischaemia. *Br J Surg* 91(8):948-955, 2004.
30. Saper JR, Dodick DW, Silberstein SD, et al: Occipital nerve stimulation for the treatment of intractable chronic migraine headache: ONSTIM feasibility study. *Cephalalgia* 31(3):271-285, 2011.
31. Henderson J, Schade C, Sasaki J, et al: Prevention of mechanical failures in implanted spinal cord stimulation systems. *Neuromodulation* 9(3):183-191, 2006.
32. Hassenusch SJ, Stanton-Hicks M, Schoppa D, Walsh JG, Covington EC: Long-term results of peripheral nerve stimulation for reflex sympathetic dystrophy. *J Neurosurg* 84(3):415-423, 1996 Mar.
33. Ochani TD Almirante J, Siddiqui A, Kaplan R: Allergic reaction to spinal cord Stimulator. *Clin J Pain* (16)178-180, 2000.
34. Schwedt TJ, Dodick D, Hentz J, Trentman TL, Zimmerman RS: Occipital nerve stimulation for chronic headache-long-term safety and efficacy. *Cephalalgia* 27:153-157, 2007.

35. Verrillis P, Vivian D, Mitchell B, Barnard A: Peripheral Nerve Stimulation for Chronic Pain: 100 cases and Review of the Literature. *Pain Medicine* 12:1395-1405, 2011.

36. Beer GM, Wallner H: Prevention of Seroma after Abdominoplasty. *Aesthetic Surgery Journal* 30(3)414-417, 2010.

37. Jasper J, Hayek S: Implanted Occipital Nerve Stimulator. *Pain Physician* 11:187-200, 2008.

38. Kumar K, Buchser E, Linderoth B, Meglio M, Van Buyten JP: Avoiding Complications From Spinal Cord Stimulation: Practical Management Recommendations an International Panel of Experts. *Neuromodulaton* 10:24-33, 2007.

39. Turner JA, Loeser JD, Deyo RA, Sanders SB: Spinal Cord Stimulation for with Failed back Surgery Syndrome or complex Regional Pain Syndrome: a systematic review of effectiveness and complications. *Pain* 108:137-147, 2004.

40. Cameron T: Safety and efficacy of spinal cord stimulation for the treatment of chronic pain: a 20-year literature review. *J Neurosurg* 100:254-267, 2004.

41. New York School of Regional Anesthesia: Complications of peripheral nerve blocks. 2009. Retrieved January 31, 2010 from http://www.nysora.com/regional_anesthesia/other_topics/3132-compliations_of_regional_anesthesia.html.

42. Auroy Y, Narchi P, Messiah A, et al: Serious complications related to regional anesthesia: Results of a prospective survey in France. *Anesthesiology* 87(3):479-486, 1997.

43. Auroy Y, Benhamou D, Bargues L, et al: Major complications of regional anesthesia in France: The SOS Regional Anesthesia Hotline Service. *Anesthesiology* 97(5):1274-1280, 2002.

3 Complications of Cranial Nerve Stimulation

Jason E. Pope

CHAPTER OVERVIEW

Chapter Synopsis: Cranial nerve stimulation has been used to treat an array of pain syndromes, including many types of headache. But the technique has also been applied for conditions as diverse as depression and congestive heart failure. Most common are stimulation of the peripheral branch of the trigeminal nerve (including the trigeminocervical complex) and the vagus nerve. As with other peripheral nerve stimulation techniques, most complications of trigeminal and vagus nerve stimulation arise from electrode lead migration, infection, or hardware malfunction. One must also consider the lifelong nature of follow-up care required for continued stimulation, which requires battery replacement and possible surgical revision or reprogramming.

Important Points:

- Appropriate Accreditation Council for Graduate Medical Education mentored subspecialty training in interventional pain management is vital to ensure patient-centered care.
- Accurate and expertly placed needles in appropriately selected patients are essential to ensure accurate diagnosis and successful treatment.
- Stimulation of the trigeminocervical complex is the most described cranial nerve stimulation target to treat pain syndromes.
- The most common complication for occipital nerve stimulation is lead migration, which may by mitigated by paddle lead choice, retromastoid position lead placement, or implantable pulse generator location in the abdomen or infraclavicular site.
- The most common complication with peripheral branch trigeminal stimulation is wound erosion and infection.
- Vagal nerve stimulation is used to treat refractory depression and epilepsy, although the applications for pain are evolving. Special surgical training is suggested for dissection and device placement.

Introduction

Cranial nerve stimulation strategies have been used to treat a variety of diverse conditions that sometimes prove to be unresponsive to conservative medical therapies. These range from depression to seizure to congestive heart failure.[1-3] More specifically, some other indications include atypical facial pain, terminal branch neuralgias, a variety of headache disorders (i.e., cluster, migraine, trigeminal autonomic cephalalgias, cervicogenic headache, hemicrania continua, trigeminal neuralgia), depression, and postherpetic neuralgia.[1,4-24] Stimulation technology has also been used in a case series to treat central hypoventilation syndrome by stimulation of the phrenic nerve.

This chapter focuses on complications reported during peripheral (distal) stimulation of cranial nerves, namely the terminal branches of the trigeminal nerve, the trigeminocervical complex, and the vagus nerve. Although epidural trigeminocervical complex stimulation has been reported to treat trigeminal neuralgia,[25] the reader is directed to Chapter 1 for discussion of complications of epidural spinal cord stimulation (SCS).

Experience with cranial nerve stimulation, compared to SCS or deep brain stimulation, is in its infancy, as suggested by the paucity of literature. Stimulation of the trigeminocervical complex via the occipital nerve, on the other hand, is well described. As one can expect, correlates can be made to patient selection for peripheral cranial nerve stimulation and SCS. The procedure is contraindicated in patients with local infection near the injection site, coagulopathy, allergy to injectate or components of the device, comorbidities or conditions that prevent fluoroscopic needle guidance, or an inability to provide consent. Furthermore, future requirement for magnetic resonance imaging should be elicited.

Although a review of the American Society of Regional Anesthesia's 2010 guidelines for neuraxial interventions may not directly be applicable to peripheral branch of cranial nerve stimulation interventions, concurrent use of anticoagulants before surgery may increase the bleeding risk. Therefore it is advised that readers familiarize themselves with these guidelines, as well as the guideline statements of perioperative use of anticoagulant therapy.[26]

Patient selection guides treatment success. Psychometric testing for neuromodulation candidacy deserves special mention. It is well established that concurrent psychiatric illness reduces interventional treatment success rates[27] and that approximately 20% to 45% of pain patients have accompanying psychopathology.[28] Therefore it is essential that appropriate measures be taken to diagnose, treat, or exclude unsuitable candidates. Instruments described to aid in identifying the presence of clinically significant psychopathology include the Symptom Checklist 90 (SCL-90-R) and the Minnesota Multiphasic Personality Inventory (MMPI-2). Poor treatment outcome was identified in patients with presurgical somatization, depression, anxiety, and poor coping.[29]

Of paramount significance, and similar to SCS, the current constraints and limitations of the current neuromodulatory technology requires vigilance and as a consequence of changes in impedance and battery life, either reprogramming or surgical revision. Simply stated, these devices require long-term management because these are lifelong therapies.

Furthermore, appropriate training within Accreditation Council for Graduate Medical Education (ACGME) accredited programs and mentorship is essential to ensure treatment success and limit iatrogenic morbidity; inadequately trained providers attempting to use these therapies will not only potentially harm their patients but will also broadly limit access to these therapies by undermining patient outcomes.

Background

Trigeminal stimulation techniques have been described both centrally and peripherally; however, more reliable stimulation has been achieved in the latter.[4] Furthermore, because overall complications of central trigeminal gasserian stimulation have been reported to be near 30% to 40%[30-32] and with reduced complications with peripheral branch stimulation, enthusiasm for central stimulation has dwindled. The trigeminal nuclear systems are bilateral structures that span from the midbrain to the medulla. The caudal-most portion, the trigeminal nucleus caudalis, may extend down as far as the second or third cervical level, which has both anatomic and clinical implications. Goadsby[33] demonstrated the presence of convergence between the cervical and trigeminal system, forming a trigeminocervical complex. This was characterized by Anthony[34] and helped form the basis for greater occipital nerve stimulation for treatment of headache (**Fig. 3-1**). Traditionally, stimulation was achieved by using either implanted cylindrical or paddle leads. There are some reports of using a small implantable device without the traditional implantable pulse generator (IPG) placement[10] along with transcutaneous electrical nerve stimulation unit applications.[11]

Peripherally, the trigeminal nerve terminates as the supraorbital and supratrochlear nerve from V1, the infraorbital nerve from V2, and the mental nerve from V3. These sites lend themselves to subcutaneous neurostimulatory targets (**Fig. 3-2**).[4,6,12,17,18,24,35,36]

Vagal nerve stimulation (VNS) has been approved for drug-refractory epilepsy and is a viable option for those who decline surgery or nonsurgical candidates. Its safety and efficacy have been well established.[37] Furthermore, it has been used in the treatment of people with treatment-resistant depression. Commonly, the left vagus nerve is stimulated, not with the commonly used spinal cord stimulator but via a NeuroCybernetic Prosthesis.[38] The exact mechanism of action is unknown, although it is postulated to involve vagal sensory afferents. Whereas high-frequency stimulation causes electroencephalographic desynchronization, low-frequency stimulation causes synchronization.[39] Typically, the VNS is positioned on the left side because right-sided stimulation causes more cardiac slowing as a consequence of sinoatrial (SA) node stimulation.[40] Although this is not commonly used to treat pain, the scope is broadening.[35,41,42] Therefore, VNS is discussed here briefly for completeness.

Although there is commonality with these approaches to cranial nerve stimulation, their indications, operative considerations, and surgical approaches are divergent. Therefore occipital nerve stimulation, peripheral trigeminal nerve stimulation, and VNS are considered here separately and sequentially.

Selected Complications

Greater Occipital Nerve Stimulation (Table 3-1)
Lead Tip Erosion   Trentman et al[43] in 2008 reported on two cases of lead erosion after greater occipital nerve stimulation occurring months after implantation. One patient was a 27-year-old woman who had intended weight loss after gastric bypass surgery

of 52 kilograms; the other case did not have any identifiable risk factors, including smoking, diabetes, or infection. The authors contended that care needs to be emphasized when implanting the paddle or percutaneous electrode, not placing the lead tip too superficial or lateral, lessened by avoiding the lateral decubitus position during implant. Furthermore, extreme weight reduction or patients with very low body mass indexes may be susceptible to eventual lead migration.[43]

Management of lead tip erosion of occipital stimulation leads centers on infection management and revision. Infectious management includes assessment of extent and depth of infection. Generally, two approaches can be used: attempt to salvage the lead and system or explant and reimplant at a future date. Because many patients have greater occipital nerve stimulators secondary to a medically intractable headache, many patients request lead salvage strategies. Trentman et al[43] described resection of granulomatous tissue around eroded lead and was sutured to the fascia and closed primarily along with a concurrent postoperative course of appropriately selected bacteria-sensitive antibiotics by culture.

Infection   As one can appreciate, a superficial or deep subcutaneous infection and its management, from a subcutaneously placed lead, are drastically different than an epidural abscess from an epidural lead. That being said, the potential for leads placed near the nuchal ridge can theoretically spread intracranially via the emissary veins.[44] As illustrated, device salvage has been described for peripheral nerve (or peripheral branch of cranial nerve) stimulation.

Surgical site wound prevention, however, is largely the same.[45] As with any surgical procedure, antimicrobial prophylaxis should occur within 30 minutes of skin incision and cover the most commonly implicated organisms. The decision to provide postoperative prophylactic antibiotics continues to be a controversial topic because many practitioners continue to do so despite only anecdotal evidence. Surgical preparation includes optimizing and mitigating patient comorbidities that increase infectious risk, ensuring proper scrub, and promoting a sterile and accessible operative field.[46] Hair removal should be performed immediately before the procedure, and hair should be clipped because shaving increases the chance of infection secondary to microabrasion. Skin preparation is usually accomplished by chlorhexidine gluconate, povidone–iodine, or alcohol-based solutions. Intraoperative strategies to reduce infection include meticulous sterile technique, layered wound closure to avoid dead space, appropriate hemostasis, avoidance of placing sutures overlying the device, and nonpressured irrigation (in clean uncontaminated surgeries).

If infection is suspected, it is usually heralded by erythema, induration, a temperature of greater than 101.4°F, purulent discharge, or wound dehiscence. If systemic signs or symptoms are present or suspected, an infectious disease consultation is mandatory, and all the hardware (IPG and leads) should be removed. If reimplantation is desirable, it should not be considered until the patient is infection free and medically stable for at least 12 weeks.

Lead Migration   Lead migration rates after greater occipital nerve peripheral nerve stimulation have varied in the literature, although it remains the most common complication described. The rate of lead migration seems to be dependent on follow-up length after implant. Schwedt et al[47] implanted 15 patients using cylindrical leads placed at C1, with the extension connector placed near the periscapular region and IPG placement in the upper buttocks, abdomen, or infraclavicular region. They reported lead migration of 33% at 6 months to 100% at 3 years follow-up and

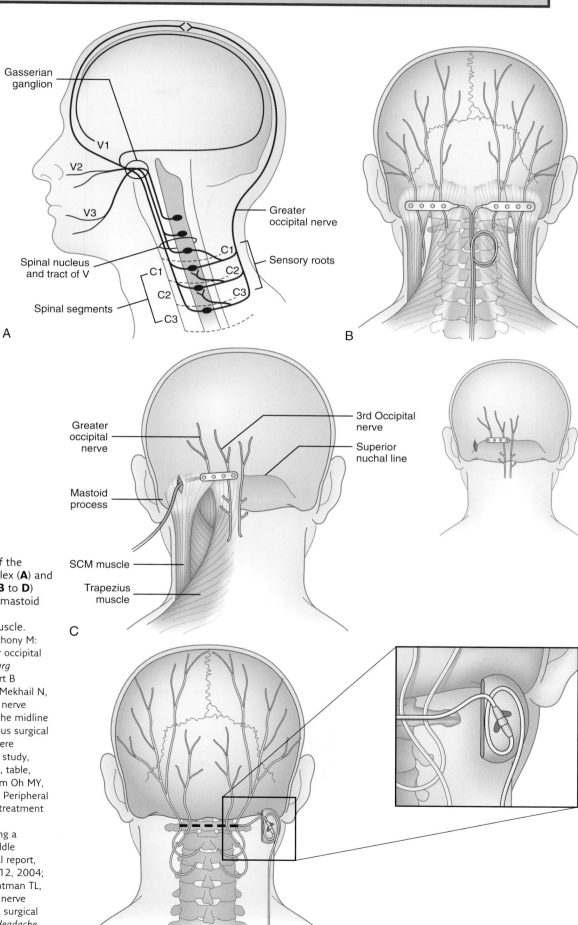

Fig. 3-1 Illustration of the trigeminocervical complex (**A**) and stimulator placement (**B** to **D**) using midline and retromastoid approaches. SCM, sternocleidomastoid muscle. (Part A modified from Anthony M: Headache and the greater occipital nerve, *Clin Neurol Neurosurg* 94(4):297-301, 1992; part B modified from Kapural L, Mekhail N, Hayek SM, et al: Occipital nerve electrical stimulation via the midline approach and subcutaneous surgical leads for treatment of severe occipital neuralgia: a pilot study, *Anesth Analg* 10:171-174, table, 2005; part C modified from Oh MY, Ortega J, Bellotte JB, et al: Peripheral nerve stimulation for the treatment of occipital neuralgia and transformed migraine using a C1-2-3 subcutaneous paddle style electrode: a technical report, *Neuromodulation* 7:103-112, 2004; part D modified from Trentman TL, Zimmerman RS: Occipital nerve stimulation: technical and surgical aspects of implantation, *Headache Currents* 48(2)319-327, 2008.)

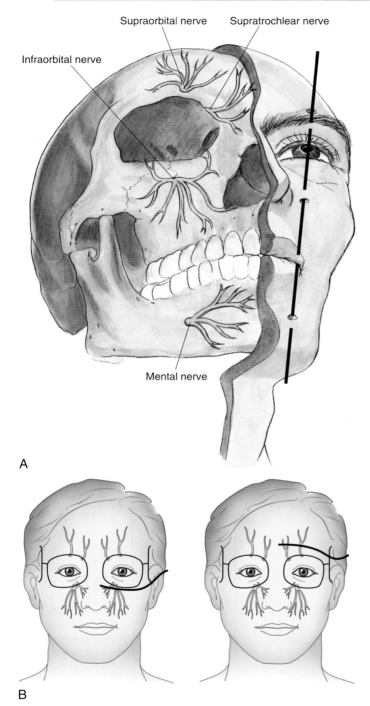

Fig. 3-2 **A,** Terminal branches of the trigeminal nerve. (From Brown DL: *Atlas of regional anesthesia*, ed 3, Philadelphia, WB Saunders, 2006.) **B,** Stimulator lead placement. (Modified from Slavin KV, Wess C: Trigeminal branch stimulation for intractable neuropathic pain: technical note, *Neuromodulation* 8(1):7-13, 2005.)

Table 3-1: Reported Greater Occipital Nerve Stimulation Complications

Complication	Frequency
Lead tip erosion	Two reported[43]
Lead migration	27.3%,[38] 33%[47]*
Hardware malfunction	1.7%,[38] 1/8[19]
Infection	5.9%,[38] 2/7,[65] 3/16[6]
Lead fracture or disconnect	2.6%[38]
Allergy	0.8%[38]
Explant	2.6%[38]
Contact dermatitis	7%[47]
Neck stiffness	13%[47]
Pain over the device (IPG or lead)	1/10,[22] 3/15,[20] 7%[47]
Myofascial pain	1/11,[66] 1/15,[20] five case reports,[44] 7%[47]
Battery depletion	42% at 3 years[47]
Stimulation tolerance	Case report[53]
Overstimulation	3/6[10]

*Reported 100% lead migration at 3 years.
IPG, implantable pulse generator.

infraclavicular, buttock, or low abdominal region, serial external surface measurements. Flexion and extension pathway changes in the infraclavicular and abdominal sites were associated with less length changes than the periscapular and gluteal sites, respectively. Furthermore, retromastoid lead insertion was hypothesized to reduce lead pathway changes.[48]

Paddle leads were hypothesized to mitigate migration.[49] In a recent review, lead migration was reported to have occurred at approximately a rate of 36% for cylindrical leads, where paddle leads migrated in approximately 5.7%.[38] Gofeld[50] suggested a distal anchor to reduce percutaneous lead migration. Midline and retromastoid techniques have been described, with a paucity of prospective data regarding migration prevalence. Oh et al[22] demonstrated in their review that placing paddle leads significantly reduced migration and loss of therapeutic stimulation. Postulated reasons include anteriorly unidirectional current application and surface area of the lead.

Similarities can be drawn to SCS. Lead migration has been reported to be 11% to 13%.[51] Cervical lead migration occurs more often than lumbar or thoracic lead migration, hypothesized to be because of higher mobility in the cervical region. Innately, because the lead placement and anchoring are anatomically in different tissue planes, this is likely as far as the comparison can be made. Regarding SCS, contradictory evidence exists between migration rates of paddle versus percutaneous leads, although the abdominal wall IPG placement fared better than the gluteal region.[52]

Hardware Malfunction Hardware malfunctions for ONS have been reported to approximately 2.6%, with lead fracture or disconnects occurring 2.6% of the time,[38] which is comparable to spinal cord stimulation (2.9%).[52]

Battery Depletion Implantable pulse generator battery depletion is expected when using the device constantly for headache treatment. Schewdt et al[47] demonstrated that 42% of implanted

estimated that "most patients" are expected to have lead migration at 1 year. No comparisons were drawn between the rate and IPG battery site placement.

In an attempt to reduce migration, Trentman et al[48] in 2010 investigated the implant pathway associated with the least length change, from occipital lead position to IPG implantation site in the

nonrechargeable batteries are depleted by 3 years. Trentman et al[53] consider battery depletion of less than 1 year a "complication" and suggest a rechargeable IPG to match the potentially required energy requirement.

Muscle Spasm   Muscle spasm associated with occipital nerve stimulation has been reported to occur in as many as 7% of cases.[47] Hayek at al[33] in 2009 described five cases of unpleasant muscle recruitment causing spasm with reimplantation at the nuchal line as opposed to the C1-C2 level. In all cases, therapeutic stimulation was achieved, and muscle recruitment was stopped. Highlighting the technical considerations of depth of subcutaneous placement, placement that is too superficial may increase propensity for lead erosion and unpleasant burning sensations, and placement that is too deep may cause unpleasant muscle spasms.

Nuchal ridge placement was hypothesized to be superior to the more caudal, traditional C1-C2 placement because less muscle stimulation may be evident when the lead is placed over the aponeurosis of the semispinalis capitis as opposed to the muscle belly.[51]

Allergy   In Jasper et al's[38] review of occipital nerve stimulation, allergy was reported in 0.8% of those studied (115 patients). However, the patient thought she was allergic to the metal because of development of severe pain at the pulse generator site.[22] Commonly, allergy manifests as skin reactions from components of the stimulator device.[54,55]

Overstimulation   Overstimulation was reported in three of six patients treated for headache disorders and implanted with a bion device, two of which resolved by 4 months of follow-up.[10] As stimulation parameters change with distance from the target nerve, recumbence may increase the strength of stimulation. Reprogramming or surgical revision may be required to resolve the stimulation difficulty. The higher the voltage or current programmed, the greater the chance for aberrant structure.

Pain Over the Device   Pain over the device is a relatively common complication, having been reported to be approximately 7%.[8,47] Treatment can involve topical or injection therapy, although

it typically requires revision. Mitigation of device site pain includes avoidance of placement around friction-generating sites; ensuring adequate distance from osteal structures; and most importantly, a clear consensus with the patient regarding IPG placement preoperatively.

Stimulation Tolerance   Although mentioned in a relatively recent review, peripheral nerve stimulation has not been associated with loss of therapeutic stimulation, or "tolerance" observed in SCS.[6]

Vascular Injury   The greater occipital nerve is consistently lateral to the occipital artery at the level of the greater occipital protuberance and vascular injury is a theoretical concern. It has not been reported in the literature; however, using ultrasound guidance with Doppler may be done to reduce the chance of vascular injury.

Peripheral Trigeminal Nerve Stimulation (Table 3-2)

Lead Erosion and Infection   In a case series reported by Amin et al,[6] cylindrical lead stimulation placement for supraorbital neuralgia (**Fig. 3-3**) was complicated by infection in 20% of cases. Interestingly, the infections occurred at the retroauricular connector and extension leads. The authors postulate that the thin dermal and subcutaneous layers results in erosion and skin breakdown.

Similarly, Johnson et al[56] reported three complications requiring surgical intervention in 10 patients implanted with four

Table 3-2: Reported Complications of Peripheral Trigeminal Nerve Stimulation

Complication	Frequency
Lead erosion	1/8[4]
Explant*	1/8[4]
Infection	2/10[6]

*Loss of therapeutic stimulation after 26 months.

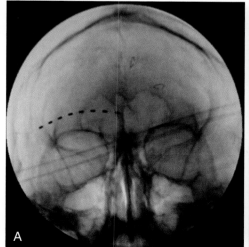
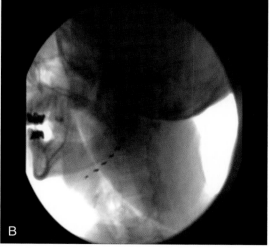

Fig. 3-3   A, Supraorbital cylindrical lead. (From Amin S, Buvanendran A, Park KS, et al: Peripheral nerve stimulator for the treatment of supraorbital neuralgia: a retrospective case series, *Cephalalgia* 28:355-359, 2008.) **B,** V3 cylindrical lead stimulation. (From Yakovlev AE, Resch BE. Treatment of chronic intractable atypical facial pain using peripheral subcutaneous field stimulation, *Neuromodulation* 13:137-140, 2010.)

contact percutaneous cylindrical leads with an infraclavicular IPG placement site for trigeminal postherpetic and posttraumatic neuropathic pain. All of the complications were located around the retroauricular position of the extension lead and the connector. Two had infection and wound breakdown, and the third patient had pain overlying the site requiring lengthening of the extension.[56]

Vagal Nerve Stimulation

Overall complication rates of VNS (**Table 3-3**) have been described to be approximately 13.3%.[2] Selected complications are described below.

Hoarseness Hoarseness associated with VNS typically improves with stimulation titration and is a consequence of activation of the recurrent laryngeal nerve.[57] The recurrent laryngeal nerve supplies motor efferents to all intrinsic muscles of the larynx, excluding the cricothyroid muscle. Delayed onset hoarseness and palsy are rare.[58-61] Tran et al[57] describe a case of traumatic delayed transient vocal cord dysfunction after blunt neck trauma.

Cardiac Arrhythmia Iriarte et al[62] described a report of delayed onset periodic asystole after VNS approximately 9 years later, presenting with dizziness discovered to be stimulation-induced second-degree heart block. This resolved after

Table 3-3: Reported Complications of Vagal Stimulation	
Complication	**Frequency**
Voice alteration	24.1% at 3 mo, 24.8% >12 mo,[2] 63%,[37] 66%[40]
Cough	10.7% at 3 mo,[2] 26%[37]
Respiratory complications	5/15[63]
Pain	20.8% at 3 mo, 10.7% at >12 mo,[1] 1/90[2]
Dyspnea	5.1% at 3 mo,[1] 10%[37]
Recurrent depression*	5.6%[1]
Infection	7.7%,[1] 7%[6]
Interruption of the electrode secondary to trauma	3/90[2]
Technical malfunction of generator	1/90[2]
Cardiac arrhythmia	Case report
Lead fracture	Case report[64]
Vocal cord palsy	1/90,[2] case reports[57-61]
Mania	1/59[37]

*Indication for implantation.

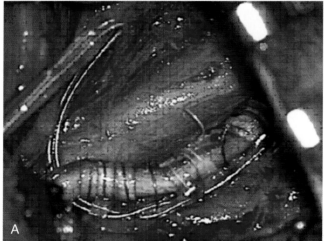

Fig. 3-4 A, Intraoperative image of vagal stimulation. (From Broggi G, Messina G, Marras C, Dones I, Franzini A: Neuromodulation for refractory headaches, *Neurol Sci* 29(suppl 1):S87-S92, 2010.) **B,** Diagram of vagal stimulation.

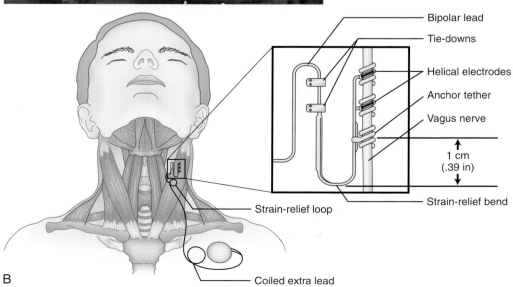

Bipolar lead
Tie-downs
Helical electrodes
Anchor tether
Vagus nerve
1 cm (.39 in)
Strain-relief bend
Strain-relief loop
Coiled extra lead

subsequent explant. Commonly, the parasympathetic, efferent vagal contribution to the atrioventricular node is supplied anatomically by the left vagus nerve (**Fig. 3-4**), and the right supplies the SA node. Retrograde stimulation is the most plausible explanation.

Dyspnea and Respiratory Complications Dyspnea from VNS may be related to less mobility of the vocal cords secondary to denervations from chronic nerve stimulation.[40] In a study by Marzec et al,[63] five of 15 patients developed clinically significant obstructive sleep apnea after device placement. These patients were treated with 9 cm of continuous positive airway pressure.[40,63]

Hardware Malfunction Historically, hardware malfunction was largely attributed to lead fracture.[57,60] Redesign improved the fracture rate but did not eliminate it. Spitz et al[64] reported a discontinuity in the silicone insulation over an electrode of a left vagus nerve stimulator, allowing aberrant leak of current. Ramsay et al[61] described a case of an aberrant and intense stimulation-caused permanent vocal cord paralysis.

Spitz et al[64] reported a woman that described phonation and breathing difficulty with VNS placement. Surgical exploration revealed silicone insulation disruption, which was adjacent to the phrenic nerve and scalene muscles. The symptoms resolved after lead revision.

Psychiatric Complications Bajbouj et al[1] investigated 2-year follow-up after vagal stimulation for treatment resistant depression, and although 27 patients (of 72) reported 39 adverse events, including worsening depression (33.3%), infection, suicide attempt (5.1%), and overdose (5.1%), 53.1% demonstrated significant improvement in depression via the Hamilton Rating Scale for Depression reduction (>50%) with no escalation in population-specific fatal adverse events.

Bajbouj et al[1] described two patients that required explantation in the 2-year follow-up for vagal stimulation for refractory depression. Kuba et al[2] investigated 5-year follow-up for patients with VNS for refractory seizure treatment. The study demonstrated a reduction in seizure intensity and frequency, and adverse events occurred in 13.3%, with explant in one patient because of "local complication."

Vocal Cord Paralysis Tran et al reported a 19-year-old woman with generalized tonic clonic seizures that was well controlled with VNS who suffered blunt neck trauma. She then had return of previous seizure activity. Interrogation of the device suggested lead fracture; operative findings confirmed the suspicion, with evidence of left vocal cord palsy and compression injury of left vagus nerve. Kalakanis et al[58] reported two cases of vagal cord nerve traction injury after manipulation of the IPG in developmentally delayed adults.

Factors to reduce the vocal cord malfunction during VNS therapy include preoperative laryngeal testing before surgery, preservation of the vasa vasorum during dissection of the vagus nerve and placement of the helical electrodes, placement of size appropriate electrode array, and intraoperative stimulation.[57]

Summary

Cranial nerve stimulation is a vital component of the armamentarium to treat a multitude of chronic pain complaints. Success of using the therapy is contingent on appropriate patient selection, careful surgical placement, and ongoing management. It cannot be overstated that the device will invariably need reprogramming or revision, innate to the deficiencies in the current technology.

References

1. Bajbouj M, Merkl A, Schlaepfer TE, et al: Two-year outcome of vagus nerve stimulation in treatment-resistant depression. *J Clin Psychopharmacol* 30:273-281, 2010.
2. Kuba R, Brazedil M, Kalina M, et al: Vagus nerve stimulation: longitudinal follow-up of patients treated for 5 years. *Seizure* 18:269-274, 2009.
3. De Ferrari GM, Sanzo A, Schwartz PJ: Chronic vagal stimulation in patients with congestive heart failure. *Conf Proc IEEE Eng Med Biol Soc* 2037-2039, 2009.
4. Slavin KV, Wess C: Trigeminal branch stimulation for intractable neuropathic pain: technical note. *Neuromodulation* 8(1):7-13, 2005.
5. Aderjan D, Stankewitz A, May A: Neuronal mechanisms during repetitive trigemino-nociceptive stimulation in migraine patients. *Pain* 151(1)97-103, 2010.
6. Amin S, Buvanendran A, Park KS, et al: Peripheral nerve stimulator for the treatment of supraorbital neuralgia: a retrospective case series. *Cephalalgia* 28:355-359, 2008.
7. Asensio-Samper JM, Villanueva VL, Perez AV, et al: Peripheral neurostimulation in supraorbital neuralgia refractory to conventional therapy. *Pain Pract* 8(2):120-124, 2008.
8. Bartsch T, Paemeleire K, Goadsby PJ: Neurostimulation approaches to primary headache disorders. *Curr Opin Neurol* 22:262-268, 2009.
9. Broggi G, Messina G, Franzini A: Cluster headache and TACs: rationale for central and peripheral neuromodulation. *Neurol Sci* 30(suppl 1):S72-S79, 2009.
10. Burns B, Watkins L, Goadsby PJ: Treatment of hemicrania continua by occipital nerve stimulation with a bion device: long-term follow-up of a crossover study. *Lancet Neurol* 7:1001-1012, 2008.
11. Drummend PD, Treleaven-Hassard S: Electrical stimulation decreases neuralgic pain after trigeminal deafferentation. *Cephalagia* 28:782-785, 2008.
12. Dunteman E: Peripheral nerve stimulation for unremitting ophthalmic postherpetic neuralgia. *Neuromodulation* 5(1):32-37, 2002.
13. Finocchi C, Villani V, Casucci G: Therapeutic strategies in migraine patients with mood and anxiety disorders: clinical evidence. *Neurol Sci* 31(supp 1):S95-S98, 2010.
14. Schoenen J, Allena M, Magis D: Neurostimulation therapy in intractable headaches. *Handb Clin Neurol* 97:443-450, 2010.
15. Reed KL, Black SB, Banta CJ, 2nd, Will KR: Combined occipital and supraorbital neurostimulation for the treatment of chronic migraine headaches: initial experience. *Cephalalgia* 3:257-259, 2010.
16. Dafer RM: Neurostimulation in headache disorders. *Neurol Clin* 28(4):835-841, 2010.
17. Popeney CA, Alò KM: Peripheral neurostimulation for the treatment of chronic disabling transformed migraine. *Headache* 43:369-375, 2003.
18. Weiner RL, Reed KL: Peripheral neurostimulation for control of intractable occipital neuralgia. *Neuromodulation* 2:217-221, 1999.
19. Burns B, Watkins L, Goadsby PJ: Treatment of medically intractable cluster headache by occipital nerve stimulation: long-term follow-up of eight patients. *Lancet* 369:1099-1106, 2007.
20. Schwedt TJ, Dodick DW, Hentz J, et al: Occipital nerve stimulation for chronic headache—long-term safety and efficacy. *Cephalalgia* 27:153-157, 2007.
21. Slavin KV, Nersesyan H, Wess C: Peripheral neurostimulation for treatment of intractable occipital neuralgia. *Neurosurgery* 58:112-119, 2006.
22. Oh MY, Ortega J, Bellotte JB, et al: Peripheral nerve stimulation for the treatment of occipital neuralgia and transformed migraine using a C1-2-3 subcutaneous paddle style electrode: a technical report. *Neuromodulation* 7:103-112, 2004.
23. Magis D, Allena M, Bolla M, et al: Occipital nerve stimulation for drug-resistant chronic cluster headache: a prospective pilot study. *Lancet Neurol* 6:314-321, 2007.

24. Holsheimer J: Electrical stimulation of the trigeminal tract in chronic, intractable facial neuralgia. *Arch Physiol Biochem* 4:304-308, 2001.

25. Tomycz ND, Deibert CP, Moossy JJ: Cervicomedullary junction spinal cord stimulation for head and facial pain. *Headache* 51:418-425, 2011.

26. Horlocker TT, Rowlingson JC, Enneking FK, et al: Regional anesthesia in the patient receiving antithrombotic or thrombolytic therapy: American Society of Regional Anesthesia and Pain Medicine Evidence-Based Guidelines (Third Edition). *Reg Anesth Pain Med* 35(1):64-101, 2010.

27. Fishbain D, Goldberg M, Meagher BR, et al: Male and female chronic pain patients characterized by DSMIII psychiatric diagnostic criteria. *Pain* 26:181-197, 1986.

28. Gallagher R: Primary care and pain medicine: a community solution to the public health problem of chronic pain. *Med Clin North Am* 83:555-583, 1999.

29. Celstin J, Edwards RR, Jamison RN: Pretreatment psychosocial variables as predictors of outcomes following lumbar surgery and spinal cord stimulation: a systematic review and literature synthesis. *Pain Med* 10(4):639-653, 2009.

30. Meglio M: Percutaneously implantable chronic electrode for radio-frequency stimulation of the Gasserian ganglion: a perspective in the management of trigeminal pain. *Acta Neurochir (Wien)* 33(suppl):521-525, 1984.

31. Meyerson BA, Håkansson S: Alleviation of atypical trigeminal pain by stimulation of the Gasserian ganglion via an implanted electrode. *Acta Neurochir (Wien)* 30(suppl):303-309, 1980.

32. Taub E, Munuz M, Tasker RR: Chronic electrical stimulation of the gasserian ganglion for the relief of pain in a series of 34 patients. *J Neurosurg* 86:197-202, 1997.

33. Goadsby PJ, Hoskin KL: The distribution of trigeminovascular afferents in the nonhuman primate brain Macaca nemestrina: a c-fos immunocytochemical study. *J Anat* 190:367-375, 1997.

34. Anthony M: Headache and the greater occipital nerve. *Clin Neurol Neurosurg* 94(4):297-301, 1992.

35. Zitnik RJ: Treatment of chronic inflammatory diseases with implantable medical devices. *Ann Rheum Dis* 70(suppl 1):67-70, 2011.

36. Levin M: Nerve Bocks in the Treatment of Headache. *Neurotherapeutics* 7(2):197-203, 2010.

37. Schlaepfer TE, Frick C, Zobel A, et al: Vagus nerve stimulation for depression: efficacy and safety in a European Study. *Psychol Med* 38:651-661, 2008.

38. Jasper J, Hayek S: Implanted occiptal nerve stimulator. *Pain Physician* 11:187-200, 2008.

39. Trescher WH, Lesser RP: Epilepsies. In *Bradley (5th ed) Neurology in Clinical Practice*, ed 5, Oxford, UK, 2008, Butterworth-Heinemann.

40. Fahy BG: Intraoperative perioperative complications with a vagus nerve stimulation device. *Clin Anesthes* 22(3):213-222, 2010.

41. Multon S, Schoenen J: Pain control by vagus nerve stimulation: from animal to man … and back. *Acta Neurol Belg*, 105:62-67, 2005.

42. Multon S, Schoenen J: Pain control by vagus stimulation: from animal to man … and back. *Acta Neurol Belg* 105:62-67, 2005.

43. Trentman TL, Dodick DW, Zimmerman RS, Birch BD: Percutaneous occipital stimulation lead tip erosion: report of 2 cases. *Pain Physician* 11:253-256, 2008.

44. Hayek SM, Jasper JF, Deer TR, Narouze SN: Occipital neurostimulation-induced muscle spasms: implications for lead placement. *Pain Physician* 12:867-876, 2009.

45. Mangram AJ, Horan TC, Pearson ML, et al: The Hospital Infection Control Practices Advisory Committee. Guideline for prevention of surgical site infection 1999. *Infect Control Hosp Epidemiol* 20:247-280, 1999.

46. Lim HB, Hunt K: Anesthetic management for surgical placement of greater occipital nerve stimulators in the treatment of primary headache disorders. *J Neurosurg Anesthesiol* 19:120-124, 2007.

47. Schwedt TJ, Dodick D, Hentz J, et al: Occipital nerve stimulation for chronic headache—long-term safety and efficacy. *Cephalalgia* 27:153-157, 2007.

48. Trentman TL, Mueller JT, Shah DM, et al: Occipital nerve stimulator lead pathway length changes with volunteer movement: an in vitro study. *Pain Pract* 10(1):42-48, 2010.

49. Kapural L, Mekhail N, Hayek SM, et al: Occipital nerve electrical stimulation via the midline approach and subcutaneous surgical leads for treatment of severe occipital neuralgia: a pilot study. *Anesth Analg* 10:171-174, table, 2005.

50. Gofeld M: Anchoring of suboccipital lead: case report and technical note. *Pain Pract* 4:307-309, 2004.

51. Kumar K, Buchser E, Linderoth B, et al: Avoiding complications from spinal cord stimulation: practical management recommendations an international panel of experts. *Neuromodulation* 10:24-33, 2007.

52. Cameron T: Safety and efficacy of spinal cord stimulation for the treatment of chronic pain: a 20-year literature review. *J Neurosurg* 100:254-267, 2004.

53. Trentman TL, Zimmerman RS: Occipital nerve stimulation: technical and surgical aspects of implantation. *Headache Currents* 48(2)319-327, 2008.

54. McKenna KE, McCleane G: Dermatitis induced by a spinal cord stimulator implant. *Contact Dermatitis* 41:279, 1999.

55. Ochani TD, Almirante J, Siddiqui A, Kaplan R: Allergic reaction to spinal cord stimulator. *Clin J Pain* 16:178-180, 2000.

56. Johnson MD, Burchiel KJ: Peripheral stimulation for treatment of trigeminal post-herpetic neuralgia and trigeminal posttraumatic neuropathic pain: a pilot study. *Neurosurgery* 55:135-142, 2004.

57. Tran Y, Shah A, Mittal S: Lead breakage and vocal cord paralysis following blunt neck trauma in a patient with vagal nerve stimulator. *J Neurol Sci* 304:132-135, 2011.

58. Kalkanis JG, Krishna P, Espinosa JA, Naritoku DK: Self-inflicted vocal cord paralysis in patients with vagus nerve stimulators. Report of two cases. *J Neurosurg* 96(5):949-951, 2002.

59. Pearl PL, Conry JA, Yaun A, et al: Misidentification of vagus nerve stimulator for intravenous access and other major adverse events. *Pediatr Neurol* 38(4):248-251, 2008.

60. Rijkers K, Berfelo MW, Cornips EM, Majoie HJ: Hardware failure in vagus nerve stimulation therapy. *Acta Neurochir* 150:403-405, 2008.

61. Ramsay RE, Uthman BM, Augustinsson LE, et al: Vagus nerve stimulation for treatment of partial seizures: 2. Safety, side effects, and tolerability. First International Vagus Nerve Stimulation Study Group. *Epilepsia* 35(3):627-636, 1994.

62. Iriarte J, Urrestarazu E, Alegre M, et al: Late-onset periodic asystolia during vagus nerve stimulation. *Epilepsia* 50:928-932, 2009.

63. Marzec M, Edwards J, Sagher O, et al: Effects of vagus nerve stimulation on sleep-related breathing in epilepsy patients. *Epilepsia* 44:930-935, 2003.

64. Spitz CM, Winston KR, Maa EH, Ojemann SG: Insulation deformity in a vagus nerve stimulator lead: treatable cause of intolerable stimulation-related symptoms. *J Neurosurg* 112(4):829-831, 2010.

65. Johnstone CSH, Sundaraj R: Occipital nerve stimulation for the treatment of occipital neuralgia—eight case studies. *Neuromodulation* 9:41-47, 2006.

66. Melvin EA, Jr, Jordan FR, Weiner RL, Primm D: Using peripheral stimulation to reduce the pain of C2-mediated occipital headaches: a preliminary report. *Pain Physician* 10:453-460, 2007.

4 Avoidance, Recognition, and Treatment of Complications in Cranial Neuromodulation for Pain

Parag G. Patil

CHAPTER OVERVIEW

Chapter Synopsis: Deep brain stimulation (DBS) was initially used as a therapy for medically intractable chronic pain; the technique is not approved by the U.S. Food and Drug Administration (FDA) for this application and is rarely used today. Nevertheless, some centers have found success with DBS and with motor cortex stimulation (MCS) for pain. Similar to any invasive brain surgery, complications may arise; surgical, hardware-related, and stimulation-related risks are most notable.

Important Points:

- Although not currently labeled for use in the United States for the treatment of pain, DBS and MCS are potentially effective therapies for medically intractable pain in carefully selected patients.
- Complications of these therapies may arise during surgery from hardware complications, tissue injury, and from the undesired effects of stimulation.
- Because few patients are treated with cranial neuromodulation, the precise rates of complications are largely unknown, although the characteristics of these complications are well defined.
- Major complications of intracranial neuromodulation are hemorrhage and infection.
- Attention to surgical technique can minimize these complications.

Introduction

Cranial forms of neuromodulation for pain include deep brain stimulation (DBS), motor cortex stimulation (MCS), and non-invasive forms of electrical stimulation such as transcranial magnetic stimulation and transcranial direct-current stimulation.[1] DBS and MCS involve the surgical implantation of electrodes within the brain or in the epidural space, respectively. The DBS and MCS electrodes are then connected subcutaneously to an implantable pulse generator (IPG), most often located in the chest. As with other forms of surgical neuromodulation, careful patient selection is critical to the success of DBS and MCS for pain, and a trial of externally driven stimulation is typically performed before placement of the IPG.

Neither DBS for pain nor MCS for pain are performed with great frequency anywhere in the world. As a result, published accounts of these procedures are primarily in the form of case reports and case series. In addition, clinically significant complications in these procedures are rare, in the range of 1% to 10%. For this reason, precise estimates of rates of complications are difficult to determine for either DBS or MCS for pain, although the nature of these complications has been described well. In this chapter, the clinically significant complications of DBS and MCS are described, with emphasis on some strategies used in neurosurgical practice to avoid these adverse outcomes.

Deep Brain Stimulation for Pain

Deep brain stimulation for medically refractory pain was the first application of chronic intracranial DBS. In 1973 Hosobuchi et al[2] implanted a stimulating electrode into the ventroposteromedial (VPM) thalamus to treat facial pain. Chronic stimulation was attempted after the observation by Hosobuchi and others that acute stimulation before lesion placement resulted in pain improvement. Today, DBS for medically intractable pain typically targets two regions, the sensory ventroposterolateral (VPL)/VPM thalamus and the periaqueductal/periventricular (PAG/PVG) grey matter. Common indications for DBS for pain include chronic poststroke pain syndromes and chronic facial pain syndromes. Rates of reported efficacy for these procedures vary widely, ranging from 12% to 60%. The U.S. Food and Drug Administration (FDA) initially approved and then rescinded the approval of DBS for pain.

The clinically significant complications of DBS take the form of surgical complications, hardware-related complications, and stimulation-dependent complications.[3] Surgical complications of DBS surgery include intracranial hemorrhage and electrode misplacement. Hardware-related complications include electrode fracture, electrode erosion, and infection. Stimulation-dependent complications are the effect of undesired modulation of neural circuits adjacent to the targets of neuromodulation.

Surgical Complications and Avoidance

Intracranial Hemorrhage Symptomatic intracranial hemorrhage is the most feared complication of DBS surgery, with an incidence of approximately 1% of patients undergoing DBS surgery. A number of source factors may influence hemorrhage rates. Bleeding may occur because of direct trauma at the brain surface; injury to vessels in cortical sulci; or injury to deeper vascular-rich structures such as the ependymal surface, the choroid plexus, or friable target regions.

During surgery, careful planning is performed to avoid traversing cortical sulci because of the presence of vessels in the subarachnoid space. If the planned trajectory traverses the ventricles, the surgeon is obliged to determine that the electrode path does not pass through the location of large veins, such as the thalamostriate veins, which are located along the caudate head, or through well-vascularized structures such as the choroid plexus. Disruption of the ependymal surface through a trajectory that skims the surface of the ventricle over a distance may also be a source of intraventricular hemorrhage.

In the author's center, multiple steps are taken to minimize the risk of hemorrhage. Meticulous surgical planning is performed to plan both entry points and trajectories for DBS placement, as outlined above. Verification of positioning is performed with the minimum number of microelectrode passages, as rates of hemorrhage are believed to scale with approximately 0.2% per electrode track. Systolic blood pressure is carefully monitored and routinely maintained below 150 mm Hg. For patients taking chronic antithrombolytic therapies, aspirin and Coumadin are halted 1 week before DBS lead placement and remain off until 1 week after DBS placement.

Venous Infarction and Air Embolism Venous infarction with delayed hemorrhage is another potential complication of DBS surgery. Burr holes for DBS are placed in close proximity to the midline in the region of the coronal suture, where large cortical veins often enter the superior sagittal sinus. Disruption of these vessels or inadvertent cauterization of large veins may lead to compromised venous drainage, venous engorgement, hemorrhage, or venous infarction.

A second form of venous complication during surgery is venous air embolism. DBS surgery is most often performed in a sitting position, with the cranial opening above the level of the heart. As a result, a potential for venous air embolism exists. The rate of asymptomatic and symptomatic air embolism is not known, although coughing and transient cardiovascular changes are occasionally observed in DBS surgery.

Venous complications of DBS surgery may be minimized through planning and surgical technique. Injury to cortical veins may be avoided through the administration of contrast during preoperative imaging so that burr hole locations may be placed distant to venous confluences. If a burr hole is placed directly above a large collection of veins, a new burr hole may be placed rather than risking injury to important surface veins. In addition, meticulous attention during dural opening potentially allows entry into dural venous lakes and inadvertent injury to superficial veins. In the author's center, venous air embolism is treated prophylactically with the administration of 500 mL of normal saline to increase venous pressure at the start of the case. In addition, bone edges, where air may enter diploic veins, are waxed carefully and quickly during opening. If signs of venous air embolism are observed during surgery, irrigation of the field and, rarely, placement of the patient into a head-lowered position can often avoid worsening of the patient's cardiopulmonary status.

Electrode Misplacement Inaccurate placement of the DBS electrodes into a location where there is diminished clinical efficacy or undesirable side effects is a second concern. DBS for pain involves lead placement into deep structures through a burr hole in the skull. Because direct visualization of the target is not observable, the method of stereotactic placement is critical to placement accuracy. The most common targeting modality is frame-based stereotaxy. In this approach, a frame is affixed to the patient's skull under local anesthetic, and stereotactic magnetic resonance imaging (MRI) is performed. This MRI, together with the frame components, allows a one-to-one mapping of each location in the brain to a unique set of coordinates. Common frame systems are the Leksell Frame, the CRW Frame, the NexFrame, and STarFix systems. These systems achieve targeting accuracy by rigidly attaching the targeting mechanism to the skull. An alternative approach is to use intraoperative MRI to observe the location of the DBS lead as it is placed into the brain.

Fluoroscopic visualization allows verification with some systems. In the Leksell system, a pair of targets allows visualization of electrode location with respect to the target (**Fig. 4-1**). The position of the electrode can then be corrected before patient testing.

In addition to accurate frames, microelectrode recording can be used. Microelectrode recording allows for measuring the responsiveness of individual neurons in the brain. During placement of DBS electrodes in the VPM/VPL thalamus, recording of cellular activity while stimulating a target region of the body can confirm localization. In addition, microstimulation, applying a stimulus through the microelectrode with a patient awake, can be used to confirm that the lead trajectory is desired.

Hardware Complications and Avoidance

Infection Infection is a major concern in the placement of any neuromodulation device. With implanted hardware, colonization by bacteria can result in persistent infection that may require

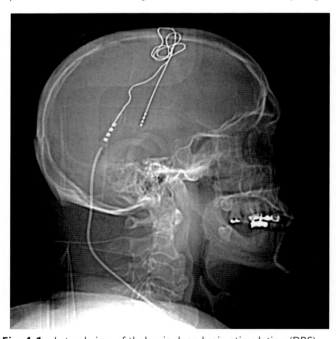

Fig. 4-1 Lateral view of thalamic deep brain stimulation (DBS). The four-contact DBS electrode located within the thalamus is secured at the skull level with a radiolucent burr hole cap. The lead terminates at a second four-contact connector to which the extension lead is attached. The extension lead then passes subcutaneously down the neck to the chest.

surgical removal of the DBS system. Rates of infection with DBS are in the range of 1% to 5%. Although many superficial infections may be successfully treated with oral antibiotics, it is unusual to successfully treat a deeper infection that has involved the implanted hardware.

Avoidance of infection requires meticulous surgical technique. Prophylactic antibiotics are given before skin incision and redosed after 4 to 6 hours. The author's center uses a three-step preparation of the surgical site that includes Betadine scrub, alcohol, and Dura-Prep. During the surgery, all personnel use double gloving when hardware is on the field. In addition, the hardware itself is handled by a minimum number of personnel, and care is taken to implant the hardware soon after package opening. Great care is taken to ensure that meticulous hemostasis is achieved to prevent the development of clots that may form a nidus for infection. Postoperatively, the author does not routinely give antibiotic prophylaxis.

Fracture or Dislocation of Electrode

An additional concern in the placement of DBS systems is fracture or displacement of the electrode after accurate placement. Displacement of the electrode can occur when excessive tensile forces are placed on the DBS lead or the extension wire or the IPG. Rates of displacement or lead fracture are in the range of 2% to 5%. In addition, leads may fracture. Lead fracture occurs when excessive focal movement occurs, allowing repeated bending of the lead at a single point, thereby weakening it.

To avoid dislocation, strain-relief coils of lead and extension wire may be placed at the burr hole at the junction between the lead and the extension wire and at the IPG. Such strain relief is only helpful when the leads do not scar into fixed position. Fracture may be avoided by allowing for movement of the lead in areas where there may be repetitive movement, such as around joints. In the case of DBS, this particularly occurs at the junction of the skull and neck.

Stimulation Complications and Avoidance

Effective stimulation requires appropriate patient selection, accurate DBS lead placement, and effective postoperative DBS programming. Complications of stimulation arise when any of these three criteria are not met. Appropriate patient selection criteria are overviewed elsewhere in this text. Some of the factors affecting accurate lead placement are discussed above.

Confirmation of accurate lead placement before securing the lead and appropriate programming of DBS leads are essential to the avoidance of stimulation complications. After the lead has been placed into the desired anatomic location based on MRI imaging and microelectrode recording, stimulation may be tested before the patient leaves the operating room. Unlike DBS for movement disorders, in which the goals of intraoperative stimulation are well designed, intraoperative DBS stimulation is less clear for pain applications. In VPM/VPL stimulation, paresthesias are felt with stimulation in the region of pain, indicating accurate anatomic localization. Untoward side effects may also be monitored. PAG/PVG stimulation can produce side effects because of stimulation of neural pathways adjacent to the aqueduct. These include diplopia, nausea, vertical gaze palsy, blurred vision, nystagmus, and oscillopsia.

Motor Cortex Stimulation for Pain

Motor cortex stimulation for pain involves the surgical placement of stimulating electrodes in the epidural space overlying the primary motor cortex (precentral gyrus). Application of stimulation to the sensory cortex (postcentral gyrus) alone is ineffective in the treatment of pain. The paddle leads used are those designed for epidural spinal placement and may be oriented either along the precentral gyrus, parallel to the central sulcus, or bridging the precentral and postcentral gyri perpendicular to the central sulcus. MCS for the treatment of thalamic pain syndrome was reported first by Tsubokawa et al[4] in 1991. Today the most common indications for MCS are trigeminal neuropathic pain and thalamic pain syndromes, although the therapy has been applied on a more limited basis to many other painful processes. For thalamic post-stroke pain, approximately two-thirds of patients are reported to achieve adequate relief from the therapy. For trigeminal neuropathic pain, impressive response rates of up to 75% to 100% have been reported in some studies. As with DBS for pain, the FDA has not approved MCS as a therapy for pain, reflecting the difficulties of patient selection and treatment efficacy for this therapy.

MCS has appeal for its reduced invasiveness compared with other intracranial ablative and neuromodulation surgeries. The majority of studies of MCS have reported no complications of the therapy. However, occasional complications are known to occur. As with DBS, clinically significant complications may be categorized as surgical, hardware related, and stimulation related. Surgical complications of MCS involve epidural hematoma and electrode misplacement. Hardware complications include infection and fracture or dislocation of the lead. Stimulation-related complications of MCS include undesirable paresthesias and seizures.

Surgical Complications and Avoidance

Epidural Hematoma   The postoperative accumulation of blood in the epidural space can produce mass effect on the brain and compromise stimulation efficiency and efficacy. Two surgical techniques are used for the placement of MCS electrodes into the epidural space. In the first approach, a craniotomy that is 4 to 5 cm in diameter is created, with removal of the bone flap and care taken to strip the dura from the underside of the bone flap during elevation to avoid dural tearing. During the procedure, the MCS leads are secured to the dura, and the bone is replaced atop the leads and then secured into position with titanium plates. In the second (and less invasive) approach, a burr hole is placed to access the epidural space, and a dural separator is used to expand a small epidural pocket adjacent to the burr hole into which the lead may be placed.

To minimize the development of postoperative epidural hematoma, care is taken to reduce the size of the epidural potential space. In the case of craniotomy, dural tack-up sutures may be placed to reapproximate the dura to the bone flap during closure. When burr holes are placed, limiting dural stripping to the size of the implanted electrode, so that the electrode itself fills the potential space, is believed to reduce the incidence of epidural hematoma. A postoperative computed tomography (CT) scan 4 to 8 hours after the surgery can be a useful tool to evaluate the accumulation of any epidural blood.

Electrode Misplacement

As in any other form of neuromodulation, the anatomic placement of the electrode is of critical importance to the success of the therapy. MCS is no exception. What is difficult in MCS is that the optimal electrode location is not known with certainty. In practice, MCS electrodes are targeted to cover the portion of the anatomic homunculus where the patient is experiencing pain. However, the relationship of electrode placement to therapeutic efficacy remains a subject of study and discussion.

Several techniques allow identification of the sensory and motor cortex during surgery. In the author's center, a stereotactic MRI and

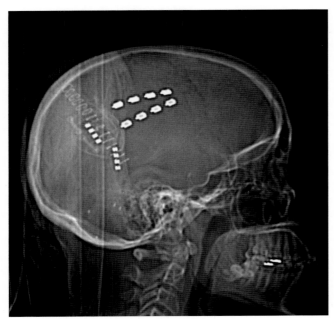

Fig. 4-2 Lateral view of motor cortex stimulation. Two four-contact paddle leads are placed through adjacent burr holes and located in the epidural space with the anterior two contacts overlying the primary motor cortex and the posterior two contacts overlying the primary sensory cortex. Somatotopically, the superior lead is overlying the hand area, and the inferior lead is overlying the face area in this patient with centralized trigeminal pain.

frameless stereotaxy are used to identify the location of the central sulcus. With a frameless imaging system, the location of the electrode with respect to the underlying brain may be directly evaluated. Ultrasound imaging of the cortical surface may also be used if an appropriately sized ultrasound probe is available. When a burr hole is used and therefore the location of the electrode cannot be directly visualized, fluoroscopy can be used to evaluate the precise location of the epidural lead (**Fig. 4-2**).

As in DBS surgery, electrophysiologic recording can also provide insight into physiologic lead location. Electrophysiologic pulsatile stimulation of the median nerve of the contralateral upper extremity evokes a negative postcentral N20 wave and a positive precentral P20 evoked potential.[5] These sensory-evoked potentials can be used reliably to identify the location of the electrophysiologic border between sensory and motor cortical regions, allowing the lead to be placed over the motor cortex. A volumetric postoperative CT scan co-registered to a preoperative MRI can additionally allow simultaneous visualization of the brain and electrode contacts, verifying electrode locations with respect to the brain surface.

Hardware Complications and Avoidance
Infection The same careful attention to infection prevention in DBS surgery also applies in MCS surgery. Infection of the MCS electrode can produce an epidural abscess. Bacteria may potentially penetrate the dura, producing subdural empyema, a potentially life-threatening complication. Furthermore, the presence of a nonvascularized bone flap overlying the electrode introduces the risk of calvarial osteomyelitis. Prevention of infection is therefore an important priority during surgery. Techniques for infection avoidance are identical to those described for DBS.

Lead Breakage and Displacement In MCS, the epidural lead lies parallel to the skull surface and is largely restricted in terms of movement. Areas of potential lead compromise and breakage occur where the lead exits the skull if the wire takes a sharp turn. Additional breakage may occur at the cranial–cervical junction if the lead has scarred in an area of repetitive movement. Displacement of the lead may occur because of tensile forces on the lead. Lead breakage and displacement may be reduced by incorporating strain-relief loops when securing the lead, affixing the lead firmly to the skull using titanium plates, minimizing tensile forces, or securing the lead directly to the dura.

Stimulation Complications and Avoidance
Seizures Stimulation at the cortical surface can produce seizures and MCS for pain has significant potential to produce seizures. Although MCS has not been associated with the development of chronic epilepsy, seizure prophylaxis with antiepileptic medications is typically used in patients treated with MCS. Typically, stimulation parameters are set at 20% to 80% of the motor threshold of stimulation to minimize the risk of seizures.

Undesirable Paresthesias Although the motor cortex and sensory cortex receive subthreshold stimulation, the dura and scalp are richly innervated; therefore patients may occasionally experience undesirable paresthesias with stimulation through epidural leads. Incising and reclosing the region underlying the stimulating electrode may accomplish denervation of the dura, thereby reducing undesirable paresthesias. Alternatively, stimulation parameters may be adjusted to fall below the stimulation threshold.

Conclusion

Deep brain stimulation and MSC are cranial neuromodulation options in the treatment of pain. Neither approach carries the approval of the FDA, and the rare complications of these procedures can be significant. However, in carefully selected patients who have exhausted other options, both DBS and MCS may be reasonable therapeutic strategies for the treatment of medically intractable pain syndromes.

References

1. Levy R, Deer TR, Henderson J: Intracranial neurostimulation for pain control. *Pain Physician* 13:157-165, 2010.
2. Hosobuchi Y, Adams JE, Rutkin B: Chronic thalamic stimulation for the control of facial anesthesia dolorosa. *Arch Neurol* 29:158-161, 1973.
3. Lyons K, Koller W, Wilkinson S, et al: Surgical and hardware complications of subthalamic stimulation. *Neurology* 63:612-616, 2004.
4. Tsubokawa T, Katayama Y, Yamamoto T, et al: Chronic motor cortex stimulation for the treatment of central pain. *Acta Neurochir (Wein)* 52:137-139, 1991.
5. Brown JA, Pilitsis JG: Motor cortex stimulation. *Pain Med* 7(suppl):S140-S145, 2006.

II Intrathecal Drug Delivery Systems

Chapter 5 Complications of Intrathecal Drug Delivery Systems

5 Complications of Intrathecal Drug Delivery Systems

Matthew T. Ranson

CHAPTER OVERVIEW

Chapter Synopsis: Similar to any sort of implantation therapy for chronic pain, intrathecal drug delivery (ITDD) carries risks and can benefit from careful patient selection. A highly trained physician should always perform the operation because misplacement of needles in the intrathecal space can produce devastating consequences. Bleeding, infection, and neurologic damage account for the most serious complications, but drug reactions are also of concern.

Important Points:
- ITDD implantation should only be performed by well-trained physicians.
- ITDD can lead to permanent neurologic sequelae and death.
- Complications can arise from medications as well as needle placement and may develop over years.
- Suspicion of epidural hematoma or abscess formation require immediate magnetic resonance imaging and surgical consultation.
- Any infection of the device requires prompt evaluation and consideration of explantation.

Introduction

Physicians implanting medical devices in the intrathecal space should undergo extensive training in the placement of needles in the intrathecal space as well as in proper surgical technique. Careful preoperative evaluation of the patient to undergo intrathecal drug delivery (ITDD) implantation is mandatory and should include at a minimum laboratory evaluation including coagulation studies, screening for the presence of obstructive sleep apnea, diseases associated with immunocompromised state, and other diseases that may make continuous opioid treatment a significant risk to the patient. Despite careful preoperative evaluation and excellent training, even the most experienced physician may have significant complications when implanting ITDD devices. In this chapter, complications are organized into procedure related, medication related, and complications associated with comorbidities.

Complications of Needle Placement in the Intrathecal Space

Bleeding

During the placement of an intrathecal catheter, the needle typically passes through the epidural space with little trauma. However, in anticoagulated patients and in patients with bleeding dyscrasias, epidural bleeding and resultant epidural hematomas are a significant risk (**Table 5-1**). Epidural bleeding is likely common but usually goes unnoticed in the absence of postoperative imaging studies. Rarely, an epidural bleed may produce a clinically significant epidural hematoma. Untreated, an epidural hematoma can progress and result in numbness, weakness, increased pain, and

ultimately paralysis. If the development of an epidural hematoma is suspected, the patient should undergo immediate magnetic resonance imaging (MRI) and surgical evaluation. Prompt hematoma evacuation should be performed within 12 hours of the onset of symptoms because evacuation within this time frame has been associated with better neurological outcomes. Any patient complaining of weakness in the postoperative period should undergo immediate evaluation for the presence of an epidural hematoma (**Box 5-1**).

Recommendations for Avoiding Bleeding-Associated Complications Today physicians encounter many patients that are anticoagulated with medications such as antifibrinolytic and antiplatelet agents. Discontinuing antifibrinolytic medications for 7 to 10 days has previously been recommended, but there are no data to establish when it is safe to perform neuraxial procedures in patients treated with these medications.[1] Additionally, there has never been a clear relationship established between aspirin and nonsteroidal administration and epidural hematoma formation. Most physicians do not require patients to discontinue low-dose aspirin and nonsteroidal antiinflammatory medications before undergoing implantation of an ITDD device. Recommendations published by the American Society of Regional Anesthesia and Pain Management attempt to provide guidelines for discontinuing anticoagulation in patients who are to undergo neuraxial procedures.[1]

Infection

Epidural abscess formation can result in compression of neurologic structures and symptoms similar to those of epidural hematoma

Table 5-1: Commonly Used Drugs That May Result in Increased Risk of Bleeding Complications

Brand Name	Generic
Angiomax	Bivalirudin
Arixtra	Fondaparinux
Jantoven	Coumadin
Fragmin	Dalteparin
Innohep	Tinzaparin
Lovenox	Enoxaparin
Argatroban	Argatroban
ATryn	Antithrombin
None	Heparin
Iprivask	Desirudin
Refludan	Lepirudin
Thrombate	Antithrombin
Pradaxa	Dabigatran
Aggrenox	Aspirin/dipyridamole
Effient	Prasugrel
Plavix	Clopidogrel
Pletal	Cilostazol
ReoPro	Abciximab
Ticlid	Ticlopidine
Aggrastat	Tirofiban
Agrylin	Anagrelide
Integrilin	Eptifibatide
Persantine	Dipyridamole

Box 5-1: Warning Signs of Epidural Hematoma

Postoperative weakness (red flag and early indicator)
Numbness
Back and leg pain
Bowel and bladder incontinence

Box 5-2: Risk Factors for Infection

Immunocompromised state such as HIV infection or cancer
History of methicillin-resistant *Staphylococcus aureus* infection
Organ transplantation with immunosuppression therapy
Diabetes
Skin infection at the time of implantation

consultation is mandatory in any patient suspected of having an epidural abscess.

Risks factors for infection include any patient with a history of immunocompromised state such as HIV infection, history of methicillin-resistant *Staphylococcus aureus* infection, organ transplantation, cancer, diabetes mellitus, and skin infections at the time of implantation (**Box 5-2**). Transverse myelitis is uncommon but is seen with catheter infections and may not be present with known infection.[2] Routine laboratory studies, including C-reactive protein (CRP), complete blood count (CBC) with differential, and erythrocyte sedimentation rate (ESR), should be obtained in patients with clinical symptoms of infection.

Recommendations for Avoiding Complications From Infection Preoperative antibiotics should be given at least 30 minutes before any surgical procedure. Recommendations for antibiotic selection should be sought from the pharmacists in the hospital where the implantation is to be performed because bacterial resistance certainly may vary by region and possibly among hospitals in the same area. In the absence of pharmacy recommendations, advice may be sought from orthopedic surgeons who routinely perform joint replacements in the hospital. In addition to prophylactic antibiotics, careful attention to strict aseptic technique is mandatory. Physicians who perform implantations should be well trained in good surgical technique. Good hemostasis, wound closure, and adherence to operating room sterile technique require extensive surgical training, which cannot be learned in a weekend course.

Neurologic Injury

Damage to spinal neurologic structures may result from direct needle trauma during intrathecal needle placement. The conus medullaris is located at the L1–L2 level in most adults with the cauda equina floating freely in the cerebrospinal fluid (CSF) below. Thus it is recommended that needle placement occur below the L1–L2 level. Monitored anesthesia care is recommended with the patient freely arousable and communicating with the surgeon during needle placement. However, it is important to realize that catheter placement in the conus medullaris is possible in an awake patient without the patient complaining of pain. In some patients, particularly very ill cancer patients, it is necessary to perform the implantation under general anesthesia. In these patients, needle placement should be performed well below the conus medullaris.

A paramedian approach with a needle entry angle of 30 to 45 degrees should minimize the chance of inadvertent penetration of the spinal cord. Additionally, obtaining later fluoroscopic images during the advancement of the needle into the intrathecal space may minimize the possibility of neurologic trauma because a steep needle angle is more easily recognized in the lateral view.

It is advisable to examine the patient in the postanesthesia recovery unit and document either the absence or the presence of new focal neurologic findings. If neurologic injury is suspected, the physician should obtain an MRI as soon as practical with the

formation. Although the risk of epidural abscess formation is probably less than one in 1000, any patient who complains of increasing pain at the catheter insertion site, develops a clinically significant fever over 101°F or greater, or complains of weakness or numbness should undergo urgent MRI with proper precautions and surgical evaluation if warranted. It is important for the physician to be aware that epidural abscess may initially present as pain around the catheter insertion point and may evolve to include severe radiating pain if the infection invades the neural foramen or compresses the spinal cord.

Discitis and meningitis are serious complications that must undergo immediate treatment if suspected. Superficial wound infections are much more common but still require prompt attention to prevent penetration of the deep tissue layers and involvement of the implant. It is recommended that an infectious disease consultation be obtained in any infection that is suspected of penetrating beyond the superficial layers. Prompt neurosurgical

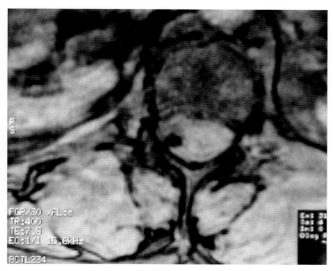

Fig. 5-1 Intrathecal granuloma.

Table 5-2: Maximum Drug Concentrations and Doses		
Drug	**Maximum Concentration**	**Maximum dose per day**
Morphine	20 mg/cc	15 mg
Hydromorphone	10 mg/cc	4 mg
Fentanyl	2 mg/cc	No upper limit
Sufentanil	50 µg/cc	No upper limit
Bupivacaine	40 mg/cc	30 mg
Clonidine	2 mg/cc	1 mg
Ziconotide	100 µg/cc	19.2 µg

appropriate precautions. Additionally, an electromyogram and nerve conduction study may be useful to characterize the extent of neurologic damage but may not show any abnormalities for several days after the insult. Many patients suspected of neurologic injury may have a contusion of neuritis that usually resolves in time with conservative treatment and observation. Finally, administration of intravenous steroids should be considered in the immediate postoperative period in any patient suspected of neurologic injury.

Postpuncture dural headache (PDPH) may result from dural tear during intrathecal needle placement. A persistent CSF leak and hygroma are other complications that can result in significant patient discomfort and eventual neurologic injury if not managed properly. Many physicians advocate placement of purse-string sutures deep within the fascia surrounding the needle and catheter before removal of the catheter. This may compress the tissue around the catheter and prevent persistent dural leak and hygroma formation. Additionally, abdominal binders should be placed in the immediate postoperative period. PDPHs are usually managed successfully with conservative treatments consisting of hydration, caffeine, and intramuscular sumatriptan in refractory cases. A neurologic consultation should be considered in any patient exhibiting evidence of cranial nerve palsy.

Catheter-Associated Complications

Infectious Complications
Infectious complications as they relate to needle placement in the intrathecal space were discussed earlier in this chapter and are essentially the same for intrathecal catheters.

Granuloma Formation
Aside from infection, the development of catheter granulomas is one of the most serious complications associated with intrathecal catheters. First reported in 1999, granulomas (**Fig. 5-1**) appear to be inflammatory, fibrotic, noninfectious masses that develop at the tip of the catheter.[3] The mass formation usually develops over months to years and is more likely to form in patients receiving high concentrations of morphine and hydromorphone.[4] Consensus recommendations have suggested limiting morphine to 20 mg/cc and hydromorphone to 10 mg/cc (**Table 5-2**).

Granuloma should be suspected when granulomagenic medications are employed intrathecally, especially outside the maximum concentration or daily dose recommendations, and heralded by a change in analgesia, new sensory or motor deficits, and often times is accompanied by an abnormal catheter evaluation. Although some physicians routinely obtain computed tomography (CT) scans to screen for asymptomatic granulomas, there is insufficient evidence to recommend surveillance CT scans or MRIs. Any patient suspected of a granuloma should undergo a T1-weighted MRI with and without gadolinium.

Mechanical Complications
Catheter fracture may occur throughout the length of the catheter but frequently occurs at points of higher stress, which include the site of anchor, catheter splice junctions such as in two-piece catheters, and on the nipple of the reservoir. Catheter failure has been reported to be 4.5% during the first nine months following implantation.[5] It is important to obtain control of the distal piece of the fractured catheter that typically occurs at the anchoring site. This can be accomplished by opening the anchor incision first and removing the distal catheter before opening the reservoir pocket. In some cases, catheter fracture may be managed with a splicing kit. If the distal catheter piece is irretrievable, a neurosurgical consultation should be obtained.

Another possible complication may result from migration of the catheter from the intrathecal space (**Fig. 5-2**). This obviously requires catheter revision and can result in side effects that range from the mundane to the serious. Migration into the epidural space may lead to CSF leak with resultant headache, loss of analgesia, and possibly hygroma formation. It is possible for the catheter to migrate into the neural foramen, which may lead to nerve root irritation and the development of radicular symptoms. Migration into the spinal cord is possible with the development of severe neurologic deficits. Any patient suspected of catheter malfunction should undergo plane radiographic imaging to assess for catheter integrity and MRI imaging with appropriate precautions if migration is suspected. Improper catheter anchoring techniques, such as failure to anchor to the thoracolumbar fascia, increase the likelihood of catheter migration.

Placement of intrathecal catheters under deep sedation or general endotracheal anesthesia may result in intraparenchymal needle and catheter placement. For this reason, it is recommended that catheter placement be placed under monitored anesthesia care.

Reservoir Pocket and Anchor Incision Complications

Infection
Infectious complications of the pocket and anchor site incisions related to ITDD devices have been reported to range from 2.5% to 9.0% and represent the most common type of infectious complications that the physician implanter is likely to encounter.[6] Risk

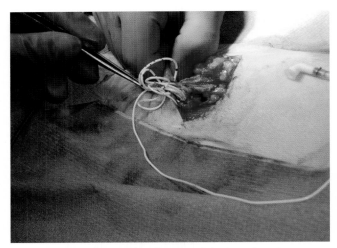

Fig. 5-2 Catheter migration out of the intrathecal space.

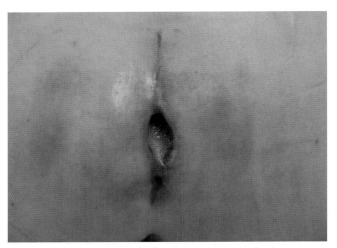

Fig. 5-3 Wound dehiscence caused by infection.

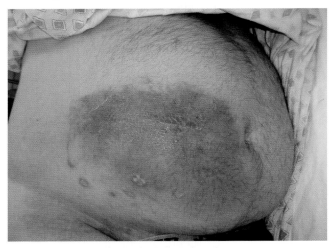

Fig. 5-4 Infected pocket.

factors for infections of the reservoir pocket and anchor site are the same as discussed previously regarding catheter-related infections. Any patient presenting with pain over the incision site, swelling, rubor, or purulent discharge should be suspected of infection (**Figs. 5-3** and **5-4**). Aggressive management of superficial infections may prevent penetration into the subfascial layers and compromise of the device.

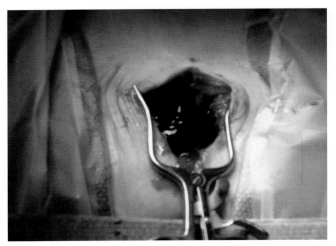

Fig. 5-5 Wound hematoma.

In addition to obtaining wound cultures for antibiotic selection, prudent physicians may choose to perform an incision and drainage procedure with pulsed lavage. It is important to inspect the incision for evidence of compromise of the deep fascial planes. In patients suspected of fascial compromise, explantation of the device should be considered as the safest course of management. Chronic slowly growing infections are possible in patients who appear to initially respond to antibiotic treatment and are often accompanied by recurrent clinical fever. Routine laboratory values, including CRP, CBC with differential, and ESR, should be obtained in any patient suspected of wound infection. Additionally, physicians should consider an infectious disease consultation in patients with infection penetrating the deep fascial layers.

Hematoma
Careful attention to wound hemostasis, including meticulous tissue dissection, suturing of arterial bleeding, and use of coagulation for small vessel bleeding, may prevent the development of wound hematomas. The physician implanter should assess the patient's risk of bleeding preoperatively. If a wound hematoma develops (**Fig. 5-5**), the physician should consider prompt evacuation and correction of any bleeding diathesis to prevent wound dehiscence and loss of the implant. Additionally, hematomas may predispose the implant to infection.

Seromas
Some patients my develop redness and swelling of the wound resulting from the buildup of serosanguineous fluid. Seromas are sterile and typically present with lack of fever and normal white blood cell count. Typically, seromas can be managed conservatively and can be prevented by using careful surgical dissection, meticulous wound hemostasis, and placement of an abdominal binder, and in rare cases, a patient with a seroma may develop a fever, which necessitates surgical evaluation of the wound with Gram stain and culture to rule out an infectious process. Fortunately, most cases of seroma formation do not lead to device removal.

Painful Reservoir Site
Pain in the reservoir site usually results from tissue irritation because of improper size or location selection. Placement of the reservoir over or near bony landmarks, especially near the inferior subchondral region, may predispose the patient to pain around the reservoir pocket. Failure to anchor the pump, especially when placed in an oversized pocket, may result in tissue irritation, pain,

and the development of a pocket seroma. It is strongly recommended that nonabsorbable anchoring sutures placed in the fascia be used to secure the pump in place. Neuroma formation, although rare, may result in significant pain surrounding the reservoir pocket and may be prevented by careful surgical dissection. The presence of complex regional pain syndrome may also be a risk factor for development of chronic postoperative pain in the pocket. Management of the painful pocket includes local anesthetic or steroid injection, Lidoderm patches or compounding cream, and revision in refractory cases.

Complications Associated with Intrathecal Medications

Currently, morphine and ziconotide are the only two medications approved by the Food and Drug Administration for intrathecal use. Bupivacaine, fentanyl, sufentanil, hydromorphone, and clonidine are frequently used off label for intrathecal infusions in the treatment of chronic and cancer pain. Side effects of intrathecal opioid medications include nausea, constipation, urinary retention, confusion, dizziness, impotence and decreased libido, hypotension, pruritus, allergic reaction, somnolence, respiratory depression, and weight gain (**Table 5-3**).[5,7] Adjunctive medications such as bupivacaine and clonidine may cause hypotension. As discussed previously, granulomas likely result from high concentrations of primarily intrathecal morphine and hydromorphone.[4] The incidence of peripheral edema has been reported to range from 1% to 20% and is thought to result from the effect of opioids on the pituitary adrenal axis.[8]

Recently, Coffey et al[9] retrospectively investigated mortality and intrathecal drug delivery for non-cancer pain. Although they reported a 3.89% mortality rate at 1 year after implantation of an ITDD device, the deaths described can be attributed to a lack of vigilance and poor insight into the predictable consequences of

Table 5-3: Reported Complications of Intrathecal Drug Delivery

Author, Year	Reported Complications
Duse et al,[10] 2009	None observed
Doleys et al,[11] 2006[11][11]	None observed
Penn and Paice,[12] 1987	None observed
Atli et al,[13] 2010	14 complications of 57 patients reported: one with wound infection, two with granulomas, two with pocket seromas, three with catheter fracture; overall complication rate, 20%; failure of treatment, 24%
Ilias et al,[14] 2008	No serious adverse outcomes reported; 92 patients reported 181 complications; 16% were pump programming related and resolved with reprogramming; 32% were drug related and benign
Ellis et al,[15] 2008	Side effects related to ziconotide were reported in 147 of 155 patients; the most common reported side effect was confusion; 39.4% of patients discontinued treatment because of side effects
Shaladi et al,[16] 2007	One patient with reported delayed wound healing and one with wound infection; some patients reported drug-related side effects
Thimineur et al,[2] 2004	One patient developed transverse myelitis with permanent neurologic sequelae; one patient had catheter kinking, and two developed wound infections
Deer et al,[17] 2004	Patient-reported complication rates were infection, 2.2%; migration, 1.5%; CSF leak, 0.7%; catheter kinking, 1.5%; catheter fracture, 0.7%; reaction to medication, 5.1%; overall, 23 patients reported complications, and 21 required surgical revision
Rauck et al,[18] 2003	40 of 119 patients implanted with IT pumps reported complications: seven developed device failures, and 36 had procedure-related complications
Deer et al,[19] 2002	Patient-reported medication side effects included peripheral edema and paresthesias; no long-term ill effects of IT reported
Smith et al,[20] 2002	194 serious complications reported in 202 patients; 16 procedure-related adverse events reported of which six were device related, five were insertion related, and five were catheter related; 10 patients required surgical revision, and 1 pump was explanted because of infection
Rainov et al,[21] 2001	26 patients were implanted with IT pump; there were two device-related complications reported as catheter leakage and leakage; one pump was filled incorrectly, leading to damage to the reservoir septum and medication leakage
Becker et al,[22] 2000	Five patients reported IT pump-related complications: one pocket hematoma, one postoperative case of pneumonia, and three catheter-related complications
Roberts et al,[23] 2001	40% (32) of patients developed technical complications primarily related to the catheter requiring surgical revision
Anderson and Burchiel[24] 1999	No serious complications reported; two patients developed PDPHs, two patients had pump malfunctions, five patients required revision of the pump because of device-related issues, and one pump was programmed incorrectly
Winkelmuller and Winkelmuller,[5] 1996	31 of 120 patients implanted with IT pumps were considered treatment failures; 14 pumps required surgical revision
Onofrio and Yaksh,[25] 1990	Human error lead to five pumps running out of medication

PDPH, postdural puncture headache; IT, intrathecal therapy.

mismanaged intrathecal therapy (i.e., respiratory depression). This report underscores the importance of vigilance in reducing iatrogenic error.

Conclusion

Complications associated with intrathecal pumps are often avoidable by careful patient selection and proper training of the physician implanter.[26] Physicians performing the implantation of ITDD devices should receive formalized training during residency and fellowship in both the access of the neuraxis as well as surgical techniques. Particular diligence is required by the physician implanter to avoid especially detrimental complications and permanent neurologic sequelae.

References

1. Horlocker TT, Wedel DJ, Benzon H, et al: Regional anesthesia in the anticoagulated patient: defining the risks (the second ASRA Consensus Conference on Neuraxial Anesthesia and Anticoagulation). *Reg Anesth Pain Med* 28(3):172-197, 2003.
2. Thimineur MA, Kravitz E, Vodapally MS: Intrathecal opioid treatment for chronic non-malignant pain: a 3-year prospective study. *Pain* 109(3):242-249, 2004.
3. North RB: Spinal cord compression by catheter granulomas in high-dose intrathecal morphine therapy: case report. *Neurosurgery* 44(3):691, 1999.
4. Coffey RJ, Burchiel K: Inflammatory mass lesions associated with intrathecal drug infusion catheters: report and observations on 41 patients. *Neurosurgery* 50(1):78-86; discussion 86-87, 2002.
5. Winkelmuller M, Winkelmuller W: Long-term effects of continuous intrathecal opioid treatment in chronic pain of nonmalignant etiology. *J Neurosurg* 85(3):458-467, 1996.
6. Follett KA, Boortz-Marx RL, Drake JM, et al: Prevention and management of intrathecal drug delivery and spinal cord stimulation system infections. *Anesthesiology* 100(6):1582-1594, 2004.
7. Paice JA, Penn RD, Shott S: Intraspinal morphine for chronic pain: a retrospective, multicenter study. *J Pain Symptom Manage* 11(2):71-80, 1996.
8. Aldrete JA, Couto DA, Silva JM: Leg edema from intrathecal opiate infusions. *Eur J Pain* 4(4):361-365, 2000.
9. Coffey RJ, Owens ML, Broste SK, et al: Mortality associated with implantation and management of intrathecal opioid drug infusion systems to treat noncancer pain. *Anesthesiology* 111(4):881-891, 2009.
10. Duse G, Davia G, White PF: Improvement in psychosocial outcomes in chronic pain patients receiving intrathecal morphine infusions. *Anesth Analg* 109(6):1981-1986, 2009.
11. Doleys D, Brown JL, Ness T: Multidimensional outcomes analysis of intrathecal, oral opioid, and behavioral-functional restoration therapy for failed back surgery syndrome: a retrospective study with 4 years' follow-up. *Neuromodulation* 9(4):270-283, 2006.
12. Penn RD, Paice JA: Chronic intrathecal morphine for intractable pain. *J Neurosurg* 67(2):182-186, 1987.
13. Atli A, Theodore BR, Turk DC, Loeser JD: Intrathecal opioid therapy for chronic nonmalignant pain: a retrospective cohort study with 3-year follow-up. *Pain Med* 11(7):1010-1016, 2010.
14. Ilias W, le Polain B, Buchser E, Demartini L: oPTiMa study group: Patient-controlled analgesia in chronic pain patients: experience with a new device designed to be used with implanted programmable pumps. *Pain Pract* 8(3):164-170, 2008.
15. Ellis D, Dissanayake S, McGuire D, et al: Continuous intrathecal infusion of ziconotide for treatment of chronic malignant and nonmalignant pain over 12 months: a prospective, open-label study. *Neuromodulation* 11(1):40-49, 2008.
16. Shaladi A, Saltari MR, Piva B, et al: Continuous intrathecal morphine infusion in patients with vertebral fractures due to osteoporosis. *Clin J Pain* 23(6):511-517, 2007.
17. Deer T, Chapple I, Classen A, et al: Intrathecal drug delivery for treatment of chronic low back pain: report from the National Outcomes Registry for Low Back Pain. *Pain Med* 5(1):6-13, 2004.
18. Rauck RL, Cherry D, Boyer MF, et al: Long-term intrathecal opioid therapy with a patient-activated, implanted delivery system for the treatment of refractory cancer pain. *J Pain* 4(8):441-447, 2003.
19. Deer TR, Caraway DL, Kim CK, et al: Clinical experience with intrathecal bupivacaine in combination with opioid for the treatment of chronic pain related to failed back surgery syndrome and metastatic cancer pain of the spine. *Spine J* 2(4):274-278, 2002.
20. Smith TJ, Staats PS, Deer T, et al: Implantable Drug Delivery Systems Study Group: Randomized clinical trial of an implantable drug delivery system compared with comprehensive medical management for refractory cancer pain: impact on pain, drug-related toxicity, and survival. *J Clin Oncol* 20(19):4040-4049, 2002.
21. Rainov NG, Heidecke V, Burkert W: Long-term intrathecal infusion of drug combinations for chronic back and leg pain. *J Pain Symptom Manage* 22(4):862-871, 2001.
22. Becker R, Jakob D, Uhle EI, et al: The significance of intrathecal opioid therapy for the treatment of neuropathic cancer pain conditions. *Stereotact Funct Neurosurg* 75:16-26, 2000.
23. Roberts LJ, Finch PM, Goucke CR, Price LM: Outcome of intrathecal opioids in chronic non-cancer pain. *Eur J Pain* 5(4):353-361, 2001.
24. Anderson VC, Burchiel KJ: A prospective study of long-term intrathecal morphine in the management of chronic nonmalignant pain. *Neurosurgery* 44(2):289-300; discussion 300-301, 1999.
25. Onofrio BM, Yaksh TL: Long-term pain relief produced by intrathecal morphine infusion in 53 patients. *J Neurosurg* 72(2):200-209, 1990.

III Discogenic Pain Procedures

6 Complications of Therapeutic Minimally Invasive Intradiscal Procedures

Tory L. McJunkin, Paul J. Lynch, and Christi Makas

CHAPTER OVERVIEW

Chapter Synopsis: Pain that originates in the discs is a significant source of chronic, debilitating back pain. Several newly developed minimally invasive techniques allow for treatment of discogenic pain when conservative treatments fail with reduced risks compared with open surgical interventions. The techniques include chemonucleolysis, intradiscal electrothermal therapy (IDET), and biacuplasty, among others. Bleeding, nerve trauma, spinal cord injury, and infection are the most common complication risks. Although rare, catastrophic sequelae can occur, including intradisc infection or heat-related damage. Extensive understanding of spinal anatomy and fluoroscopic guidance can reduce the risk of complications.

Important Points:

- Spinal pain that originates from the disc is thought to be a major cause of severe and chronic back pain.
- Discogenic pain may be caused by herniated and bulging discs, as well as internal disc disruption (IDD), which may be caused by annular tears that irritate small nociceptive nerve fibers within the outer layer of the annulus fibrosis.
- People presenting with discogenic pain are typically treated with conservative modalities, including physical therapy, chiropractic care, proper activity performance, and antiinflammatory and over-the-counter medications.
- If conservative care fails to provide relief, other diagnostic and therapeutic modalities may be performed, including epidural steroid injections, selective nerve root blocks, discography, and facet-related interventions.
- However, if conservative diagnostic and therapeutic interventions do not alleviate discogenic pain, minimally invasive intradiscal procedures are often considered.
- Some of these minimally invasive intradiscal treatments include chemonucleolysis, IDET, biacuplasty, Disc Dekompressor, nucleoplasty, percutaneous laser disc decompression, and injectable treatments such as methylene blue and tumor necrosis factor α. Each of these procedures addresses a key element in disc pathology.
- Although some of these minimally invasive treatments are new and research is limited, they typically involve fewer risks and quicker recovery times compared with traditional open surgical practices.
- Minimally invasive intradiscal procedures are designed to lower risks, but as in any spine-related procedure, specific and sometimes catastrophic sequelae do occur.
- Because these procedures penetrate the protective skin barrier and are placed near critical spinal structures, complications may include bleeding; nerve trauma; spinal cord injury; infection; and damage to vital structures, including vessels, nerve roots, vertebral endplates, the spinal cord, and organs.
- A potentially catastrophic type of infection from intradiscal procedure is discitis, or infection within the disc.
- Another potentially serious complication that may be related to infection is transverse myelitis, which involves inflammation of the spinal cord. It has been reported to occur in conjunction with chemonucleolysis.
- Allergic reaction can be caused by preoperative skin preparations, antibiotics, local anesthesia, and latex.
- Another complication of intradiscal procedures is bleeding in and around the spine, which can lead to epidural, subdural, muscular, and superficial hematomas.
- A common type of structural trauma associated with intradiscal procedures is a dural tear, or tearing of the outermost of the three meninges surrounding the spinal cord.
- Various intradiscal procedures use heat, leading to risk of heat damage to surrounding structures. One potentially serious complication that has been reported in conjunction with these high-heat intradiscal procedures is osteonecrosis, which may result in a painful fracture that requires surgery or percutaneous vertebral augmentation.
- Physicians can hope to avoid complications associated with intradiscal procedures through extensive knowledge of anatomy, use of fluoroscopy and other visualization methods, and meticulous sterile technique, as well as administration of perioperative antibiotics.
- If a patient appears to be experiencing a complication after an intradiscal procedure, the practitioner should quickly consider its possible etiologies and in particular rule out neurologic insult and infection.

Introduction

Chronic spinal pain is one of the most common reasons why people seek out medical attention. Between 70% and 90% of the population will experience back pain at some point in their lives,[1,2] but thankfully, 80% to 90% of these people will recover from acute episodes with conservative therapy within 3 months.[3,4] But for those who continue to suffer with chronic pain, performing activities of daily living can be excruciating. This ongoing turmoil leads to frequent absence from work, loss of employment, opioid dependence, and ever-increasing disability. Spinal pain that originates from the disc, or intradiscal pain, is thought to be a major cause of severe and chronic pain in this population. Over the past 50 years, researchers have been attempting to identify and treat the various sources of spinal pain. In fact, many procedures have been developed to identify the source of one's pain. Some of the more commonly performed diagnostic procedures include medial branch blocks, selective nerve root blocks, and discography. After the source of one's pain is located, disc-related procedures may be considered to relieve the pain.

Surgery, typically involving laminectomy and microdiscectomy, has been shown to produce excellent clinical outcomes in patients with disc extrusion and neurologic deficits. However, patients with disc herniation smaller than 6 mm have fair or poor surgical outcomes.[5] In addition, conventional open disc surgery can be associated with complications from general anesthesia, nerve damage, epidural fibrosis, chronic postoperative pain syndrome, and adjacent spinal instability. Intradiscal procedures aim to address key issues in disc pathology. Bulging, herniation, prolapse, and disc tears (internal disc disruption [IDD]) are some of the most common causes of spine pain. Disc bulging or herniation can cause pain, numbness, or weakness by mechanical irritation and compression of an adjacent nerve root. When this occurs, pain presents typically in a radicular pattern. Herniation is caused when fluid from the nucleus does not leak out of the annulus but bulges against it (**Fig. 6-1**). This can cause compression of nerve roots as well as stretching of annular fibers.

Various studies have shown that disc herniation disrupts the capsule around the dorsal root ganglion (DRG) (**Fig. 6-1**), allowing permeation of large molecules such as albumin, subsequently followed by edema, scarring, and inflammation.[6] When an inflammatory reaction occurs, chemical irritation of an adjacent DRG or nerve root can occur, often causing axial or radicular pain.

Conversely, discogenic pain can occur without a disc bulge or prolapse. Such pain may originate from within the disc itself and is thought to be caused by tears and fissures in the annular layer of the disc.[7] This type of pain is often called IDD or simply "discogenic pain" and is diagnosed by concordant pain on a provocative discography. IDD is believed to be caused by the lamellar fibers of the posterior annulus that are weaker than the anterior. This allows more flexion and extension of the lower lumbar spine but also predisposes the area to tears and herniations.[8] Current thought suggests that discogenic pain may stem from irritation of small nociceptive nerve fibers within the outer third of the annulus fibrosis. The annulus is innervated by gray rami laterally, lateral ventral rami anteriorly, and sinuvertebral nerves posteriorly.[9,10] People with nerve penetration deeper than the initial third of the annulus may be at higher risk for IDD pain problems.[11] Additionally, as people age, the discs between the vertebrae lose water content and become brittle (degenerative disc disease).[12] This can cause small tears in the annulus fibrosis, allowing some of the nucleus pulposus to leak out and causing irritation of the nociceptive fibers, local sympathetic nerves, and afferent nerve roots. Many irritating fluids are found within this space, including glycosaminoglycans and lactic acid. Pain signals also release irritating chemical mediators such as phospholipase A2, prostaglandin E, tumor necrosis factor α (TNF-α), nitric oxide (NO), substance P, and many others.[13-15]

Disc-related pain from a disc herniation or IDD can take many forms. Pain can be sharp and shooting with radiation along a dermatomal distribution with corresponding magnetic resonance imaging (MRI) disc findings, or it can be more complex with radiation into other structures (e.g., groin pain from L5–S1). As we learn about pain pathways from nerve roots, the adjacent DRGs, the spinal cord, and the brain, our understanding of the complex pain patterns experienced by patients is growing. For instance, research has shown that pain signals from the lower lumbar discs travel from lower DRGs along the sympathetic nerves of the gray rami communicans to higher DRGs. There may also be a convergence of lower level lumbar disc-related pain signals to the L2 DRG.[16,17] This may explain the nondermatomal pain patterns that some patients experience. Some treatments are now being directed at the DRG as opposed to intradiscal for discogenic pain from IDD.[18-20] Another treatment consideration is use of an investigational device from Spinal Modulation, Inc., which offers hardware that applies DRG neurostimulation for pain relief.[21]

Disc pathology can also cause localized pain; for instance, discogenic low back pain is often described as "a belt of pain across my low back." People presenting with these types of pain symptoms are typically treated with conservative care, including physical therapy, chiropractic care, proper activity performance, over-the-counter medications, and antiinflammatory medications.[22] If conservative care fails to provide relief, imaging is typically performed at this stage if it has not already been done. If the disc is believed to be responsible for the pain symptoms, epidural steroid injections are often performed based on the imaging and patient's pain pattern. Other diagnostic and therapeutic modalities may be performed based on the patient's pain complaints. These treatments may include epidural steroid injections, selective nerve root blocks,

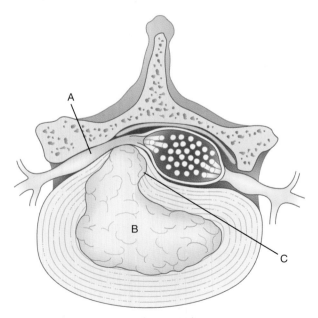

A. Compression of adjacent level DRG
B. Herniation of nucleus pulposus
C. Disruption of annular capsule

Fig. 6-1 Disc herniation showing disruption of annular capsule near the dorsal root ganglion.

discography, facet-related interventions, and others. If a patient fails to respond to conservative therapy and pain interventions, minimally invasive intradiscal procedures or surgery is often considered.

Because many spine surgeries involve extensive recovery times and numerous potential risks, many minimally invasive alternatives have emerged. Many of these procedures are designed specifically to treat disc-related pathologies. Although some of these treatments are new and research is limited, many patients choose to have minimally invasive intradiscal procedures because they typically involve fewer risks and a much more rapid recovery time compared with traditional open surgical practices.

Some of these minimally invasive intradiscal treatments include chemonucleolysis, intradiscal electrothermal therapy (IDET), biacuplasty, Disc Dekompressor, nucleoplasty, percutaneous laser disc decompression (PLDD), and injectable treatments such as methylene blue and TNF-α. Each of these procedures addresses a key element in disc pathology. Whereas positive studies on intradiscal procedures have shown reductions in pain scores and opioid use, negative studies refute the efficacy of intradiscal procedures.

Many intradiscal procedures are no longer widely used because they are labeled "experimental" and frequently denied by insurance companies. More recently, the use of intradiscal biologic agents is being trialed for IDD, although current research on these emerging procedures has not been widely published.

Inclusion Criteria

Because of the wide range of symptomatology and comorbid factors, there has been difficulty in designing a specific set of inclusion criteria for study population recruitment. Most studies agree patients should have failed previous conservative care, pain should be severe or have lasted longer than 6 months and involve confirmed axial or leg dermatomal pain, and disc height should be greater than 50% as confirmed by MRI. Additionally, all disc herniations must be contained. These procedures may not be appropriate if there is already extravasation of nuclear contents or disc sequestration. If a patient has weakness or bowel deficits, many surgeons prefer an open surgical technique or one guided by microscope to prevent any difficulties that could result in further compression. Discography and selective nerve root blocks are often performed before the patient undergoes these procedures in an attempt to target the source of pain.

Review of Intradiscal Procedures

Chemonucleolysis

Chemonucleolysis is one of oldest of all intradiscal procedures and has been performed in humans since 1963. Initially used for sciatica, chemonucleolysis is used to treat disc protrusions. The active enzyme, chymopapain, was derived from papaya fruit and was found to dissolve the nucleus pulposus when injected within the disc. When the nucleus pulposus dissolves, the disc begins to shrink. Since then, it has been shown that chymopapain works by depolymerizing proteoglycan and glycoprotein molecules. Chemonucleolysis is performed after a provocative discogram elicits concordant pain and is used in patients with disc herniations and radicular pain. Chymopapain is injected within the nucleus pulposus of the affected disc in the same fashion that contrast is injected during a discogram. The procedure has been performed in cervical, thoracic, and lumbar discs. The procedure is controversial despite its long track record and Food and Drug Administration approval because of anaphylactic reactions experienced in 1% of those who

underwent the procedure. Preoperative hypersensitivity testing and pretreatment with antihistamine medications has made allergic complications related to the procedure relatively rare. Chemonucleolysis is currently not widely used despite studies that show successes achieved in 70% of patients and higher. Chymopapain is not currently distributed within the United States.

A study by Hoogland and Scheckenback[23] supporting the efficacy of low-dose chemonucleolysis showed good or excellent results in 19 of 22 patients with obvious preoperative cervical disc herniation with predominantly radicular pain over a follow-up period of at least 1 year. In one patient, a fair result was obtained, and in two patients, the symptoms were unchanged; one of these patients subsequently underwent discectomy and anterior cervical spine fusion. No intra- or postoperative complications were noted. Furthermore, the authors of a review of 105 consecutive cases of chymopapain chemonucleolysis for single-level lumbar disc herniation concluded "the advantages of chemonucleolysis are well recognized."[24] Of the studies included in the review, mean follow-up was 12.2 years (range, 10 to 15.3 years). Eighty-seven patients were assessed using the Oswestry Disability Questionnaire during follow-up. An excellent or good response occurred in 58 patients (67%); four patients (4.5%) had a moderate response but were only minimally disabled. The treatment failed in 25 patients (28.5%), and 21 of them went on to surgery within a mean of 5.2 months (range, 3 weeks to 12 months). In 15 patients (71%), disc sequestration or lateral recess stenosis was found. Five of the remaining six patients had a large disc herniation at surgery. Surgery resulted in a significant improvement in nine cases. Discitis after chemonucleolysis occurred in six patients (5.7%). The authors of the review further concluded that chemonucleolysis is a safe and effective alternative to surgery in the treatment of herniated lumbar intervertebral discs in appropriately selected patients. The authors also noted chemonucleolysis appears to be a minimally invasive technique that has little traumatic effect on surrounding structures and is safer than surgery. They also remarked chemonucleolysis requires less operative time and postoperative hospital stay than discectomy and can be performed under local anesthesia, although all of the patients in this series had general anesthesia.

Intradiscal Electrothermal Therapy (Annuloplasty)

Intradiscal electrothermal therapy was first developed by Saal and Saal[9] in 2000. The underlying theory is that intradiscal pain is caused by irritation of small nerves within the annulus fibrosis and that destroying those nerves will relieve the patient's pain.[9,25] IDET is designed to address the pain from annular tears, something very few procedures are designed to do. This procedure was meant to be a less invasive and safer alternative to spinal fusion for discogenic pain.

Intradiscal electrothermal therapy is performed under fluoroscopy and conscious sedation. It consists of a needle being inserted into the posterior lateral disc (**Fig. 6-2**) and a catheter being threaded into the disc (**Fig. 6-3**). This catheter has a special thermal coil that converts radiofrequency energy to heat. This coil is threaded through the disc in a circular fashion and is positioned adjacent to the tear or nerve distribution area in the posterior lateral aspect of the disc.[3] Proper positioning is the key to a good result. The catheter should span the entire lesion and should be positioned near the pedicles on each side of the posterior annulus.[26,27] Subsequently, the tip is heated, through radiofrequency, to 90°C, modifying the collagen matrix, and breaking the triple helix bonds, causing thickening, contraction, and a 10% decrease in disc volume.[27] Heat is transferred through the coil to the surrounding tissues by conduction. The surrounding vascular

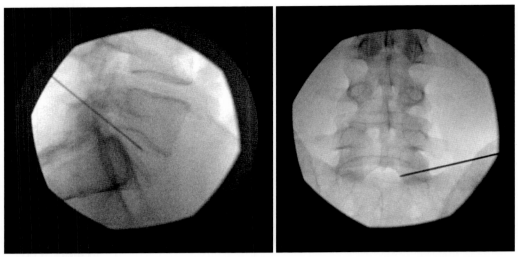

Fig. 6-2 Correct angle of approach for intradiscal electrothermal therapy trocar as seen on lateral and anteroposterior views.

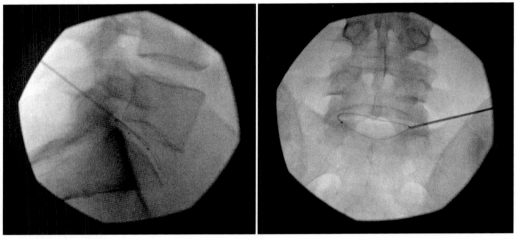

Fig. 6-3 Intradiscal electrothermal therapy cannula placed into the disc as seen on lateral and anteroposterior views.

areas act as a heat sink, preventing damage to tissues beyond the desired region.[9,27] The heating seals the tear if present and causes thermal injury to all intradiscal nerve fibers in close proximity, effectively destroying pain transmission.[27,28]

The heating, thickening, and contraction process in IDET is believed to enhance the structural integrity of the disc, stabilizing intradiscal fissures and decreasing new nerve growth, although as of yet there are no studies to support this thought.[9,26] However, studies using an electron microscope have been able to show visible shrinking of collagen molecules, giving credibility to this theory.[27]

Of concern with IDET is that the heating coil extends 5 cm through the heating probe; if poorly positioned, this can place heating elements near adjacent spinal nerves or into the spinal canal. Patients must be kept alert through this procedure to make sure there are no signs of radicular pain.

Biacuplasty

Biacuplasty is a newer technique developed by Baylis Medical to address intradiscal back pain produced by irritation of intradiscal nerve fibers.[28,29] This procedure is considered by many to be safer than IDET because its bipolar design system allows for internal cooling of the radiofrequency transfer of heat between electrodes. The bipolar design pinpoints the area of treatment and prevents

outside structures from being heated. Cooling is accomplished by running cool sterile water through an adjacent channel inside the probe. This prevents tissue closest to the probes from being scorched and protects spinal nerves outside the desired region from being heated by conduction through the hot probe. If needed, this system can treat an area of up to 4 cm.[28,29] Unlike IDET, biacuplasty uses a lower temperature, at 40° to 50°C. This range is sufficient for thermoregulating nerves but may be insufficient for repairing annular tears, thus limiting its scope. The procedure consists of two radiofrequency probes placed under fluoroscopy posterior laterally into the annulus fibrosis with one on each side.[29,30] Because the probes only need to be placed opposite each other, another advantage to this procedure is how easy it is to position the probes into the appropriate place. Whereas IDET requires threading a catheter and using fluoroscopy to make sure it is near the desired area, biacuplasty uses two adjacent probes coming from opposite sides of the vertebrae toward each other (**Fig. 6-4**), allowing for much easier placement.[29,31]

Subsequently, current is passed between the two probes, causing them to warm. The heat destroys the surrounding annular nerve fibers, and the probes are removed. Karaman et al[30] and other physicians performing this technique recommend that patients wear an external stabilizing back brace for 6 to 8 weeks after the

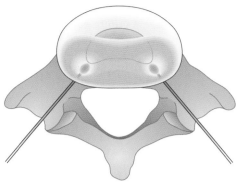

Fig. 6-4   Dual-probe system in biacuplasty.

NUCLEOPLASTY CHANNELING

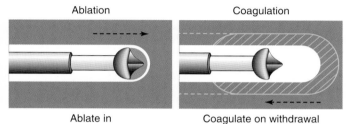

Fig. 6-5   The nucleoplasty wand ablates when advanced and coagulates as it is withdrawn.

procedure to prevent injury to the area before stabilization of the disc can occur.[29]

Nucleoplasty

Another intradiscal technique is nucleoplasty. This procedure is fundamentally different than IDET and biacuplasty in that it treats disc herniation. It was first used in 2000 and is effective in mild to moderate herniation of discs.[3,32] Herniation is problematic in that it not only causes stretching of intradiscal fibers but also can compress adjacent nerve roots, causing radicular pain. Nucleoplasty may be the most commonly used form of disc decompression. The procedure differs from IDET and biacuplasty in that the wand is placed into the nucleus pulposus and not into the annulus. It also uses radiofrequency waves. Heating the gel-like matrix of the nucleus to about 40° to 70°C, it breaks the bonds and vaporizes the matrix. The vaporized matrix gases are then removed through the probe. The wand is moved back and forth throughout the gel, creating channels that allow for a creation of space (**Fig. 6-5**). The vaporization and retraction of matrix causes a vacuum in those channels that produces subsequent contraction in the rest of the disc.[32] This central vacuum is believed to allow space for the herniated disc section to contract back into the disc, consequentially relieving compression on the adjacent nerve roots. In total, about 1 mL of gel is removed (**Fig. 6-6**).[32,33] Because the probe acts within the nucleus pulposus, it is relatively unlikely to cause injury to surrounding structures. Although existing studies are limited and are mostly observational, level II evidence exists for pain relief and improved functional outcomes.[33,34] Available studies show nucleoplasty to be an encouraging procedure with few complications, decrease in pain, and rapid recovery time postoperatively.[34] Li et al[35] presented a study done in England with 126 patients undergoing cervical nucleoplasty, finding favorable results in 83% of patients. The only reported complication was a broken wand.

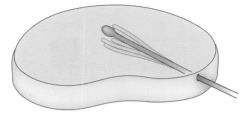

Fig. 6-6   Multiple channels created in a disc through multiple passes of the nucleoplasty wand.

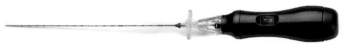

Fig. 6-7   Wand used in nucleoplasty. (Copyright ©2010 Stryker Corporation.)

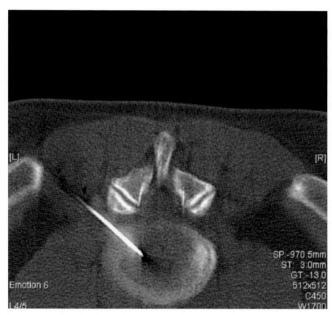

Fig. 6-8   Disc Dekompressor placed into the nucleus pulposus as seen on a computed tomography scan.

Disc Dekompressor

The Disc Dekompressor, created in 2002, is a handheld device also designed to treat herniated discs by aspirating disc material. It consists of a disposable helical probe with an outer shell and an inner rotating probe (**Fig. 6-7**). The Dekompressor is placed posterior laterally into the nucleus pulposus under fluoroscopic guidance (**Fig. 6-8**). The rotating probe mines out a designated amount of matrix, creating channels similar to those created in the nucleoplasty procedure (**Figs. 6-9** and **6-10**).[36,37] These channels retract, causing contraction of the disc and effectively shrinking the herniated portion. This releases compression of the nerve root and adjacent annular nerves as in nucleoplasty. Studies are limited with this new technique. A review of four studies done in 2009 by Singh et al[38] found that all of the studies produced favorable results and were able to achieve level III evidence. It was thought that the studies could have been more conclusive if they were nonrandomized and nonblinded and entailed longer follow-up times. Alò et al[37] studied 50 patients and found 88% satisfaction at 1-year follow-up with a 78.6% decrease in analgesic intake. No complications were reported in their study. Although the existing literature on the Disc Dekompressor is promising, much more research needs to be completed.

Percutaneous Laser Disc Decompression

Percutaneous laser disc decompression was used by Choy and Ascher in 1986[39] and has made a tumultuous entry into the medical field. Similar to many other intradiscal procedures, data are lacking in prospective randomized controlled studies.[38,40] However, despite the paucity of studies, the procedure has been consistently performed with success for more than 2 decades. Since its inception, a variety of lasers have been used, including yttrium aluminium garnet (YAG), potassium-titanyl-phosphate, holmium, argon, and CO_2. However, most physicians prefer the Nd:YAG (neodymium-doped YAG) laser because of its optimal wavelength for PLDD and applicability to other types of commonly performed laser procedures.[40,41]

Percutaneous laser disc decompression is similar in approach to other intradiscal procedures and some use the procedure for disc herniations, but others use the procedure to perform laser annuloplasty for discogenic pain and disc tears. It starts with sterile technique, and a needle is introduced under direct fluoroscopy into the nucleus pulposus posterior laterally. A laser fiber is advanced through the needle, extending 1 cm beyond the tip (**Figs. 6-11** and **6-12**).[41] Laser pulses of 20 to 40 W deliver 1000 to 2000 J of energy into the nucleus, converting light into heat, vaporizing the water, and relieving intradiscal pressure.[41,42] In addition to the vaporization, the laser also destroys the chemical bonds within the matrix,

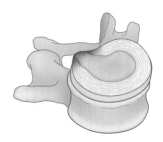

Herniated disc before procedure

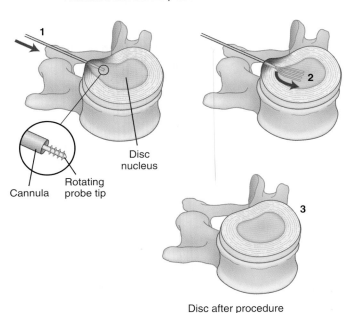

Disc after procedure

Fig. 6-9   Disc Dekompressor.

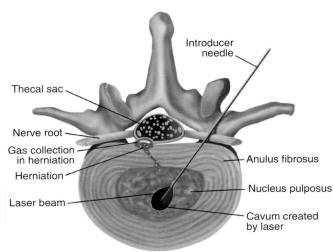

Fig. 6-11   Percutaneous laser disc decompression. (From Brouwer P, Schenk B: Percutaneous intradiscal therapies. In Pope TL Jr, editor. *Imaging of the musculoskeletal system*, Philadelphia, 2008, Elsevier.)

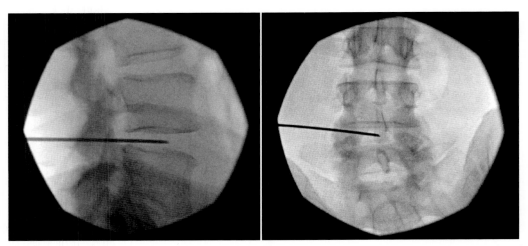

Fig. 6-10   Disc Dekompressor trocar in place at the L4–L5 level shown in both lateral and anteroposterior views.

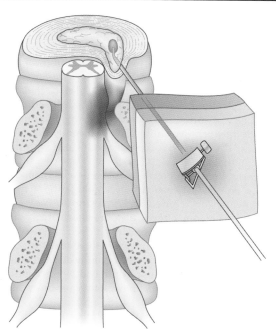

Fig. 6-12 Percutaneous laser disc decompression.

causing protein denaturation and a definitive change that will not allow the nucleus to absorb further water in the future. This prevents the disc from swelling back to its previous size and again causing the herniation that the procedure sought to eliminate[39,43] After the procedure is finished, the patient is monitored for 30 minutes and released.

A problem with this procedure is that laser thermal energy is difficult to control. Temperatures can reach up to 250°C and have the potential to burn adjacent tissues, causing scarring and inflammatory reactions.[42,43] Conversely, problems also seem to arise when studies fail to use laser intensity strong enough to denature the matrix, succeeding only in vaporizing the water. If the matrix is not changed, then the nucleus over time will reabsorb the water volume lost in the procedure, and the herniation will return.

Initial studies in PLDD by Choy[39] reported a 91% success rate at 1-year follow up, and Gupta et al[42] reported an 85% success rate as far as a 7-year follow up for their study of 40 patients. Despite favorable clinical trials, however, strong evidence of the efficacy of this procedure is still missing.[43] Gibson and Waddell[44] performed one of the most extensive reviews of the literature available and found that the evidence for the efficacy of surgical correction for disc prolapse is still unresolved. Through their review of more than 40 articles, only level II evidence could be demonstrated.

Methylene Blue

Methylene blue, used widely as a histologic stain, is considered by some to have a viable role in the treatment of discogenic pain. This is attributed to its weak neurolytic effects and ability to block synthesis of NO, which has been implicated in the inflammatory processes associated with disc pain and degeneration.[45,46]

A 72-patient Chinese study in the injection of methylene blue to relieve discogenic pain called the treatment "revolutionary"[46] and "extraordinary"[47] and yielded highly encouraging results. According to the authors of this trial, methylene blue proved to be a safe, effective, and minimally invasive method with significantly better outcomes over placebo for the treatment of intractable and

incapacitating discogenic low back pain.[48] Patients in a methylene injection group showed a mean reduction in pain measured by numerical rating scale of 52.50, a mean reduction in Oswestry Disability Index (ODI) scores of 35.58, and satisfaction rates of 91.6% compared with 0.70%, 1.68%, and 14.3%, respectively, in a placebo treatment group ($P < .001$, $P < .001$, and $P < .001$, respectively). No adverse effects or complications were found in the group of patients treated with intradiscal methylene blue injection.

The efficacy of methylene blue for discogenic back pain is likewise supported by a preliminary report of a clinical trial.[49] According to the authors, 24 patients with chronic discogenic low back pain who met criteria for lumbar interbody fusion surgery were treated instead with an intradiscal injection of methylene blue for pain relief; of these patients, 21 (87%) reported a disappearance or marked alleviation of low back pain and experienced a definite improvement in physical function. A statistically significant and clinically meaningful improvement in the changes in ODI and the Visual Analog Scale scores were obtained in the patients with chronic discogenic low back pain after the treatment.

Tumor Necrosis Factor α Inhibitors

The cytokine TNF-α, a potent influencer of the inflammatory response, is believed to contribute significantly to radiculopathy and discogenic pain of the lumbosacral spine. Because of this belief, agents that block TNF-α have been used experimentally to treat discogenic pain in patients whose pain is refractory to nonsteroidal antiinflammatory drugs. Two such inhibitors are etanercept and infliximab, which bind TNF-α receptors.

Although anti-TNF-α medications are frequently prescribed for low back pain, very few randomized controlled clinical trials back their effectiveness in this capacity. For example, a double-blind, placebo-controlled pilot study found a single low dose of intradiscal etanercept did not seem to be an effective treatment for chronic radicular or discogenic low back pain.[50] Six patients received 0.1, 0.25, 0.5, 0.75, 1.0, or 1.5 mg etanercept intradiscally in pain-generating discs, and in each escalating dose group of six patients, one patient received placebo. Neurologic examinations and post-procedure leukocyte counts were performed in all patients at 1-month follow-up visits. In patients who experienced significant improvement in pain scores and function, follow-up visits were conducted 3 and 6 months after the procedure. At 1-month follow-up, no differences were found for pain scores or disability scores between or within groups for any dose range or subgroup of patients. Furthermore, only eight patients remained in the study after 1 month and elected to forego further treatment. No complications were reported, and no differences were noted between pre- and postprocedure leukocyte counts. Although the study failed to find efficacy in TNF-α–blocking medications, no adverse effects were reported.

However, a study in pigs found these two anti-TNF-α medications prevented the reduction of nerve conduction velocity and also seemed to limit nerve fiber injury, intracapillary thrombus formation, and intraneural edema formation in the animals' spines.[51] The authors of the study further concluded that TNF-α is clearly involved in the basic pathophysiologic events leading to structural and functional changes in the nerve root.

Contraindications

Intradiscal procedures are similar to most other invasive procedures in that they are absolutely contraindicated in patients who are pregnant, cannot follow instructions, have an active infection, or have a bleeding disorder that prevents surgery.[4]

Relative contraindications include the presence of other sources of pain such as spinal stenosis, spinal fracture, spondylolisthesis, or spinal tumors. Patients may also be excluded if they have problems at more than two levels or have significant comorbidities or psychiatric problems.[37-39] Morbid obesity can also be a relative contraindication because it is an impediment to accomplishing the procedure. Instrumentation comes in specific sizes and may not be of adequate length to place probes in the desired area. Additionally, IDET and biacuplasty are contraindicated in cervical and thoracic disc spaces because the discs are not large enough to accommodate the catheters used in theses procedures.[52] Nucleoplasty and Disc Dekompressor are contraindicated in patients with greater than 50% loss of vertebral height or severe disc degeneration because further reduction of the disc risks more harm than benefit.[38,53]

Selected Complications

Minimally invasive intradiscal procedures are designed to lower risks, but as in any spine-related procedure, specific and sometimes catastrophic sequelae do occur. Consequently, physicians must be knowledgeable of the complications, prepared to avoid pitfalls, and ready to manage difficult challenges. Physicians can hope to avoid complications with thorough knowledge of anatomy, assistance of fluoroscopy and other visualization methods, and meticulous use of sterile technique. However, development of complications is still possible even with extensive preventative measures and years of practitioner experience.

All intradiscal procedures share many of the same risks because the instruments are placed into the disc in a similar fashion for each procedure (e.g., anteromedial for cervical and posterolateral for thoracic and lumbar); conversely, each intradiscal procedure poses unique risks. Because these procedures penetrate the protective skin barrier and are placed near critical spinal structures, they may result in bleeding, nerve trauma, spinal cord injury, infection, and damage to vital structures (e.g., vessels, nerve roots, vertebral endplates, the spinal cord, and organs).

Infection

One of the most common complications of intradiscal procedures is infection of involved skin or deeper structures. Signs and symptoms of postprocedural infection may include pain, swelling, rubor, purulent drainage, fever, nausea, vomiting, and chills. Of particular concern are signs of advanced infection, including elevated white blood cell, C-reactive protein, and erythrocyte sedimentation rate counts.

Because infection is a known risk of intradiscal procedures, the practitioner should endeavor to lower the incidence of topical and systemic infection in the patient. Prophylactic antibiotics may be given intravenously (e.g., 1 g of cefazolin), particularly in intradiscal procedures that involve injection or insertion of foreign materials into the body.[54] Beyond administration of antibiotics, screening patients for topical infections, immunocompromised status, and systemic conditions, the most important measure against infection is meticulous surgical technique. To achieve this, iodine or chlorhexidine should be used as a surgical preparation with a wide area of the back prepared because a variety of angles of approach may be used. In many intradiscal procedures, sterile drapes should be placed over the patient, and measures such as a surgical scrub and use of masks and gowns should be incorporated when appropriate. One must remember that the disc is the largest structure in the body without its own circulation and therefore has an increased risk of severe and catastrophic infections.

Discitis

A potentially catastrophic type of infection from intradiscal procedure is discitis (**Fig. 6-13**), or infection within the disc. It presents as worsening back pain after an intradiscal procedure and is most commonly caused by *Staphylococcus aureus*.[55,56] Discitis can also present with nausea, vomiting, fever, chills, malaise, or any other complaints commonly associated with infections. The possibility of intradiscal infection is why administration of prophylactic preoperative antibiotics is currently the standard of care and why discography is typically performed with intradiscal antibiotic administration.[56,57] Classen et al[58] prospectively monitored timing of antibiotic prophylaxis and development of surgical wound infections in 2847 patients undergoing surgical procedures. Among patients who received antibiotics up to 24 hours before surgery, 2 hours before surgery, 3 hours after surgery, and more than 3 hours after surgery, those who received antibiotics 2 hours before surgery had the lowest rates of subsequent surgical wound infections. Some studies recommend intradiscal injection of antibiotics after procedures, but this recommendation is controversial.[4] Before the commencement of preoperative and intradiscal antibiotics, vertebral osteonecrosis and epidural abscesses were reported. Thankfully, most infectious complications can be avoided with meticulous use of sterile surgical technique. Unfortunately, discitis can also be aseptic, the result of inflammatory changes in the disc secondary to heat damage. This consequence may be prevented with precision of location of procedure and is also better controlled in techniques such as biacuplasty in which there is an internal cooling system.

Transverse Myelitis

Another potentially serious complication that may be related to infection is transverse myelitis, which has been reported to occur in conjunction with chemonucleolysis. Transverse myelitis, which involves inflammation of the spinal cord caused by a range of etiologies, may result in diminished or absent sensation below the

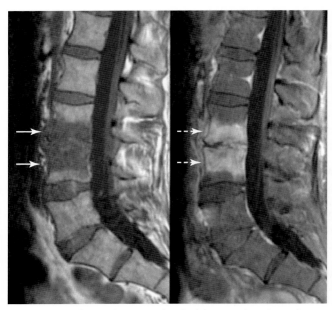

Fig. 6-13 Discitis at the L3–L4 level with extension through endplates and spread into adjacent level vertebral bodies.

injury. It may arise as a complication from an intradiscal procedure as a result of infection, autoimmune reaction, or thrombosis of spinal arteries. A case report describes mild paraplegia secondary to transverse myelitis in a 48-year-old male patient who underwent chemonucleolysis for disc degeneration and radiculopathy.[59] However, no specific source of infection was found in his case, which suggested that the patient's transverse myelitis may have been caused by an autoimmune reaction or a thrombosis of the anterior spinal artery.

Allergic Reactions

Most intradiscal procedures are done under conscious sedation, minimizing risks for sedation-related side effects. Allergic reaction can be caused by preoperative skin preparations, antibiotics, local anesthesia, and latex. Because the patient may be unaware of any allergies surrounding these products, the physician should remain vigilant for development of allergic sequelae during the procedure. For example, local anesthetics or antibiotics are common elicitors of adverse reactions with clinical symptoms such as anaphylaxis with tachycardia; hypotension; and subjective feelings of weakness, heat, or vertigo.[60] Latex can also produce allergic reactions as serious as anaphylaxis.[60,61] Physicians and staff should always be vigilant about monitoring the patient for deleterious events. Local pain is frequently reported at the catheter or probe insertion site, but most patients remain comfortable throughout the entire procedure. Occasionally, muscle spasm can also occur but is usually short lived.

Increased Postprocedure Pain

Greater than expected postprocedural pain is one of the most common complications reported after any intradiscal procedure, although it is usually benign and self-limiting. If the pain is severe or any new neurologic deficits are reported, more severe complications must be suspected and quickly ruled out.

Bleeding or Spinal Hematoma

Another feared but infrequently reported complication of intradiscal procedures is bleeding in and around the spine, which can lead to epidural, subdural, muscular, and superficial hematomas. Although rare, spinal hematomas can occur because needles pass precariously close to spinal nerve roots and blood vessels. Subarachnoid hemorrhage is an infrequent and unexplained finding that has been reported with a chemonucleolysis patient. A report of clinical and postmortem findings in a 42-year-old man who died 5 days after chemonucleolysis at the L4–5 and L5–S1 disc spaces found the predominant histologic abnormality was a severe inflammatory arteritis of a medium-sized artery at the upper cervical level with disruption of the vessel wall. The potential causative role of chymopapain in this situation and the correlation of a vascular basis for many of the complications found after inadvertent intrathecal chymopapain injection remain topics of discussion.[62]

Dural Puncture and Spinal Cord or Nerve Root Damage

Because of the location of the procedure, the risk of puncturing the dura and damage to the thecal sac is also possible. One case of cauda equina syndrome was reported with IDET caused by improper needle and catheter placement by the physician.[63] With PLDD, there was one reported case of subacute cauda equina syndrome from an internist performing PLDD on a patient with lumbar spinal stenosis.[64] Cauda equina syndrome was resolved after the patient underwent a hemilaminectomy and discectomy 2 months later by a neurosurgeon. All of these problems are usually

avoided by use of fluoroscopy during the procedure and being performed by one well versed in interventional techniques, spinal anatomy, and spinal fluoroscopy. A thorough knowledge of vertebral anatomy and proper technique drastically minimize these risks. All five procedures use a posterolateral spinal approach in the lumbar spine, and many believe this is the best angle to use to minimize injury. However, there is still a risk of injuring nerve roots and vessel damage, including the radiculomedullary artery of Adamkiewicz (**Fig. 6-14**). In addition, patients are also kept under light sedation so they can tell the physician if they experience any radicular pain. Finally, because of the location of the procedure, the potential for intrathecal placement of the device is possible along with spinal headache, but as of yet, no studies have reported patients with this complication. If any of the procedures are attempted in the cervical or thoracic region in which IDET is contraindicated, new risks are associated with the placement of the surgical instrumentation via the typically used paramedian anterior approach.

Damage to Surrounding Structures

A more common complication of intradiscal procedures is structural damage to tissues, such as damage to the endplate, a structure that plays a crucial role in nutritional supply to the intervertebral disc. When structural damage from an intradiscal procedure does occur, it is normally caused by complications from the instruments used in these procedures. One common instrument-related complication is catheter or probe breakage. Each intradiscal procedure uses instrumentation with fine-tipped devices. Poor positioning or difficult anatomy can force these tips against the edges of the

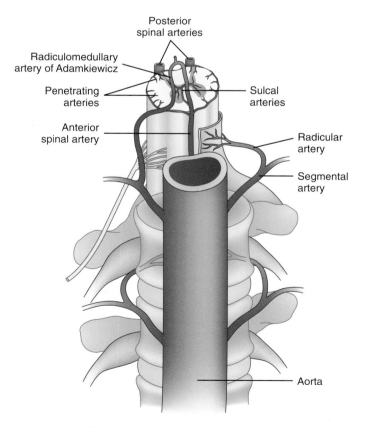

Fig. 6-14 Major arteries of the spine.

vertebrae or the posterior or anterior longitudinal ligaments, causing trauma. Most commonly, this results in the need to surgically remove the probe from the disc. Li et al[36] presented one case in which a probe fractured off during nucleoplasty. The probe was unable to be retrieved, and it was therefore left inside the patient. No subsequent complications were reported from the patient during follow-up. However, current guidelines do not recommend leaving the probe tip unless removal proves to be more dangerous than leaving the tip in place. Additionally, the IDET catheter is subject to damage of its insulation with frequent repositioning. Therefore, if the catheter must be repeatedly moved, caution should be taken, and at any sign of kinking, the catheter should be removed and replaced. Three studies reported breakage of the Disc Dekompressor during a procedure; however, in each instance, the part was able to be successfully removed surgically with no additional complications.[4] Physicians performing these procedures should be trained by manufacturers to correctly use the device. Likewise, performance of the technique should be done as directed to minimize the potential for damage to the probes and subsequent patient injury. Multiplanar fluoroscopic views should be used throughout the procedure to ensure positioning and advancement.

Osteonecrosis and Heating Complications

Biacuplasty, IDET, nucleoplasty, and PLDD all use heat as part of the procedure, leading to a risk of heat damage to surrounding structures. Osteonecrosis is a potentially serious complication that has been reported in conjunction with these high-heat intradiscal procedures. Osteonecrosis of the spine may result in a painful fracture that requires further intervention in the form of surgery or percutaneous vertebral augmentation to stabilize the injury and relieve the pain.[65]

Intradiscal electrothermal therapy and PLDD in particular have been reported to expose cortical and cancellous bone to temperatures well within the range reported to induce necrosis.[66,67] IDET presents the greatest risk of producing this outcome if the physician is not careful with exact catheter placement. Because the heating element in IDET extends 5 cm, improper placement can position this heating element near spinal nerve roots. Proper orientation on radiography is crucial. Furthermore, in IDET, nucleoplasty, and PLDD, the needle used to place the catheter is not insulated. Therefore, care must be taken to ensure that the probe is not touching the needle when the heating element is activated or the needle will heat risking damage to structures outside the desired area along the needle path. Biacuplasty and the injectable therapies may be the safest of the techniques with regard to this problem. Biacuplasty's bipolar water cooling system prevents elements outside the desired area from being heated by conduction. Fortunately, in all heat-generating procedures, the nucleus of the disc itself has high water content and acts as a heat sink, absorbing much of the heat. If done properly, the heat is absorbed and presents minimal risk to adjacent structures external to the disc.

Nucleoplasty carries with it an added risk of wand failure because it vaporizes the matrix and removes the gases. Rarely, chunks of the matrix may occlude the probe, causing blockage and leading to failed completion of the procedure.[13] Another nucleoplasty complication reported by Cohen et al[68] was an incidence (15%) of minor new-onset neurologic symptoms occurring in patients, including numbness and twitching in the distal lower extremities. A total of 4% of patients reported new-onset low back pain different than previous, but all new low back pain resolved within 2 weeks.

Biacuplasty studies reported minimal complications of 1 to 2 days of low back pain after the procedure that resolved spontaneously.[29,30] Many believe that the increased pain is related to inflammatory changes secondary to thermal injury, and pain resolves with the passing of the inflammation. One incidence of vasovagal reaction was also noted. In this instance, the patient was treated with fluid support and released the same day.[30] Some studies have reported recurrence of pain over time.

Percutaneous laser disc decompression (PLDD) carries with it a unique set of complications, including safety risks to the physician and staff performing the procedure. Safety goggles must be worn at all times by the physician, patient, and other staff. If pointed toward the eyes, the laser can cause significant retinal damage. Many facilities and hospitals using this procedure have a designated laser safety technician who is in charge of ensuring that safety procedures are observed.[40,43] Likewise, all physicians using these lasers should be trained by the manufacturers on how to avoid errors that can be costly to patients and staff. All lasers use high levels of heat, and care must be taken to prevent adjacent nerve root injury. One study reported four cases of thermal nerve root damage because of accidental heating of the cannula by CO_2 laser.[69]

Complication Prevention

Recommendations to avoid potential complications in intradiscal procedures (**Table 6-1**) include meticulous observation of aseptic technique and administration of preprocedural antibiotics to lower the incidence of postprocedural infection and extensive knowledge of relevant anatomy to promote accurate placement of instruments and injected medications and to avoid structural damage of the spine and nervous tissues. If a patient appears to be experiencing a complication after an intradiscal procedure, the practitioner should quickly consider its possible etiologies and in particular rule out neurologic insult and infection. A thorough neurologic examination should be performed and documented. Typically, an MRI or computed tomography scan with contrast is used to assess structural damage and may be beneficial in identifying edema or infection in late cases. If neurologic insult is suspected, surgical consultation should be obtained immediately. If an infection is suspected, hospitalization is recommended with an infectious disease and surgical consultation. If a complication is recognized early in its course, more serious insult may be avoided by early recognition and intervention when appropriate.

Conclusion

Although more invasive procedures may be appropriate to treat discogenic pain in patients refractory to conservative treatments, minimally invasive intradiscal therapies can offer substantial benefits with potentially fewer and more manageable complications. Complications of intradiscal interventions designed to correct spinal pain are generally considered to be minimal if performed on carefully selected patients by experienced physicians.

Although no procedure is without its inherent risks, these procedures and the studies associated with them note mostly theoretical complications with few actual reports of problems. Of the cases in which complications arose, most were able to be fully resolved in a timely manner, and the overall outcome of the procedure still showed benefit to the patient. Attention to detail and proper technique by the physician are most important in minimizing the risk to the patient and maximizing the effectiveness of these innovative procedures.

Table 6-1: Potential Complications from Intradiscal Procedures

Intradiscal Procedure	Cervical	Thoracic	Lumbar
IDET or biacuplasty	Not recommended	Not recommended	Trauma to the paraspinal blood vessels (including the anterior segmental medullary arteries or the artery of Adamkiewicz), spinal canal, spinal cord, or spinal nerve roots while accessing the posterior lateral disc Disc disruption with disc migration, spinal cord injury, nerve root injury, CSF leak, or vessel penetration (including the aorta or vena cava and iliac vessels) during the procedure Discitis, epidural hematoma, or neurologic sequelae (e.g., cauda equina syndrome, paralysis) after the procedure
Nucleoplasty or Dekompressor	Trauma to the carotid artery, internal jugular vein, thoracic duct, trachea, or esophagus while accessing the anterior disc Disc disruption with posterior disc migration; spinal cord compression, penetration, or injury; nerve root injury; CSF leak; or deep vessel penetration during the procedure Discitis, epidural hematoma, abscess, or neurologic sequelae after the procedure	Trauma to the lung space (pneumothorax), paraspinal blood vessels (including the anterior segmental medullary arteries or the artery of Adamkiewicz), thoracic duct, spinal canal, spinal cord, or spinal nerve roots while accessing the posterior lateral disc Disc disruption with disc migration; spinal cord compression, penetration, or injury; nerve root injury; CSF leak; or vessel penetration (including the aorta or vena cava) during the procedure Discitis, epidural hematoma, abscess, or neurologic sequelae after the procedure	Trauma to the paraspinal blood vessels (including the anterior segmental medullary arteries or the artery of Adamkiewicz), spinal canal, spinal cord, or spinal nerve roots while accessing the posterior lateral disc Disc disruption with disc migration, spinal cord injury, nerve root injury, CSF leak, or vessel penetration (including the aorta or vena cava and iliac vessels) during the procedure Discitis, epidural hematoma, abscess, or neurologic sequelae after the procedure
Laser (PLDD)	Trauma to the carotid artery, internal jugular vein, thoracic duct, trachea, or esophagus while accessing the anterior disc Disc disruption with posterior disc migration; spinal cord compression, penetration, or injury; nerve root injury; CSF leak; or deep vessel penetration during the procedure Discitis, epidural hematoma, or neurologic sequelae after the procedure	Trauma to the lung space (pneumothorax), paraspinal blood vessels (including the anterior segmental medullary arteries or the artery of Adamkiewicz), hemothorax, thoracic duct, spinal canal, spinal cord, or spinal nerve roots while accessing the posterior lateral disc Disc disruption with disc migration; spinal cord compression, penetration, or injury; nerve root injury; CSF leak; or vessel penetration (including aortic) during the procedure Discitis, epidural hematoma, or neurologic sequelae after the procedure	Trauma to the paraspinal blood vessels (including the anterior segmental medullary arteries or the artery of Adamkiewicz), spinal canal, spinal cord, or spinal nerve roots while accessing the posterior lateral disc Disc disruption with disc migration; spinal cord compression, penetration, or injury; nerve root injury; CSF leak; or vessel penetration (including the aorta or vena cava and iliac vessels) during the procedure Discitis, epidural hematoma, neurologic sequelae, osteonecrosis, or vertebral endplate damage after the procedure

Continued

Table 6-1: Potential Complications from Intradiscal Procedures—cont'd

Intradiscal Procedure	Cervical	Thoracic	Lumbar
Chemonucleolysis	Trauma to the carotid artery, internal jugular vein, thoracic duct, trachea, or esophagus while accessing the anterior disc Disc disruption with posterior disc migration; spinal cord compression, penetration, or injury; nerve root injury; CSF leak; or deep vessel penetration, during the procedure Discitis, epidural hematoma, abscess, or neurologic sequelae after the procedure Transverse myelitis, subarachnoid hemorrhage, anaphylactic allergic reaction, or neurotoxicity	Trauma to the lung space (pneumothorax), paraspinal blood vessels (including the anterior segmental medullary arteries or the artery of Adamkiewicz), hemothorax, thoracic duct, spinal canal, spinal cord, or spinal nerve roots while accessing the posterior lateral disc Disc disruption with disc migration; spinal cord compression, penetration, or injury; nerve root injury; CSF leak; or vessel penetration (including aortic) during the procedure Discitis, epidural hematoma, abscess, or neurologic sequelae after the procedure Transverse myelitis, subarachnoid hemorrhage, anaphylactic allergic reaction, or neurotoxicity	Trauma to the paraspinal blood vessels (including the anterior segmental medullary arteries or the artery of Adamkiewicz), spinal canal, spinal cord, or spinal nerve roots while accessing the posterior lateral disc Disc disruption with disc migration; spinal cord compression, penetration, or injury; nerve root injury; CSF leak; or vessel penetration (including the aorta or vena cava and iliac vessels) during the procedure Discitis, epidural hematoma, abscess, or neurologic sequelae after the procedure Transverse myelitis, subarachnoid hemorrhage, anaphylactic allergic reaction, or neurotoxicity
Methylene blue or TNF-α	Unknown	Unknown	Trauma to the paraspinal blood vessels (including the anterior segmental medullary arteries or the artery of Adamkiewicz), spinal canal, spinal cord, or spinal nerve roots while accessing the posterior lateral disc Disc disruption with disc migration; spinal cord compression, penetration, or injury; nerve root injury; CSF leak; or vessel penetration (including the aorta or vena cava and iliac vessels) during the procedure Discitis, epidural hematoma, or neurologic sequelae after the procedure

CSF, cerebrospinal fluid; IDET, intradiscal electrothermal therapy; PLDD, percutaneous laser disc decompression; TNF, tumor necrosis factor.

References

1. Kennedy M: IDET: A new approach to treating lower back pain. *WMJ* 98:18-20, 1999.
2. Andersson GBJ: Epidemiological features of chromic low back pain. *Lancet* 354:581-585, 1999.
3. Raj PP, Lou L, Erdine S, et al: Percutaneous therapeutic procedures for disc lesions. In Ruiz-Lopez R, Pichot C, editors: *Interventional pain management: image guided procedures*, Philadelphia, 2008, Saunders Elsevier, pp 539-558.
4. Fenton D, Czervionke L: Intradiscal electrothermal therapy (IDET). In Fenton D, Czervionke L, editors: *Image guided spine intervention*, Philadelphia, 2003, Saunders, pp 257-284.
5. Carragee EJ, Kim DH: A prospective analysis of magnetic resonance imaging findings in patients with sciatica and lumbar disc herniation. Correlation of outcomes with disc fragment and canal morphology. *Spine* 22(14):1650-1660, 1997.
6. Murata Y, Rydevik B, Takahashi K, et al: Incision of the intervertebral disc induces permeability of the dorsal root ganglion capsule. *Spine* 30(15):1712, 2005.
7. Maroon J: Current concepts in minimally invasive discectomy. *Neurosurgery* 51(5):137-145, 2002.
8. Peng B, Hou S, Wu W, et al: The pathogenesis and clinical significance of a high intensity zone (HIZ) of lumbar intervertebral disc on MR imaging in the patient with discogenic low back pain. *Eur Spine J* 15(5):583-587, 2006.
9. Saal JS, Saal JA: Management of chronic discogenic low back pain with a thermal intradiscal catheter: a preliminary report. *Spine* 25(3):382-388, 2000.
10. Cohen SP, Larkin TM, Barna SA, et al: Lumbar discography: a comprehensive review of outcome studies, diagnostic accuracy, and principles. *Reg Anesth Pain Med* 30:163-184, 2005.
11. Deramond H, Debussche C, Pruvo JP, Galibert P: La vertebroplastie. *Feuillets Radiol* 30:262-268, 1990.

12. Nachemson A: Measurement of intradiscal pressure. *Acta Orthop Scand* 28:269-289, 1959.

13. Singh V, Derby R: Percutaneous lumbar disc decompression. *Pain Physician* 9(2):139-146, 2006.

14. Freemont A, Peacock T, Goupille P, et al: Nerve in-growth into diseased intervertebral disc in chronic low back pain. *Lancet* 350:178-181, 1997.

15. Jimbo K, Park JS, Yokosuka K, et al: Positive feedback loop of interluken-1 beta upregulation production of inflammatory mediators in human intervertebral disc cells in vitro. *J Neurosurg Spine* 2(5):589, 2005.

16. Morinaga T, Takahashi Y, Yamagata M, et al: Sensory innervation of the anterior portion of the lumbar intervertebral disk in rats. *Spine* 21:1848-1851, 1996.

17. Ohtori S, Takahashi Y, Takahashi K, et al: Sensory innervation of the dorsal portion of the lumbar intervertebral disc in rats. *Spine* 24:2295-2299, 1999.

18. Oh WS, Shim JC: A randomized controlled trial of radiofrequency denervation fo the ramus communicans nerve for chronic discogenic low back pain. *Clin J Pain* 20(1):55-60, 2004.

19. Simopoulos T, Malik A, Sial K, et al: Radiofrequency lesioning of the L2 ramus communicans in managing discogenic low back pain. *Pain Physician J* 8:61-65, 2005.

20. Menedez R, Bailey S, Paine G, et al: Evaluation of the L2 spinal nerve root infiltration as a diagnostic tool for discogenic low back pain. *Pain Physician J* 8:55-59, 2005.

21. Caraway D, Deer T, Levy R: *Results from a prospective, multicenter dorsal root ganglion (DRG) stimulation clinical trial.* Presentation at the North American Neuromodulation Society meeting, Las Vegas, Nevada, December 2010.

22. Benzon HT, Rathmell J, Wu C, et al: Intradiskal procedures for the management of low back pain. In Gretter B, Mekhail N, editors: *Raj's practical management of pain,* ed 4, Philadelphia, 2008, Mosby Elsevier, pp 1112-1117.

23. Hoogland T, Scheckenbach C: Low-dose Chemonucleolysis combined with percutaneous nucleotomy in herniated cervical disks. *J Spinal Disord* 8(3):228-232, 1995.

24. Poynton A, O'Farrell D, Mulcahy N, et al: Chymopapain chemonucleolysis: a review of 105 cases. *J R Coll Surg Edinb* 43:407-409, 1998.

25. Broadkey JS, Miyazaki Y, Ervin FR, et al: Reversible heat lesions with radiofrequency current. *J Neurosurg* 21:49-53, 1964.

26. Waldman S: Intradiscal electrothermal annuloplasty, percutaneous laser diskectomy. In Whitworth M, editor: *Pain management,* Philadelphia, 2007, Saunders, pp 1484-1499.

27. *Intradiscal electrothermal (IDET) therapy training course syllabus,* Menlo Park, CA, 2006, Oratec Interventions Inc.

28. Deen HG, Fenton DS, Lamer TJ: Minimally invasive procedures for disorders of the lumbar spine. *Mayo Clinic Proc* 78(10):1249-1256, 2003.

29. Kapural L, Cata J, Narouze S: Successful treatment of lumbar discogenic pain using intradiscal biacuplasty in previously discectomized disc. *Pain Pract* 9(2):130-134, 2009.

30. Karaman H, Tufek A, Kavak GO, et al: 6 month results of transdiscal biacuplasty on patients with discogenic low back pain: preliminary findings. *Int J Med Sci* 8(1):1-8, 2011.

31. Benzon H, Raja S, Molloy R, et al: Intradiscal techniques: intradiscal electrothermal therapy and nucleoplasty. In Walega D, editor: *Essentials of pain medicine and regional anesthesia,* ed 2, Philadelphia, 2005, Elsevier Churchill Livingstone, pp 485-493.

32. Singh V, Piryani C, Liao K, Nieschultz S: Percutaneous disc decompression using Coblation (Nucleoplasty) in the treatment of chronic discogenic pain. *Pain Physician* 5:250-259, 2002.

33. Gerges F, Lipsitz S, Nedeljkovic S: A systematic review of the effectiveness of nucleoplasty procedure for discogenic pain. *Pain Physician* 13(1):117-132, 2010.

34. Yakovlev A, Tamimi M, Liang H, Eristavi M: Outcomes of percutaneous disc decompression utilizing nucleoplasty for the treatment of chronic discogenic pain. *Pain Physician* 10(1):319-327, 2007.

35. Li J, Yan D, Zhang Z: Percutaneous cervical nucleoplasty in the treatment of cervical disc herniation. *Eur Spine J* 17(1):1664-1669, 2008.

36. Stryker Corp: Dekompressor for clinicians. *Interventional Pain, Kalamazoo, MI,* Stryker Corp, 2004.

37. Alò KM, Wright RE, Sutcliffe J, Brandt S: Percutaneous lumbar discectomy: one year follow-up in an initial cohort of fifty consecutive patients with chronic radicular pain. *Pain Pract* 5(2):116-124, 2005.

38. Singh V, Manchikanti L, Benyamin R, et al: Percutaneous lumbar laser disc decompression: a systematic review of current evidence. *Pain Physician* 12:573-588, 2009.

39. Choy DS, Ascher PW, et al: Percutaneous laser disc decompression: a new therapeutic modality. *Spine* 17:949-956, 1992.

40. Schenk B, Brouwer PA, Van Buchem MA: Experimental basis of percutaneous laser disc decompression (PLDD): a review of literature. *Lasers Med Sci* 21:245-249, 2006.

41. Patel J, Singh M: Laser discectomy. *eMedicine J* 3(6), 2002.

42. Gupta AK, Bodhey NK, Jayasree RS, et al: Percutaneous laser disc decompression: clinical experience at SCTIMST and long term follow up. *Neurol India* 54(2):164-167, 2006.

43. Brouwer PA, Peul WC, Brand R, et al: Effectiveness of percutaneous laser disc decompression versus conventional open discectomy in the treatment of lumbar disc herniation; design of a prospective randomized control trial. *BMC Musculoskelet Disord* 10:49, 2009.

44. Gibson JN, Waddell G: Surgical interventions for lumbar disc prolapse: updated Cochrane review. *Spine* 32:1735-1747, 2007.

45. Ballantyne J, Fishman S, Rathmell J: *Bonica's management of pain,* Philadelphia, 2009, Lippincott Williams & Wilkins, p 1481.

46. Mangrum S: A cure for back pain? Review of intradiscal methylene blue study. *Back Exercise Doctor,* 2011. Available at http://www.backexercisedoctor.com/journal/2011/1/17/a-cure-for-back-pain-review-of-intradiscal-methylene-blue-st.html.

47. Ballantyne J, Fishman S, Rathmell J: *Bonica's management of pain,* Philadelphia, 2009, Lippincott Williams & Wilkins, p 1482.

48. Peng B, Pang X, Wu Y, et al: A randomized placebo-controlled trial of intradiscal methylene blue injection for the treatment of chronic discogenic low back pain. *Pain* 149(1):124-129, 2010.

49. Peng B, Zhang Y, Hou S, et al: Intradiscal methylene blue injection for the treatment of chronic discogenic low back pain. *Eur Spine J* 16(1):33-38, 2007.

50. Cohen, S, Wenzell, D, Hurley, R, et al: A double-blind, placebo-controlled, dose-response pilot study evaluating intradiscal etanercept in patients with chronic discogenic low back pain or lumbosacral radiculopathy. *Anesthesiology* 107(1):99-105, 2007.

51. Olmarker K, Rydevik B: Selective inhibition of tumor necrosis factor-alpha prevents nucleus pulposus-induced thrombus formation, intraneural edema, and reduction of nerve conduction velocity: possible implications for future pharmacologic treatment strategies of sciatica. *Spine (Phila Pa 1976)* 26(8):863-869, 2001.

52. Derby R, Eek B, Chen Y, et al: Intradiscal electrothermal annuloplasty (IDET): A novel approach for treating chronic discogenic back pain. *Neuromodulation* 3:82-88, 2000.

53. ArthoCare Corporation: *DISC nucleoplasty overview.* Available at http://www.Nucleoplasty.com/dphy.aspx?s=0201.

54. Ruiz-Lopez R, Pichot C: Vertebroplasty. In *Interventional pain management,* ed 2, Philadelphia, 2008, Saunders, p 560.

55. Guyer RD, Collier R, Stith WJ, et al: Discitis after discography. *Spine* 13:1352-1354, 1998.

56. Silber JS, Anderson DG, Vaccaro AR, et al: Management of postprocedural discitis. *Spine* 2:279-287, 2002.

57. Rathmell JP, Lake T, Ramundo MB: Infectious risks of chronic pain treatments: injection therapy, surgical implants and intradiscal techniques. *Reg Anesth Pain Med* 31:346-352, 2006.

58. Classen DC, Evans RS, Pestotnik SL, et al: The timing of prophylactic administration of antibiotics and the risk of surgical-wound infection. *N Engl J Med* 326(5):281-286, 1992.

59. Eguro H: Transverse myelitis following chemonucleolysis. Report of a case. *J Bone Joint Surg Am* 65(9):1328-1330, 1983.

60. Ring J: Anaphylactic reactions to local anesthetics. *Chem Immunol Allergy* 95:190-200, 2010.

61. Heitz JW, Bader SO: An evidence-based approach to medication preparation for the surgical patient at risk for latex allergy: is it time to stop being stopper poppers? *J Clin Anesth* 22(6):477-483, 2010.

62. Cusick J, Khang-Cheng H, Schamberg J: Subarachnoid hemorrhage following chymopapain chemonucleolysis. *J Neurosurg* 5(66):775, 1987.

63. Hisa A, Isaac K, Katz J: Cauda equina syndrome from intradiscal electrothermal therapy. *Neurology* 55:320-322, 2000.

64. Epstein NE: Laser-assisted diskectomy performed by an internist resulting in cauda equine syndrome. *J Spinal Discord* 12(1):77, 1999.

65. Ma R, Chow R, Shen FH: Kummell's disease: delayed post-traumatic osteonecrosis of the vertebral body. *Eur Spine J* 19(7):1065-1070, 2010.

66. Scholl B, Theiss S, Lopez-Ben R, Kraft M: Vertebral osteonecrosis related to intradiscal electrothermal therapy: a case report. *Spine (Phila Pa 1976)* 28(9):E161-E164, 2003.

67. Djurasovic M, Glassman S, et al: Vertebral osteonecrosis associated with the use of intradiscal electrothermal therapy: a case report. *Spine (Phila Pa 1976)* 27(13):E325-E328, 2002.

68. Cohen S, Williams S, Kurihara C, et al: Nucleoplasty with or without intradiscal electrothermal therapy (IDET) as a treatment for lumbar herniated disc. *J Spinal Disorder Tech* 18:119-124, 2005.

69. Nerubay J, Caspi L, Levinkopf M: Percutaneous carbon dioxide laser nucleolysis with 2- to 5-year followup. *Clin Orthop Relat Res* 337:45-48, 1997.

7 Complications Related to Radiofrequency Procedures for the Treatment of Chronic Pain

Jonathan D. Carlson and Patrick W. Hogan

CHAPTER OVERVIEW

Chapter Synopsis: Radiofrequency ablation (RFA) for chronic pain has been used for decades, and severe complications are rare. However, because of the nature of the functions inherent to the nerves and ganglia targeted by RFA, catastrophic consequences can arise. RFA of the cervical, thoracic, and lumbar medial branches can result in pneumothorax or permanent spinal nerve damage. RFA aimed at the sympathetic ganglia or nerves can cause heart block, total spinal block, pneumothorax, meningitis, and other nerve damage–related consequences. Use of fluoroscopic guidance by a highly trained practitioner can minimize the risks associated with RFA, which should never be performed under general anesthesia.

Important Points:

- RFA can allow for reliable and discrete thermal lesioning in a desired specific neurologic location with prolonged pain relief.
- Severe complications are rare but can be as catastrophic as heart block and permanent spinal cord or brain injury.
- Adequate training and board certification of the interventional physician are ideal and could theoretically lead to greater safety measures and less chance of complications when RFA is used.
- The ability to implement lifesaving measures such as intubation, advanced cardiac life support, and management of local anesthetic toxicity as well as an extensive knowledge of the anatomy and proficiency at reading fluoroscopic images are mandatory.
- Consent; sterile technique; and a review of the patient's allergies, use of anticoagulants, and medical history (especially infection risks and indwelling pacemakers, defibrillators, or spinal cord or peripheral nerve stimulators) are essential.
- General anesthesia should be avoided; light sedation via the guidelines set forth by the American Society of Anesthesiologists for conscious sedation and monitoring can be used by properly trained personnel, but it is recommended that the patient be able to maintain meaningful communication throughout the entire procedure.
- Use of negative aspiration; myelogram-compatible contrast under live fluoroscopy; and when indicated, a test dose with local anesthetic and dilute epinephrine can mitigate risks.
- Evaluation of specific motor stimulation and, when applicable, sensory stimulation with their respective relevant responses should always be used.
- Severe complications associated with RFA of the cervical, thoracic, and lumbar medical branches include but are not limited to pneumothorax and permanent nerve or spinal cord injury.
- Severe complications associated with RFA of the sympathetic ganglion and nerves include but are not limited to heart block, total spinal blockade, pneumothorax, meningitis, major vessel injury (vertebral artery, subclavian vessels, vena cava, or aorta), blindness, spinal cord injury, and brain injury.

Introduction

Radiofrequency (RF) has been used clinically as a modality to treat chronic pain as early as the 1950s.[1,2] It is unique in that it can allow for reliable and discrete thermal lesioning in a desired specific neurologic location. The end result can produce pain relief from a prolonged duration up to 6 months or longer. RF is a low-energy, high-frequency, alternating current of which an electrical field is created between the active electrode and the grounding pad. The term *radio* was implemented because the frequency field that is used for treatment is often within the same frequency range of AM radio (300 to 500 kHz).[3] When the RF probe and dispersive grounding pad are properly placed, the body tissue completes the circuit. The uninsulated needle tip is the active portion of the electrode. The probe itself does not generate heat; rather, the frictional dissipation of current within the surrounding tissue heats the electrode.[4]

Radiofrequency can either be continuous at a temperature usually greater than 45°C or intermittently dispersed at 42°C; the latter is referred to as pulsed RF. Continuous RF ablation (RFA) is considered to be neurodestructive. Pulsed RF therapy is not fully understood but is thought to be a type of neuromodulation.[5] The active tip of the RF probe is beneficial as it also can be used for monitoring electrical impedance, sensory and motor stimulation, and real-time temperature measurement and control. The RF technique virtually eliminates undesired results such as combustion, sticking and breaking of the probe, and charring of the adjacent tissue. Other neuroablative techniques such as chemical destruction and cryotherapy do not have this luxury and are less predictable with the lesioning size. Even the use of a laser for neurodestruction has apparent limitations in creating an effective lesion compared with RF therapy.[6] Although conventional RFA for the treatment of chronic pain has proven to be an effective minimally invasive treatment option, it is not without its inherent risks and complications.

Closed Claims Cases in Pain Management and Ablative Procedures

The American Society of Anesthesiologists (ASA) Closed Claims Project in 2004 by Fitzgibbon et al[7] reported an increase in adverse chronic pain outcomes from 1979 to 1999. During the 1980s, there was a 3% increase in chronic pain claims. It increased to 10% in the 1990s. Fortunately, most of the chronic pain management claims were temporary or nondisabling injuries. Of the 276 claims related to chronic pain invasive procedures, 17 were associated with ablative procedures (chemical or thermal), making up 6.2% of the overall claims. Interestingly, only four cases were related to temperature (thermal RF or cryoablation) complications (Table 7-1).

Although this appears to be promising, the author underscores that the Closed Claims Project is devoid of denominator data and therefore cannot adequately assess the overall amount of claims related to interventional pain management. The project also evaluated a period of almost 30 years during which there was a clear change in pain management practice patterns. The ASA Closed Claims Project clearly has its limitations, but because of the paucity of complications reported in the literature, it seems to be the best tool to assess the possible incidence of complications associated with invasive pain interventions.

One of the largest confounding variables of the Closed Claims Project is that it primarily selects for cases that are of a greater severity and injury. Pursuit of cases that will likely yield less than $50,000 is not typically characteristic of plaintiff attorneys.[8] Therefore the amount of overall untoward events and complications are more than likely greater because they are not recorded from a legal standpoint or simply not reported by the pain practitioner. Thirteen of the 17 closed claims were related to chemical ablation. It is clear that chemical ablation seems to carry a higher risk of severe complications. Unfortunately, the ASA project did not further delineate between which specific complications were related to chemical versus temperature-related neurolysis (Table 7-2).

Nerve injury was the most common severe complication overall ($n = 8$). Three of the ablative nerve injury claims were associated with spinal cord injury, and one resulted in paraplegia. There was one case of pneumothorax. There were no ablative claims associated with infection even though infection comprised 13% of all invasive procedure claims. There was one case of death and brain damage with ablative procedures.

Avoidance of Radiofrequency Complications

The avoidance of theoretical and reported complications is divided into two broad categories: patient selection and interventionalist dependent. Both, of course, are interrelated and ultimately require a high degree of vigilance on the part of the pain provider to ensure patient safety.

Table 7-1: Procedures in Chronic Pain Management Claims, 1970-1999 ($n = 276$)

Claims	Number	Percentage
Invasive procedures	276	100
Injections	138	50
Epidural steroids ± local anesthetic agents	114	
Trigger point	17	
Facet	4	
Other	3	
Blocks	78	28.3
Peripheral	28	
Stellate ganglion	19	
Other autonomic	9	
Neuraxial	9	
Upper or lower extremity	7	
Axial	4	
Head and neck	2	
Ablative Procedures	17*	
Chemical (phenol, alcohol)	13	
Temperature (RF, cryoablation)	4	
Implantation or Removal of Devices	12	4.3
Implantable pump	5	
Nerve stimulator	4	
Catheter	3	
Device Maintenance	20	7.2
Other Interventions	11	4

*6.2% of all complications.
RF, radiofrequency.
Revised from Fitzgibbon DR, Posner KL, Domino KB, et al; American Society of Anesthesiologists: Chronic pain management: American Society of Anesthesiologists Closed Claims Project. *Anesthesiology* 100:98-105, 2004.

Patient Selection Factors

Proper patient selection by the pain provider is vital in mitigating risk associated with the use of electrical current and percutaneous needle placement.

Absolute contraindications include a lack of patient consent, infection at the site of RF probe placement, systemic infection, anticoagulants,* pacemaker or implantable cardioverter defibrillator (ICD),* and nonsystemic infection distant from the RF site.*

Relative contraindications include active comorbid disease, pregnancy,* poor hygiene, allergy to pertinent RF-related medication (local anesthetic, iodine, latex), anticoagulants,* pacemaker or ICD,* preexisting dorsal column or peripheral nerve stimulator,* and nonsystemic infection distant from the RF site.*

---

*Some interventional physicians disagree on whether these factors are absolute or relative contraindication; however, the author and practice colleagues believe that it is prudent to take the more conservative approach with elective chronic pain procedures when deciding on a contraindication.

Table 7-2: Primary Outcome for Invasive Pain Management Claims*

Outcome	All Invasive Procedures (n = 276)		Ablative (n = 17)†	
	n	%	n	%
Nerve injury	63	23	8	47
Pneumothorax	59	21	1	6
Infection	35	13	0	0
Death or brain damage	26	9	1	6
Headache	21	8	0	0
Increased pain or no relief	21	8	0	0
Retained catheter	9	3	0	0
None	7	3	1	6
Other	42	15	6	35

*Totals sum to more than 100% because of multiple complications in some claims.
†6.2% of all complications.
Revised from Fitzgibbon DR, Posner KL, Domino KB, et al; American Society of Anesthesiologists: Chronic pain management: American Society of Anesthesiologists Closed Claims Project. *Anesthesiology* 100:98-105, 2004.

Allergy   If applicable, avoidance of agents that cause allergic reaction should be implemented during the RFA procedure. These can include but are not limited to iodine-based sterile preparation and contrast, latex, and amide local anesthetics (rare). A thorough evaluation of the patient's past allergy history, preprocedural screening, and a preprocedure "time out" should help circumvent any serious allergic reactions.

Sedation   Conscience sedation or monitored anesthetic care during chronic pain procedures is a topic of debate among experts in the field of pain medicine. Some believe that sedation should be avoided in procedures that have an inherently higher risk of catastrophic outcome if injury to vascular or neurologic structures were to occur (e.g., cervical epidural steroid injection, stellate ganglion [SG] block). It is thought that local anesthetic only would allow for the patient to communicate marked pain related to ensuing injury to vital structures.[9] The opposing view is that if a patient has light sedation via the guidelines set forth by the ASA for conscious sedation and monitoring as well as implemented by the hands of an experienced anesthesia provider, he or she may have a more comfortable experience and is thus less likely to make sudden movements. Sudden patient movement during the procedure could significantly affect the outcome of the procedure and potentially increase the chance of an untoward event. The anesthetic goal for advocates of light sedation is to have a minimally anxious patient who is able to maintain meaningful communication throughout the entire procedure and stable vital signs. In either case, it is at the discretion of the pain and anesthesia providers to decide which patients are good candidates. Light sedation with agents that can be reversed are recommended (benzodiazepines: midazolam; short-acting opioids: fentanyl). A propofol anesthetic would be less than ideal because of the chance of (1) the patient becoming disinhibited during the procedure[10] and (2) unintentional general anesthesia could prevent the patient from alerting the physician to complications. In the United States, general anesthesia for common percutaneous chronic pain procedures is thought to be excessive and risky by most pain specialists.

Infection   Although there have been no literature reports of infection complications with RF procedures, pain practitioners should minimize this risk by postponing RF treatment with the presence of active infection or concurrent antibiotic or antimicrobial use. Consultation with an infectious disease specialist should be considered if the patient has a history of osteomyelitis or methicillin-resistant *Staphylococcus aureus*. Studies have shown that smoking cessation promotes better healing in surgical patients.[11] Although no studies have linked the abatement of smoking with patients undergoing percutaneous RFA, the practitioner may want to take this into consideration if the patient is at high risk for infection (e.g., history of infection, abscess). Providers may also want to instruct patients with poor hygiene to bathe with over-the-counter Hibiclens (4% chlorhexidine) the night before the procedure. This may decrease the chance of infection by the seeding of human skin flora via percutaneous technique.[12]

Cheng and Abdi[13] describe infection complications from several different case reports with patients undergoing intraarticular zygapophyseal (facet) joint injections. These complications include epidural abscess, septic arthritis, spondylodiscitis, and chemical meningism (thought to be related to inadvertent dural puncture with a high-dose steroid injection). These authors also report no known case reports of infections related directly to RF neurolysis; however, one could reasonably conclude that the above complications could occur with RF if confirmation of proper needle placement and sterile precautions are not used.[13]

Presence of a Pacemaker or an Implantable Cardioverter-Defibrillator Device

Radiofrequency in patients with a cardiac pacemaker or ICD is a controversial topic. Some authors believe that it is adequate to turn off the pacemaker before proceeding with RF lesioning.[14] However, the routine practice of placing of a magnet to set the pacer to an asynchronous mode should be reconsidered because of the ever-changing complexity of cardiac pacemakers. A comprehensive pre- and postprocedure evaluation should be performed by the device representative as well as intraoperative monitoring during the RF procedure itself.[15] This practice is supported by the 2002 American College of Cardiology and American Heart Association (ACC/AHA) guideline update for perioperative cardiovascular evaluation for noncardiac surgery.[16] Consulting the patient's cardiologist is advised, but one should be aware that there has been inaccurate information about pacer function given by cardiologists;[17] therefore the presence of the cardiac device representative is still advised. RFA procedures should never be done while the defibrillator function is still active, regardless of the location of the RF lesioning in the body. There are known medicolegal cases involving patients being defibrillated after RF treatment was started. There have been anecdotal reports of RF lesioning being done safely for pain patients with indwelling defibrillators, but this was done after the defibrillator function was deactivated and the ACC/AHA guidelines used; the formal literature is lacking. In the rare case that the pain practitioner decides to move forward with an RF procedure, it is advised to use extreme caution with meticulous attention to the cardiologist's direction and complete compliance with the ACC/AHA guidelines.

Implanted Dorsal Column and Peripheral Nerve Stimulators Performing RFA while an implanted neuromodulation device is in place is controversial. To date, no case reports have been published on associated complications or the safety of using RFA with a preexisting stimulator in place. There are numerous anecdotal reports of clinicians implementing RFA while the neuromodulation device is off with no untoward events.

Anticoagulation The American Society of Regional Anesthesia Consensus Guidelines for the anticoagulated patient by Horlocker et al[18] have become the gold standard when performing neuraxial procedures in anticoagulated patients. Interventionalists should have a thorough understanding of these guidelines, anticoagulant medications, and the nuances of pathology associated with a deviation from the normal clotting cascade. Adherence to these guidelines is not a fail-safe measure, and the pain specialist should always exercise vigilance when there is the possibility of an epidural hematoma.

A traumatic procedure seems to be the biggest risk factor in epidural hematoma formation.[19] The incidence of a hematoma when entering the epidural space is estimated to be one in 20,000 (traumatic) to one in 220,000 (nontraumatic).[18,20] Because of the nature of the common RF spine procedures, inadvertent needle placement in the epidural space is certainly possible. Because the epidural space is not accessed during most RF procedures, it is thought that the incidence of epidural hematoma would be much lower than with epidural steroid injections. No case reports in the literature have been associated with RFA and epidural hematoma formation. However, there have been epidural hematomas with surgical evacuation after intraarticular facet joint injections for pain.[21] The larger gauge needles used in RF procedures could have a higher propensity to cause severe bleeding if cessation of anticoagulation medications is not done. As a general rule for outpatient elective chronic pain procedures, an international normalized ratio (INR) of less than 1.3 and a platelet count greater than 100,000 (assuming no qualitative platelet dysfunction such as in end-stage renal disease) is desired, although some practitioners use an INR of less than 1.5 and platelets greater than 80,000 if the patient is asymptomatic.

Physician-Dependent Factors

It is imperative that interventional physicians be well versed in the anatomy of where the percutaneous RF procedure is done. Recognizing what vital structures are at risk for injury is paramount. Fluoroscopic guidance should be used to optimize patient safety. Current advanced cardiac life support training and a proficiency in how to manage emergent situations such as epidural hematoma,

seizure, and total spinal anesthesia are essential. Formal interventional pain fellowship training, board certification in pain management, and cadaver training laboratories are steps that a physician can take to develop the fundamental skills and knowledge required to safely perform RFA procedures. Despite appropriate training and certification, complications can occur with even the most experienced clinicians.

Infection or Abscess Poor sterile technique by the pain physician or the procedural team can certainly increase the risk of infection or abscess formation. Surgical masks can contribute to a decrease in morbidity related to infection.[12] A surgical scrub and prep with chlorhexidine with ethanol (CHE) has been shown in studies to be superior to iodine-based solutions.[22] Viable microorganisms of the human skin flora were still present on the skin of patients after preparation with iodine-based products to a level of significance ($P < .01$) compared with CHE.[23] Proper precautions by the procedural team as well as the above suggestions will decrease the likelihood of complications related to infection.

Faulty Equipment A careful examination of the insulation of the RF needles should always be done. To date, there have been four reported cases of superficial burns secondary to disrupted insulation of the probe.[24] Kornick and associates[25] described two case reports of burns related to a malfunction of the adhesion site of the grounding pad.

Radiofrequency Probe Placement and Neurolysis Fluoroscopic guidance when placing the RF needle is essential to ensure patient safety and mitigate complication risks. As mentioned above, neurologic injury was the most common severe complication related to neuroablative procedures in the ASA Closed Claims Project cases. Pneumothorax was also an issue. The application of an extensive knowledge of the anatomy along the trajectory of the needle will minimize risk to the nerves, viscera, and vascular structures. It is imperative that the fluoroscopic images have no parallax. Sharp alignment of the margins of the bilateral osseous target structures minimizes confusion of where exactly the needle is being placed. **Fig. 7-1** is a lateral fluoroscopic image that demonstrates a malalignment or parallax of bilateral osseus structures (C5) and an optimized or crisp alignment of structures (C3) in the same image; parallax of the target area increases the risk of incorrect needle placement and possible neurologic injury.

Contrast dye injected under live fluoroscopy should always be used if the needle tip is to be placed in the vicinity of a vascular structure or certain vital organs (e.g., lung, bowel). There have been no formal case reports related to RFA and nerve or viscera injury; however, Bogduk and associates[26] report two medicolegal cases involving direct spinal cord trauma. The first case of spinal cord injury involves a patient undergoing a C3–C4 RFA. The case was done under general anesthesia. The proceduralist placed the active tip of the RF probe medial to the facet joint, traversed the lamina, and into the spinal cord. This was confirmed via the intraoperative images. The patient developed Brown-Séquard syndrome subsequent to the procedure. The two key points are that (1) general anesthesia rendered the patient helpless in being able to report symptomatology related to impending cord injury and (2) the radiographic images were not properly used to ensure correct needle placement. The second case involved a patient who underwent an attempted C3 (third occipital) RFA. The anteroposterior (AP) images showed the RF probe was placed at the wrong level (C3–C4). The tip was also too medial and anterior and thus inside the foramen (**Fig. 7-2**); the result was severe neurologic injury.

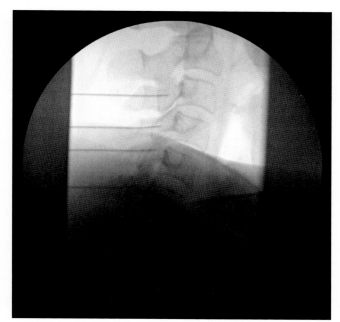

Fig. 7-1 A lateral fluoroscopic image of needle placement at C3–C6 before implementing continuous radiofrequency (RF) ablation of the left cervical medial branches. The third RF probe is placed at the lateral pillar of C5. Notice the parallax at the posterior aspect of the C5 lateral pillar. If the margins of the target structures are not in optimal alignment, it increases the chance of improper needle placement and nerve injury. The superior RF probe at C3 demonstrates optimized alignment of the margins of the C3 lateral pillar with no parallax. This patient required individual lateral pillar image alignment at each level to eliminate parallax and ensure proper RF needle placement.

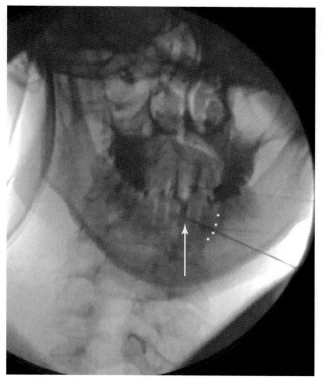

Fig. 7-2 Anteroposterior fluoroscopic image of the radiofrequency (RF) needle in position for an attempted third occipital radiofrequency ablation. The active tip of the RF probe (*arrow*) lies inside in the C3–C4 intervertebral foramen (incorrect level and too far medial). The *dots* mark the lateral aspect of the C3–C4 facet joint. (From Bogduk N, Dreyfuss P, Baker R, et al: Complications of spinal diagnostic and treatment procedures, *Pain Med* 9(suppl 1):S11-S34, 2008.)

If the probe had been correctly placed, the active tip would be at the correct level (C2–C3) and would be flush against the lateral pillar just lateral to the lateral margin of the facet joint. It was later determined that a radicular artery was coagulated via RF, which led to an infarction of the anterior spinal artery (**Fig. 7-3**).[26]

Postprocedural Pain and Neuritis These may be looked more as a part of the healing process of RF neurolysis rather than complications. Postprocedural pain is thought to be related to neuropathic pain with the ablation of the target nerve as well as injury to the adjacent soft tissue and periosteum. Symptoms associated with postprocedural pain usually resolve within 1 to 3 weeks. Neuritis typically abates in 2 to 6 weeks but may last for several months.[27]

Complications Associated with Continuous Radiofrequency Ablation

The remainder of this chapter focuses primarily on the avoidance of theoretical complications associated with the more common continuous RF procedures and their respective reported complications, if available.

Zygapophyseal (Facet) Joint Medial Branch Radiofrequency Neurolysis

The treatment of cervical, thoracic, and lumbar facet–mediated pain with medial branch RF neurolysis has a low morbidity. The most common complaint was burning or neuropathic pain that

was usually self-limited. Complaints of temporary sensory deficits consistent with the cutaneous branches of the posterior rami have been reported.[28] As mentioned previously, cases involving treatment by intraarticular facet joint blocks leading to complications such as epidural hematoma and abscess with subsequent surgical evacuation have been reported.[13,21] The proceduralist should always use vigilance when using the typically larger gauge RFA needles as well a proper sterile technique. Medicolegal cases of permanent spinal cord injury related to RFA have been described.[26]

Cervical Medial Branches

Cervical facet medical branch neurolysis is typically done via the posterolateral approach (**Fig. 7-4**). With this technique, there have been fewer complications reported.[29] A prospective pilot study by van Suijlekom and colleagues[30] reported a 30% incidence of postprocedural burning pain that usually resolved in 1 to 3 weeks.[27] Lord and Bogduk[31] reported observed or theoretical complications related to cervical RF neurolysis as outlined in **Table 7-3**.

The symptom of dizziness can occur after medial branch blocks at the higher cervical levels. Ataxia and unsteadiness may also occur. It is thought that a blockade of the cervical proprioceptive afferents may be the primary contributing factor to these transient symptoms. No prolonged cases have been reported.[32] Patients should be instructed to not drive or operate heavy or dangerous machinery subsequent to a cervical medial branch RFA, although a clear time frame has not been established. There was a higher percentage (13%) of patients reporting postprocedural pain

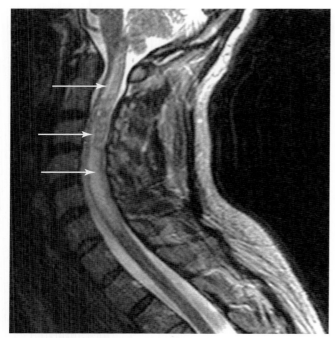

Fig. 7-3 A sagittal magnetic resonance imaging showing a spinal cord lesion after the attempted third occipital radiofrequency ablation. The *arrows* indicate severe central edema of the spinal cord, which is consistent with an infarction in the distribution of the anterior spinal artery. (From Bogduk N, Dreyfuss P, Baker R, et al: Complications of spinal diagnostic and treatment procedures, *Pain Med* 9(suppl 1):S11-S34, 2008.)

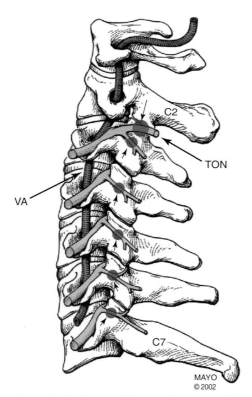

Fig. 7-4 Anatomic depiction of the usual location of the cervical medial branches (*blue dots*). (Copyright © 2002 Mayo Clinic.)

Table 7-3: Reported and Theoretical Complications from Cervical Medial Branch Ablation

	Observed Frequency/ Procedures Performed	Percentage
Allergic reactions	0/83	0
Vasovagal syncope	2/83	2
Risks associated with implanted electrical devices (pacemakers)	0/83	0
Vascular injury	0/83	0
Nerve injury	0/83	0
Burn injury	0/83	0
Postprocedural pain	81/83	97
Ataxia, unsteadiness, spatial disorientation	19/83	23
Cutaneous Numbness		
Third occipital procedures	22/25	88
C3–C4 procedures	8/10	80
Lower cervical level procedures	9/48	19
Dysesthesias		
Third occipital procedures	14/25	56
C3–C4 procedures	3/10	30
Lower cervical level procedures	8/48	17
Neurologic Complications		
Transient neuritis	2/83	2
Neuroma	0/83	0
Rare Complications		
Infection	0/83	0
Hematoma	0/83	0
Dermoid cyst	1/83	1

Adapted from Lord S, Bogduk N: Radiofrequency procedures in chronic pain, *Best Pract Res Clin Anesth* 16(4):597-617, 2002.

than reported in other studies. The pain was burning in nature and lasted 2 to 6 weeks in duration. A 4% incidence of occipital hyperesthesia was also reported, lasting approximately 3 months and thought to be related to the lesioning of the third occipital nerve.[32]

Thoracic Medial Branches

Apart from post procedural pain, pneumothorax (**Fig. 7-5**) is anecdotally the most common complication. Fluoroscopic guidance is essential to minimize this risk. The patient should be informed about the increased risk of a pneumothorax. Before discharge, the patient should be instructed to go immediately to the emergency department if he or she has difficulty breathing or if pain with inspiration ensues. If there is any question by the provider about a possible pneumothorax, a radiograph should be obtained.[29] A theoretical risk of nerve damage applies to the thoracic region as well as the other complications related to any RFA procedure.

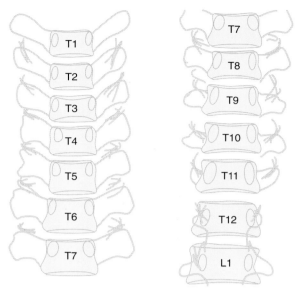

Fig. 7-5 Anatomic depiction of the location of the thoracic medial branches.

Table 7-4: Avoidance of Observed and Theoretical Complications Associated with Radiofrequency Neurolysis of the Cervical, Thoracic, and Lumbar Medial Branches and Sacroiliac Denervation

Complication	Avoidance
Postprocedural pain, neuritis, transient cutaneous numbness	Intrinsic to thermal RFA
Ataxia, dizziness, dysesthesias	Consider RF at a lower temperature, especially at higher cervical levels involving the third occipital
Pneumothorax, nerve or spinal cord injury, radiculopathy	Fluoroscopically guided probe placement, especially if needles are readjusted; avoidance of placing the probe tip too anterior in the lateral view (avoid placing in the foramen), or too lateral in the AP view; motor stimulation >1.0-3.0 V with no motor response of the associated nerve root

AP, anteroposterior; RF, radiofrequency; RFA, radiofrequency ablation.

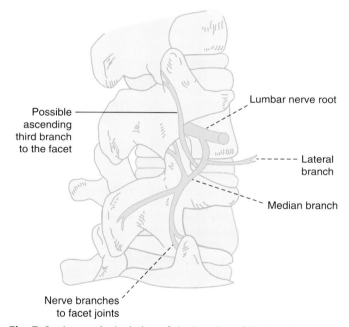

Fig. 7-6 Anatomic depiction of the location of the lumbar medial branches.

Lumbar and Sacroiliac

Kornick et al[25] did a retrospective analysis of 92 patients who had a total of 616 lumbar RF medial branch lesions (**Fig. 7-6**). There was a total 1% overall incidence of minor complications per each RF site with no major complications such as infection, bleeding, or new motor or sensory deficits. There were three cases (0.5%) of neuropathic pain lasting less than 2 weeks and three cases (0.5%) of prolonged pain lasting longer than 2 weeks.[25] Coskun and colleagues[33] reported a case of RFA nerve injury that led to lumbosacral radiculopathy. Gekht and associates[34] described a case of a patient who developed a painful medial branch neuroma after numerous lumbar RFA procedures. The mechanism is unclear, and no other reports in the literature of this type of complication exist.

The pain from the neuroma resolved completely after a surgical neurectomy. There have been no formal reports of complications related to the RF neurolysis of the sacroiliac joint innervation. There have been anecdotal findings of buttock discomfort usually lasting about 2 weeks. Numbness in the buttock region has also been reported but was typically self-limited to about 2 to 6 weeks' duration.[27]

Observed and Theoretical Complications Associated with Radiofrequency Neurolysis of the Cervical, Thoracic, and Lumbar Medial Branches and Sacroiliac Denervation
(Table 7-4)
These observed and theoretical complications include:

- Cervical: ataxia, dizziness, occipital hypoesthesia, vasovagal syncope, dysesthesias
- Thoracic: pneumothorax
- All spinal levels: nerve injury, neuritis, radiculopathy, transient cutaneous numbness, postprocedural pain, neuroma and dermoid cyst formation (both extremely rare)

Sympathetic Radiofrequency Ablation
Sympathetically mediated pain has been implicated in chronic pain syndromes of various origins. Blockade of the sympathetic nervous system has been associated with marked pain relief in syndromes such as complex regional pain syndrome (CRPS), cancer pain, vascular pain, and visceral pain.[35] When the transmission of pain via the sympathetic nervous system has been interrupted or attenuated via local anesthetics or neurolysis, it has proven to decrease the use of opioids in these patient populations.[36] Local anesthetic blockade of the sympathetic ganglia of the splanchnic and celiac plexus was first reported by Kappis in 1914, and evolved chemical neurolysis by Jones in 1957.[37] Sympathetic neurolysis has evolved to include the sphenopalatine ganglion (SPG) for facial pain; SG for pain of the cervicothoracic region, upper extremities, and face; splanchnic nerves and celiac plexus for abdominal and visceral pain; lumbar plexus for lower extremity pain; superior hypogastric plexus for pelvic pain; and ganglion impar for pain of the perineum. Although some of these structures are not made up entirely of

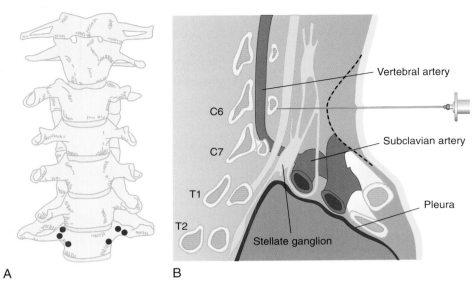

Fig. 7-7 Drawings of posteroanterior and lateral views of the cervical spine. **A,** Dots that mark the target points for radiofrequency lesioning of the cervical sympathetic nerves (stellate ganglion block) at C7. Note that these are at the junction of the medial aspect of the transverse process with the lateral aspect of its respective vertebral body. **B,** The vertebral artery directly posterior to the anterolateral aspect of the transverse process (needle at alternate target area at C6). Extreme caution should be used when placing a needle at this target area.

sympathetic nerve fibers, RF neurolysis of these structures has shown to have lasting relief in many patients with chronic sympathetically mediated pain. As with any percutaneous procedure, bleeding and infection are always concerns. Although rare, severe complications are thought to be more commonly associated with improper needle placement, but RF neurolysis can also have devastating outcomes if it is not executed properly.

Stellate Ganglion
Radiofrequency ablation of the SG has been effective in treating patients with CRPS of the upper extremity, phantom limb pain, peripheral neuropathy, Raynaud phenomenon, postherpetic neuralgia, and atypical facial pain. Posttraumatic stress disorder has been shown to be treatable by SG blockade, although the mechanism for this is poorly understood.[38] Most of the complications associated with SG RFA are related to incorrect needle placement or the spread of the local anesthetic into a precarious location. Fig. 7-7, *A* demonstrates the proper needle placement of the RF probes. Fig. 7-7, *B* demonstrates the close proximity of the vertebral artery and other vital structures close to the target area.

The most severe theoretical complication is complete heart block associated with an RFA of the SG if the patient is being treated for a bilateral sympathetic pain syndrome (**Table 7-5**). Bilateral continuous RFA, even done on separate occasions, is not recommended because of the risk of prolonged blockade of the sympathetic fibers to the sinoatrial node and cardiac accelerators. Pulsed RF treatment may be a viable option. There are case reports of even unilateral SG blockade leading to heart block. Saxena and associates[39] reported a case in which a 29-year-old woman experienced sinus arrest after a right-sided SG block. The complication of total spinal anesthesia has been reported with intrathecal spread of local anesthetic.[40] Cases of cerebral air embolisms have occurred and can easily be prevented by removal of the air from the syringe. Transient neuritis and persistent cough have been reported. A sudden death was reported after a SG block. The patient was found to have severe bleeding and bilateral pneumothorax. Paralysis

related to spinal cord injury has been a debilitating outcome.[37] One case of osteomyelitis of the cervical spine was reported in a patient who received multiple SG blocks. The patient did not appear to have any other pathology that would predispose her to develop such an infection. A complication of this nature is exceedingly rare.[41]

Splanchnic Nerves and Celiac Plexus
Saltzburg and Foley[42] reported relief of a visceral abdominal pain and pancreatic cancer pain via splanchnic nerve and celiac plexus blocks and neurolysis to be at 45% to 100% (**Fig. 7-8**). These structures include innervations to the distal third of the esophagus to the transverse colon, mesentery, pancreas, spleen, kidneys, liver, adrenals, and biliary tract.[36] Complications vary with these blocks. Transient hypotension and diarrhea are the more common complications. Cases of pneumothorax have occurred.[36] Takahashi and associates[43] reported a case of silent gastric perforation during a celiac plexus block. The use of a blunt needle may obviate the risk of visceral structures such as the stomach, liver, bowel, and kidneys as demonstrated by Heavener and Racz[44] (**Table 7-6**).[35,36] Cases of spinal cord injury and paraplegia have been reported with chemical neurolysis, but no major complications have been described with RFA.[36]

Lumbar Sympathetic Ganglion
The lumbar sympathetic block was first described by Brunn and Mandl in 1924[37] (**Fig. 7-9**). It has been implicated in the treatment of chronic pain disorders such as CRPS, postsurgical neuropathic pain, peripheral neuropathy, phantom limb pain, postherpetic neuralgia, and pain associated with peripheral vascular disease.[35,37] The concern for hypotension secondary to sympathectomy is more common with lumbar blockade; this is a transient effect, and no long-term cases are described in the literature. Intravascular injection and subarachnoid spread are always of concern, and contrast should always be used. The use of a blunt needle may decrease the risk of vital structure injury.[44] The remaining complications are described in **Table 7-7**.

Table 7-5: Avoidance of Observed and Theoretical Complications Associated with Radiofrequency Neurolysis of the Stellate Sympathetic Ganglion

Complication	Avoidance
Complete heart block	Avoid bilateral RF; 0.5-mL test dose
Total spinal or epidural injection leading to unconsciousness, apnea, and possibly bradycardia	Negative aspiration; myelogram-compatible contrast use indicating no epidural or subarachnoid spread; 0.5-mL test dose (although the patient could have this complication from < 0.5 mL of local anesthetic)
Intravascular uptake: seizure or local anesthetic toxicity from uptake into the vertebral artery or subclavian artery or vein	Negative aspiration; contrast use indicating no vascular uptake; 0.5-mL test dose (although the patient could have this complication from < 0.5 mL of local anesthetic); fluoroscopic image should be optimized; osseous contact should be made with extreme caution in not moving the needle posterolateral into the vertebral artery; needle placement at C7 or T1 may create better lesioning of the stellate ganglion, but there is a greater risk of subclavian puncture
Recurrent laryngeal nerve injury leading to hoarseness, loss of laryngeal reflexes, respiratory distress (bilateral injury)	Have the patient say "ee" while implementing motor stimulation; if there are no changes in the pronunciation, then the nerve should be preserved
Phrenic nerve injury leading to respiratory distress	Motor stimulation with no diaphragm movement
Persistent Horner syndrome	1-mL test dose or negative Horner syndrome with the local anesthetic block (although this is not a complete fail-safe method to prevent this complication)
Pneumothorax or pneumochylothorax	Fluoroscopic guidance; avoid lateral placement of the needle; use vigilance if the block is to be done below C6
Cerebral air embolism	Remove air from injectate
Paralysis from spinal cord injury	Confirm proper needle placement with fluoroscopy before RF lesioning
Retropharyngeal, cervicomediastinal, or posttracheal hematoma	Retract the carotid artery lateral if necessary; if vascular uptake is appreciated, especially if it appears arterial, close postprocedural observation is recommended

RF, radiofrequency.

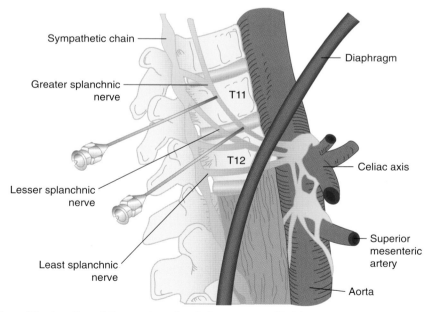

Fig. 7-8   Anatomic depiction of the location of the greater splanchnic nerve. (Modified from Waldman SD (editor): *Interventional pain management*, 2nd ed, Philadelphia, 2001, Saunders.)

Table 7-6: Avoidance of Observed and Theoretical Complications Associated with Radiofrequency of the Sympathetic Celiac Plexus or Splanchnic Nerves

Complication	Avoidance
Paraplegia, spinal cord injury, nerve damage	Negative motor stimulation ≤3.0 V with the associated nerve root; confirm proper needle placement with fluoroscopy before RF lesioning; avoid chemical neurolytic agents; avoid aortic injury to minimize risk of injury to the artery of Adamkiewicz
Intercostal neuritis	Negative motor stimulation ≤3.0 V with no response of intercostal muscle contraction; if this occurs, move the needle a few millimeters anterior
Bowel, gastric, liver, renal, ureter injury	Fluoroscopic guidance; use of a blunt needle
Pneumothorax, chylothorax	Avoid placing needle >4 cm lateral from the midline
Aortic or inferior vena cava injury	Careful needle placement not to go too anterior, but for celiac plexus block, it is an inherent risk of the procedure; use of a blunt needle
Seizure or local anesthetic toxicity from intravascular injection	Negative aspiration; myelogram-compatible contrast
Vascular embolism or plaque dislodgement	Avoid transaortic approach in high-risk patients
Retroperitoneal hematoma or abscess or peritonitis	Proper sterile technique; avoid bowel puncture by using a blunt needle
Discitis	Avoid transdiscal approach; use preprocedure antibiotics
Transient diarrhea	Common intrinsic result of block
Transient hypotension	Avoid bilateral block on the same day; fluid bolus before the procedure

RF, radiofrequency.
From Raj P, Lou L, Erdine S, et al, editors: *Interventional pain management: image-guided procedures*, ed 2, Philadelphia, 2008, Saunders.

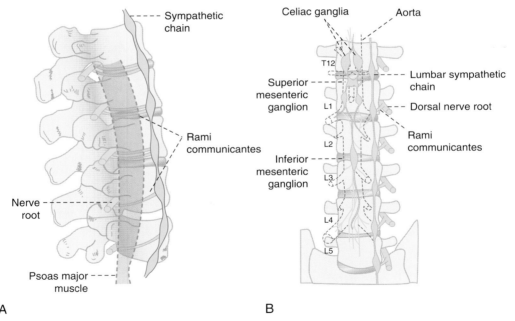

Fig. 7-9 A, The sympathetic chain as it courses the lordotic curve of the lumbar vertebrae in an anterolateral view. **B,** The course of the sympathetic chain in an anterior view. (Modified from Raj P, Lou L, Erdine S, et al (editors): *Interventional pain management: image-guided procedures*, 2nd ed, Philadelphia, 2008, Saunders.)

Superior Hypogastric Plexus

The superior hypogastric plexus block has proven to be effective in treating visceral pelvic pain (**Fig. 7-10**).[45] Chronic pain associated with pelvic pathology such as endometriosis, adhesions from surgery, interstitial cystitis, and malignancies, have been treated with RF neurolysis.[35,37] The superior hypogastric plexus innervates the descending colon to the rectum and the urogenital tract and viscera.[36] Complications such as inadvertent intravascular and subarachnoid injection should be considered as with all neuraxial procedures, and contrast should always be used. The transdiscal approach seems to be more effective with less complication risk than the classic approach.[35] The risk of discitis is the concern with this approach (**Table 7-8**).

Table 7-7: Avoidance of Observed and Theoretical Complications Associated with Radiofrequency of the Lumbar Sympathetic Ganglion

Complication	Avoidance
Seizure or local anesthetic toxicity from intravascular injection	Negative aspiration, myelogram-compatible contrast
Lumbar nerve root injury	Negative motor stimulation ≤3.0 V with the associated nerve root; confirm proper needle placement with fluoroscopy before RF lesioning; avoid chemical neurolytic agents
Lumbar plexus injury	Negative motor stimulation of the quadriceps ≤2.0 V; confirm proper needle placement with fluoroscopy before RF lesioning; avoid chemical neurolytic agents
Genitofemoral neuralgia	Negative sensory stimulation ≤3.0 V; confirm proper needle placement with fluoroscopy before RF lesioning; avoid chemical neurolytic agents
Aortic or inferior vena cava injury	Avoid needle placement going too anterior in the lateral view; use of a blunt needle
Transient hypotension (can be significant for patients who have severe aortic stenosis)	Avoid bilateral block on the same day; fluid bolus before the procedure
Renal injury	Confirm proper needle placement; use of a blunt needle
Sexual dysfunction in men (no ejaculation), especially if bilateral sympathetic blockade[37]	Avoid bilateral RF ablation; consider pulsed RF treatment

RF, radiofrequency.
Modified from Raj P, Lou L, Erdine S, et al, editors: *Interventional pain management: image-guided procedures*, ed 2, Philadelphia, 2008, Saunders.

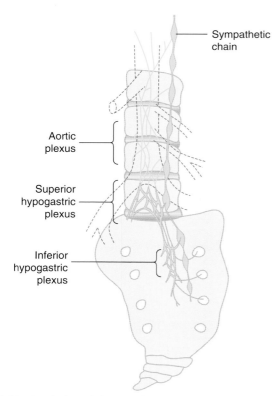

Fig. 7-10   Depiction of the superior hypogastric plexus in relation to L5 vertebral body and sacrum. (Modified from Raj P, Lou L, Erdine S, et al (editors): *Interventional pain management: image-guided procedures*, 2nd ed, Philadelphia, 2008, Saunders.)

Table 7-8: Avoidance of Observed and Theoretical Complications Associated with Radiofrequency of the Superior Hypogastric Sympathetic Plexus

Complication	Avoidance
Seizure or local anesthetic toxicity from intravascular injection	Negative aspiration, myelogram-compatible contrast
Lumbar nerve root injury	Negative motor stimulation ≤3.0 V with the associated nerve root; confirm proper needle placement with fluoroscopy before RF lesioning; avoid chemical neurolytic agents
Iliac vessel injury	Avoid needle placement going too anterior in the lateral view; use of a blunt needle
Transient hypotension (can be significant for patients that have severe aortic stenosis)	Avoid bilateral block on the same day; fluid bolus before procedure
Ureter injury	Use of a blunt needle
Sexual dysfunction in men (no ejaculation),[37] especially if bilateral sympathetic blockade	Avoid bilateral RF ablation; consider pulsed RF treatment
Discitis	Avoid transdiscal approach or use preprocedural antibiotics
Bowel or bladder incontinence (rare)	Consider pulsed RF
Rectum injury	Use of a blunt needle

RF, radiofrequency.

Ganglion Impar

The ganglion impar supplies the innervation to the perineum and rectum (**Fig. 7-11**). Patients with malignancies or coccydynia may receive prolonged relief from RFA of the terminal end of the sympathetic chain.[37] There have been case reports showing up to 100% pain relief with this block.[36] To date, there are no formal case reports on complications from RF neurolysis of the ganglion impar. **Table 7-9** includes observed and theoretical complications.

Radiofrequency Treatment for Head and Facial Pain

Sphenopalatine (Pterygopalatine) Ganglion Radiofrequency ablation of the SPG (**Fig. 7-12**) has been used as a treatment modality to treat refractory headaches and atypical facial pain. Narouze and coworkers[46] demonstrated this treatment as being an effective means to treat intractable cluster headaches. Pain practitioners have also used this method in the treatment of severe refractory headaches unresponsive to conservative therapies, migraines, and atypical facial pain.[27,37] Sphenopalatine RF procedure complications primarily involved incorrect needle placement rather than with neurolysis issues. The complication of the needle entering the superior orbital fissure has been described but not reported.[47] Careful attention to lateral and AP fluoroscopic images to confirm proper needle placement should be used (**Table 7-10**). Konen[48] reported reflex bradycardia or the oculocardiac reflex

being triggered during RFA of the SPG. Immediate procedure cessation and needle retraction and removal are recommended. Atropine or glycopyrrolate should be readily available to reverse bradycardia. Inadvertent local anesthetic vascular injection via the maxillary artery (see **Fig. 7-12**) may cause loss of consciousness or seizure. Appropriate supportive action should be taken.[27] Dryness of the ipsilateral eye and numbness of the soft palate have been associated with RF neurolysis of the SPG. If numbness of the soft palate occurs, it is usually transient, typically resolving in 4 to 6 weeks. There has been anecdotal discussion of an extremely rare complication involving taste deficiencies.[29]

Trigeminal (Gasserian) Ganglion Radiofrequency neurolysis of the trigeminal ganglion (**Fig. 7-13**) has been implicated in treatment of idiopathic trigeminal neuralgia (tic douloureux), atypical trigeminal neuralgia, atypical facial pain, intractable ocular pain, cluster headache, and cancer pain.[27,29,37] As with all invasive procedures, bleeding and infection are of concern. Numerous complications have been reported in the literature as outlined in **Table 7-11**. Overall, there is a low morbidity and no mortality with percutaneous trigeminal RF neurolysis; however, because of the close

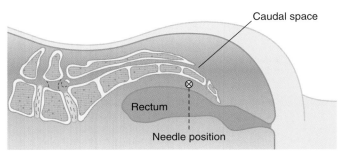

Fig. 7-11 Lateral view of the anatomical location of the ganglion impar (x) and the approximate needle placement.

Table 7-9: Avoidance of Observed and Theoretical Complications Associated with Radiofrequency of the Sympathetic Ganglion Impar

Complication	Avoidance
Seizure or local anesthetic toxicity from intravascular injection	Negative aspiration; myelogram-compatible contrast
Caudal epidural or intrathecal spread	Confirm proper needle placement with fluoroscopy and contrast before RF lesioning; avoid chemical neurolytic agents when possible
Rectum injury	Use of a blunt needle
Infection	Proper sterile technique and preparation

RF, radiofrequency.

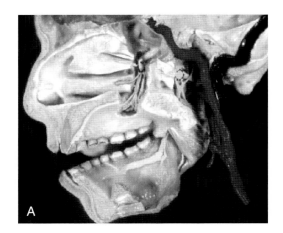

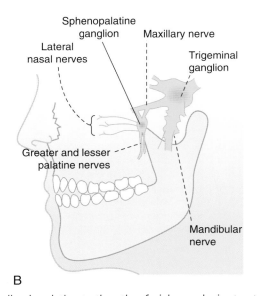

Fig. 7-12 **A,** Cadaver dissection of sphenopalatine ganglion. **B,** The ganglion in relation to the other facial neurologic structures. (Modified from Raj P, Lou L, Erdine S, et al (editors): *Interventional pain management: image-guided procedures*, 2nd ed, Philadelphia, 2008, Saunders.)

proximity to cerebral matter and the cranial nerves, it should be performed only by experienced proceduralists.[3,29]

Complications of Pulsed Radiofrequency Treatment

Pulsed RF treatment for chronic pain has been implemented as a minimally destructive means to attenuate the signals from nerve fibers that transmit pain. It is thought to be a form of neuromodulation. Small studies have demonstrated good to fair results in chronic pain relief. Vatansever and colleagues[49] demonstrated at a microscopic level that pulsed RF of peripheral nerves appeared to be less neurodestructive compared with traditional RFA. Benzon and associates[50] state that complications related to pulsed RF are lacking in the literature. Apart from similar complications related to continuous RF needle placement, there appear to be no additional anecdotal or theoretical complications associated with pulsed RF itself.

Conclusion

Radiofrequency ablation allows discrete lesioning of nerves and neurologic structures that transmit painful signals to the central nervous system. It has proven to be a vital asset in the treatment of chronic pain. The majority of the common RF-related complications seem to be of minimal impact and typically transient, primarily involving postprocedural pain and neuritis. Formal literature reports of RFA complications are rare. It is not clear if this is related to a low occurrence of complications associated with continuous RF procedures or a failure to report these types of complications

Table 7-10: Avoidance of Observed and Theoretical Complications Associated with Radiofrequency of the Sphenopalatine Ganglion

Complication	Avoidance
Loss of consciousness or seizure: uptake of local anesthetic via the maxillary artery	Use of a blunt needle; test dose; confirm proper needle placement with fluoroscopy and myelogram-compatible contrast before RF lesioning
Oculocardiac reflex or severe bradycardia	Varies; if bradycardia occurs, stop the procedure immediately; give supportive cardiac medications if necessary
Globe injury secondary to the needle or probe entering the superior orbital fissure	Use of a blunt needle; test dose; confirm proper needle placement with fluoroscopy in the AP view, incrementally each time on advancing the needle
Perforation of the perpendicular palatine bone and nasal mucosa by probe being place too medial	Confirm needle placement with the AP view; do not force the needle through any areas of resistance
Ipsilateral eye desiccation, numbness of the soft palate (usually transient), taste deficiencies (extremely rare)	Inherent risks of the procedure

AP, anteroposterior.

Table 7-11: Observed and Theoretical Complications Associated with Percutaneous Radiofrequency of the Trigeminal Ganglion

Complications
Total spinal
Meningitis
Seizure or local anesthetic toxicity
Paresthesias and facial numbness in the distribution of the trigeminal V_1, V_2, and V_3
Dysesthesia
Anesthesia dolorosa
Keratitis secondary to loss of corneal reflex
Masseter paresis or paralysis
Transient paralysis of cranial nerves III and IV[51]
Permanent palsy of the abducens nerve[52]
Mono-ocular blindness[53]

Data from Benzon H, Rathmell J, Turk D, Argoff C, editors: *Raj's practical management of pain*, ed 4, Philadelphia, 2008, Mosby-Elsevier; Neal J, Rathmell J, editors: *Complications in regional anesthesia and pain medicine*, ed 4, Philadelphia, 2006, Elsevier.

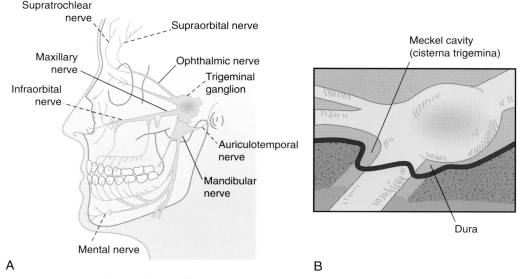

Fig. 7-13 A, The trigeminal or gasserian ganglion and its three nerve branches: (1) ophthalmic, (2) maxillary, and (3) mandibular. **B,** The ganglion within Meckel cavity (containing cerebrospinal fluid). (Modified from Raj P, Lou L, Erdine S, et al (editors): *Interventional pain management: image-guided procedures*, 2nd ed, Philadelphia, 2008, Saunders.)

by pain providers. Anecdotal and medicolegal discussion in the interventional pain community suggest the latter. Nonetheless, severe complications appear to be extremely rare. A systematic means of tracking and perhaps anonymously reporting RF-related complications would be of value. Regardless, if proper patient selection and interventional physician-dependent precautions are implemented, the benefits of radiofrequency procedures seem to far outweigh the risks.

References

1. Hunsperger R, Wyss O: Production of localized lesions in the nervous tissue by coagulation with high frequency current. *Helv Physiol Pharmacol Acta* 11:283, 1953.
2. Rosomoff H, Carrol F, Brown J, Sheptak T: Percutaneous radiofrequency cervical cordotomy: technique. *J Neurosurg* 23:639, 1965.
3. Neal J, Rathmell J, editors: *Complications in regional anesthesia and pain medicine*, ed 4, Philadelphia, 2006, Elsevier.
4. Van Zundert J, Sluijter M, van Kleef M: Thermal and pulsed radiofrequency. In Raj P, editor: *Interventional pain management: image-guided procedures*, Philadelphia, 2008, Saunders, p 58.
5. Sluijter M, Vosman E, Rittman W, van Kleef M: The effects of pulsed radiofrequency fields applied to the dorsal root ganglion—a preliminary report. *Pain Clin* 11:109-117, 1998.
6. Young R: Clinical experience with radiofrequency and laser DREZ lesions. *J Neurosurg* 72:715, 1990.
7. Fitzgibbon DR, Posner KL, Domino KB, et al: American Society of Anesthesiologists: Chronic pain management: American Society of Anesthesiologists Closed Claims Project. *Anesthesiology* 100:98-105, 2004.
8. Huycke L, Huycke M: Characteristics of potential plaintiffs in malpractice litigation. *Ann Intern Med* 120:792-798, 1994.
9. Hodges S, Castleberg R, Miller T, et al: Cervical epidural steroid injection with intrinsic spinal cord damage: two case reports. *Spine* 23(19):2137-2140, 1998.
10. Canaday B: Amorous, disinhibited behavior associated with propofol. *Clin Pharm* 12(6):449-451, 1993.
11. Møller A, Villebro N, Pedersen T, Tønnesen H: Effect of preoperative smoking intervention on postoperative complications: a randomised clinical trial. *Lancet* 359(9301):114-117, 2002.
12. Steffen P, Seeling W, Essig A, et al: Bacterial contamination of epidural catheters: microbiological examination of 502 epidural catheters used for postoperative analgesia. *J Clin Anesth* 16:92-97, 2004.
13. Cheng J, Abdi S: Complications of joint, tendon, and muscle injections. *Tech Reg Anesth Pain Manag* 11(3):141-147, 2007.
14. Rosenthal R, Starley D, Austin C: Avoiding complications from interventional spine techniques. *Pract Pain Manage* 10(2):77-87, 2010.
15. Sun D, Martin L, Honey C: Percutaneous radiofrequency trigeminal rhizotomy in a patient with an implanted cardiac pacemaker. *Anesth Analg* 99:1585-1586, 2004.
16. Eagle K, Berger PB, Calkins H, et al; American College of Cardiology/American Heart Association Task Force on Practice Guidelines: ACC/AHA guideline update for perioperative cardiovascular evaluation for noncardiac surgery. *Circulation* 105(10):1257-1267, 2002.
17. Rozner M: Pacemaker misinformation in the perioperative period: programming around the problem. *Anesth Analg* 99:1582-1584, 2004.
18. Horlocker TT, Wedel DJ, Benzon H, et al: Regional anesthesia in the anticoagulated patient: defining the risks (The Second ASRA Consensus Conference on Neuraxial Anesthesia and Anticoagulation). *Reg Anesth Pain Med* 28(3):172-197, 2003.
19. Abram S, O'Conner T: Complications associated with epidural injections. *Reg Anesth* 21:149-162, 1996.
20. Stafford-Smith M: Impaired haemostasis and regional anaesthesia. *Can J Anaesth* 43:R129-R141, 1996.
21. Nam K, Choi C, Yang M, Kang D: Spinal epidural hematoma after pain control procedure. *J Korean Neurosurg Soc* 48(3):281-284, 2010.
22. Sato S, Sakuragi T, Dan K: Human skin flora as a potential source of epidural abscess. *Anesthesiology* 85:1276-1282, 1996.
23. Kinirons B, Mimoz O, Lafendi L, et al: Chlorhexidine versus povidone iodine in preventing colonization of continuous epidural catheters in children: a randomized, controlled trial. *Anesthesiology* 94:239-244, 2001.
24. Shealy C: Percutaneous radiofrequency denervation of spinal facets. Treatment for chronic back pain and sciatica. *J Neurosurgery* 43:448-451, 1975.
25. Kornick C, Kramarich S, Lamer T, Sitzman B: Complications of lumbar facet radiofrequency denervation. *Spine* 29(12):1352-1354, 2004.
26. Bogduk N, Dreyfuss P, Baker R, et al: Complications of spinal diagnostic and treatment procedures. *Pain Med* 9(suppl 1):S11-S34, 2008.
27. Waldman S, editor: *Pain management*, Philadelphia, 2007, Elsevier.
28. Tzaan W, Tasker R: Percutaneous radiofrequency facet rhizotomy: experience with 118 procedures and reappraisal of its value. *Can J Neurol Sci* 27(2):125-130, 2000.
29. Benzon H, Rathmell J, Turk D, Argoff C, editors: *Raj's practical management of pain*, ed 4, Philadelphia, 2008, Mosby-Elsevier.
30. van Suijlekom JA, van Kleef M, Barendse G, et al: Radiofrequency cervical zygapophyseal joint neurotomy for cervicogenic headache: a prospective study in 15 patients. *Funct Neurol* 13:297-303, 1998.
31. Lord S, Bogduk N: Radiofrequency procedures in chronic pain. *Best Pract Res Clin Anesth* 16(4):597-617, 2002.
32. Vervest A, Stolker R: The treatment of cervical pain syndromes with radiofrequency procedures. *Pain Clin* 4:103-112, 1991.
33. Coskun D, Gilchrist J, Dupuy D: Lumbosacral radiculopathy following radiofrequency ablation therapy. *Muscle Nerve* 28:754-756, 2003.
34. Gekht G, Nottmeier E, Lamer T: Painful medial branch neuroma treated with minimally invasive medial branch neurectomy. *Pain Med* 11(8):1179-1182, 2010.
35. Day M: Sympathetic blocks: the evidence. *Pain Pract* 8(2):98-109, 2008.
36. Alshab A, Goldner J, Panchal S: Complications of sympathetic blocks for visceral pain. *Tech Reg Anesth Pain Med* 11:152-156, 2007.
37. Raj P, Lou L, Erdine S, et al, editors: *Interventional pain management: image-guided procedures*, ed 2, Philadelphia, 2008, Saunders.
38. Mulvaney S, McLean B, De Leeuw J: The use of stellate ganglion block in the treatment of panic/anxiety symptoms with combat-related post-traumatic stress disorder; preliminary results of long-term follow-up: a case series. *Pain Pract* 10(4):359-365, 2010.
39. Saxena A, Saxena N, Aggarwal B, Sethi A: An unusual complication of sinus arrest following right-sided stellate ganglion block: a case report. *Pain Pract* 4(3):245-248, 2004.
40. Forrest J: An unusual complication after stellate ganglion block by the paratracheal approach: a case report. *Can Anaesth Soc J* 23(4):435-439, 1976.
41. Maeda S, Murakawa K, Fu K: A case of pyogenic osteomyelitis of the cervical spine following stellate ganglion block. *Masui* 53:664-667, 2004.
42. Saltzburg D, Foley K: Management of pain in pancreatic cancer. *Surg Clin North Am* 69:629-649, 1989.
43. Takahashi M, Yoshida A, Ohara T, et al: Silent gastric perforation in pancreatic cancer patient treated with neurolytic celiac plexus block. *J Anesth* 17:196-198, 2003.
44. Heavner JE, Racz GB, Jenigiri B, et al: Sharp versus blunt needle: a comparative study of penetration of internal structures and bleeding in dogs. *Pain Pract* 3:226-231, 2003.
45. Bosscher H: Blockade of the superior hypogastric plexus for visceral pelvic pain. *Pain Pract* 1:167-170, 2001.
46. Narouze S, Kapural L, Casanova J, Mekhail N: Sphenopalatine ganglion radiofrequency ablation for the management of chronic cluster headache. *Headache* 49(4):571-577, 2009.
47. Racz G, Day M: Needle probe entering superior orbital fissure during a sphenopalatine ganglion block, verbal communication, 2009.
48. Konen A: Unexpected effects due to radiofrequency thermocoagulation of the sphenopalatine ganglion: two case reports. *Pain Digest* 10:30, 2000.

49. Vatansever D, Tekin I, Tuglu I, et al: A comparison of the neuroablative effects of conventional and pulsed radiofrequency techniques. *Clin J Pain* 24(8):717-724, 2008.

50. Benzon H, Nader A, Avram M, Moore J: *Pulsed radiofrequency ablation for chronic pain: a review of its effectiveness and complications [meeting abstract]*, San Diego, 2010, Annual American Society of Anesthesiology, p 986.

51. Kanpolat Y, Savas A, Bekar A, Berk C: Percutaneous controlled radiofrequency trigeminal rhizotomy for the treatment of idiopathic trigeminal neuralgia: 25 years experience with 1600 patients. *Neurosurgery* 38(3):524-534, 2001.

52. Kanpolat Y, Savas A, Berk C: Abducens nerve palsy after radiofrequency rhizolysis for trigeminal neuralgia: case report. *Neurosurgery* 44(6):1364, 1999.

53. Egan R, Pless M, Shults W: Monocular blindness as a complication of trigeminal radiofrequency. *Am J Ophthalmol* 131(2):237-240, 2001.

8 Complications of Lumbar Spine Fusion Surgery

Justin S. Field

CHAPTER OVERVIEW

Chapter Synopsis: Lumbar spinal fusion surgery may be used as a treatment for chronic back pain that arises from lumbar spinal stenosis when physical and drug therapies have failed. This invasive surgery carries particular risks that should be well understood by the treating physicians. Infection, dural tears, pseudoarthrosis, and adjacent segment degeneration are the most common complications, but more serious consequences can also arise, including root injury, paralysis, and death.

Important Points:

- Many patients have back and leg pain arising from lumbar spinal stenosis with or without instability.
- Conservative treatment in the form of physical therapy, chiropractic care, medications, and injections should be the first line of care. However, when conservative modalities fail and there is obvious instability or potential for instability, as well as acute neurologic changes, spinal surgery must be considered.
- Lumbar surgery often includes decompression of the soft and bony tissues contributing to central and neuroforaminal stenosis that may be compressing the spinal cord or nerve roots. This can reliably relieve pain, numbness, and weakness.
- It is crucial to understand the specific complications related to lumbar spinal fusion and to recognize and treat them immediately if they occur.
- The most commonly discussed complications directly related to lumbar spinal fusion include infection, dural tears, pseudoarthrosis, and adjacent segment degeneration.
- Rarer, more serious complications associated with lumbar spinal fusion include nerve root injury, paralysis, massive blood loss, blindness, heart attack, stroke, and death.
- Careful patient selection, meticulous surgical technique, expert intraoperative anesthetic monitoring and care, and extensive postoperative monitoring can significantly decrease many of these complications.
- Emerging surgical techniques and refinement of equipment have been directed at reducing these complications, but quality evidence is still needed to prove their efficacy.

Introduction

Back pain affects millions of people and is one of the most common reasons why patients consult with a medical professional. Many of these patients have back and or leg pain because of lumbar spinal stenosis with or without instability. Conservative treatment in the form of physical therapy, chiropractic care, medications, and injections should be the first line of care if a patient does not present with new neurologic insult. If these conservative modalities fail, then surgery must be considered.

Most lumbar spine surgery involves decompressing the soft tissue, which often includes a herniated disc (**Fig. 8-1**) or hypertrophied ligamentum flavum. Lumbar spine surgery also involves decompressing the bony elements, which can include hypertrophied facet joints, spinous processes, and lamina that make up the spinal canal. By decompressing both soft and bony tissue, spine surgery can often make patent both central and neuroforaminal narrowing that may be impinging on the spinal cord or nerve roots. Thoroughly decompressing the stenosis and nerve roots can reliably relieve leg pain and its associated symptoms of numbness and weakness. However, there are instances wherein there is obvious instability, spinal spondylolisthesis (**Fig. 8-2**), or the potential for instability. In this situation, a surgeon must consider both decompressing the stenosis along with stabilizing the affected spinal segments.

Particular ways to achieve fusion of the lumbar spine are discussed throughout the literature. Spinal fusion is a very successful procedure when chosen for patients with the correct indications for surgery. Newer surgical technologies and minimally invasive surgery have been touted to result in quicker recovery and less morbidity for the patient. However, lumbar spinal surgery and fusion with any approach has its associated relevant complications.

Some very serious complications of lumbar spine fusion have been reported, including nerve root injury, paralysis, massive blood loss, blindness, heart attack, stroke, and death. A comprehensive preoperative workup can help to stratify those patients at the most risk for medical complications. In some instances, optimization of a patient's preexisting medical conditions (e.g., untreated diabetes, hypertension, reactive airway disease) should be taken to minimize their risks before surgery. Expert intraoperative anesthetic monitoring and care, as well as postoperative monitoring, can significantly decrease many of these complications. The surgeon must work effectively and efficiently to address the patient's disease but also keep operative time as low as possible. Increased operative time often leads to increased complications, including increased blood loss, infection, and possibly blindness from being prone for too long (>8 hours).

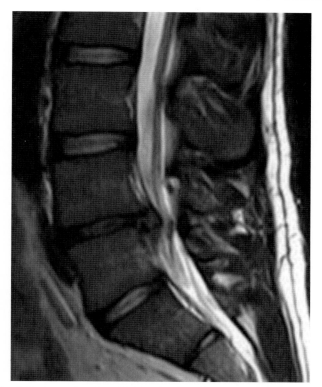

Fig. 8-1 Large herniated L4–L5 lumbar disc requiring decompressive surgery.

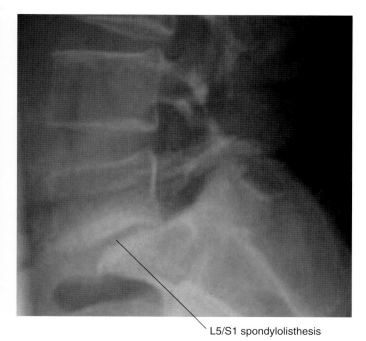

L5/S1 spondylolisthesis

Fig. 8-2 Significant L5–S1 spondylolisthesis requiring surgery.

The most commonly discussed complications directly related to lumbar spinal fusion include infections, dural tears, pseudoarthrosis, and adjacent segment degeneration (ASD). These specific complications are all important to understand, and if they occur, they must be recognized and treated rapidly, and as such will be elaborated on in more depth.

Selected Complications

Infection

Patients undergoing lumbar spinal fusion typically receive prophylactic intravenous (IV) antibiotics within 1 hour of surgery and postoperatively in several doses. This perioperative regimen, along with proper intraoperative sterility, has decreased infection rates dramatically. However, postoperative spinal wound infection is not an uncommon complication (**Fig. 8-3**). If not properly recognized and treated, a wound infection can be devastating and affect the ultimate desired surgical outcome.

A review of the literature shows that postoperative wound infections are common and range from 1% to 6% after lumbar spine fusions.[1] *Staphylococcus aureus* was the most common pathogen cultured, but some patients have multiple organisms causing an infection. Multiple studies have assessed risk factors for postoperative wound infections (**Table 8-1**).

Age greater than 60 years, smoking, diabetes, previous surgical infection, increased body mass index, and alcohol abuse were statistically significant risk factors. In addition to these factors, more complex spine procedures that involved multiple levels being fused, tumors, surgical revisions, and anterior or posterior reconstructions, also increased the rates of postoperative infections and complications.[2]

Early detection is of paramount importance for appropriate care of any postoperative infection. Patients with postoperative infection may complain of classic symptoms, including fever, chills, nausea or vomiting, erythema, and drainage from the incision. Patients also may have more insidious complaints such as an increase in pain after an initial improvement postsurgically. If an infection is suspected, it is important to have the patient urgently come to the clinic or a nearby hospital for immediate evaluation. Thankfully, suspected infection is often the result of much less serious superficial wound dehiscence. This can usually be treated with dressing changes and oral antibiotics as needed. When treating wound dehiscence, it is imperative to have the patient follow up closely for several evaluations to ensure the wound is healing appropriately. If the patient remains symptomatic and the incision is not healing, then further workup, including imaging in the form of magnetic resonance imaging (MRI) or computed tomography (CT), is warranted. This may show a postoperative abscess, seroma (fluid collection), hematoma, or even an undetected cerebrospinal fluid (CSF) leak.

If a wound infection is diagnosed after a spinal fusion, aggressive treatment is essential. Many physicians also obtain an infections blood workup, including complete blood count, erythrocyte sedimentation rate, C-reactive protein test, and blood cultures with sensitivities. MRI or CT scans with and without contrast are sometimes obtained to evaluate the underlying pathology. Suspected deep tissue infections require deep wound irrigation and debridement. At the same time, targeted wound cultures and sensitivities must be taken and sent to pathology for further analysis. Wound irrigation and debridement may be required multiple times before closure of the wound is possible.

When one has a deep infection, there is much debate on whether instrumentation needs to be removed at the time of irrigation and debridement. Instrumentation is a foreign body and thus can be a nidus for infection because bacteria can form a glycocalyx, or an extracellular adhesive slime. This bacteria-generated layer can make it difficult or impossible for antibiotics to penetrate the bacteria and rid the area of infection. If the infection is of late onset, there may be evidence of full bony fusion. In that instance, hardware may be removed. However, with earlier infection,

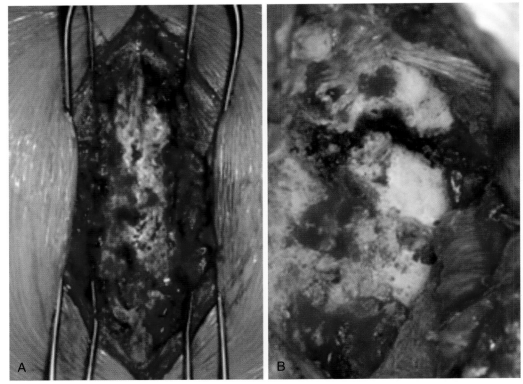

Fig. 8-3   Normal postsurgical fusion (**A**) compared with postsurgical infection (**B**).

Table 8-1: Patient and Surgical Risk Factors for Postoperative Wound Infections	
Patient Risk Factors for Postoperative Wound Infections	**Surgical Risk Factors for Postoperative Wound Infections**
>60 years of age	Complex spine procedures
Smoking	Fusing multiple levels
Diabetes	Spinal revisions
History of previous surgical infections	Anterior or posterior reconstruction
Obesity and increased body mass index	Increased operative times
Alcohol abuse	

the hardware may need to remain in place to maintain structural stability of the lumbar spine. Aggressive debridement of soft tissue, bone, and surgical hardware is obviously needed in that circumstance. In all instances of wound infection, it is important to consult a patient's primary care physician as well as infectious disease specialists. Typically, an infection requires 4 to 8 weeks of IV antibiotics through a peripherally inserted central catheter line with the choice of antibiotics chosen by an infectious disease specialist and dependent on the results of the cultures and sensitivities of the organism.

Dural Tear

Most lumbar spine fusion cases involve decompression of posterior elements. The soft tissue is often decompressed, which can include a herniated or extruded disc, excessive fat, or hypertrophied ligamentum flavum. Lumbar spine surgery also involves decompressing the bony elements, which often include hypertrophied facet joints, spinous processes, and lamina. The neural elements bathe in CSF and are contained within a thin tissue, the dura mater, before branching out into the neuroforamen to supply motor and sensory function to the body. The dural sac with its neural elements is compressed in central spinal stenosis. There exist central, lateral recess, and foraminal stenoses, and patients may have one or all three of these components comprising their stenosis. To adequately decompress the canal and ligamentum flavum, often the medial aspect of hypertrophied facets joints are excised. In the process of accomplishing this, dural tears may occur secondary to the bone and soft tissue being adherent to the dura from longer standing stenosis or a large herniated disc (**Fig. 8-4**). While performing a posterior decompression of the lumbar spinal canal, bony spicules may also pierce the dural sac, causing CSF leaks. As a rule, the more severe the spinal stenosis, the higher the likelihood of a dural tear occurring as a result of surgery. In addition, patients who have had previous lumbar spine surgery and have recurrent stenosis also have an increased risk of a dural tear because of formation and adherence of scar tissue.

Dural tears are a common complication of lumbar spine surgery (**Fig. 8-5**). Khan et al[3] reviewed a total of 3183 degenerative lumbar spine cases at one institution, and cases complicated by dural tears were identified. They found that the incidence of dural tears during a primary lumbar surgery was 7.6%. This was significant but appreciably lower than the 15.9% dural tear risk seen with the surgical revision cases. Cammisa et al[4] reviewed a total of 2144 patients and found that dural tears occurred in 3.1% of patients during spinal surgery. The incidence of dural tears varied according to the specific procedure performed but was again highest in the group that underwent revision surgery.

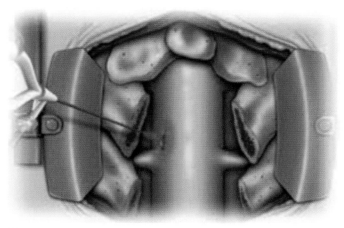

Fig. 8-4 Dural tear occurring after medial aspect of hypertrophied facets joints are excised.

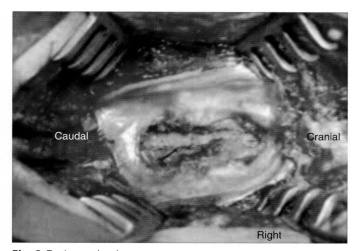

Caudal   Cranial

Right

Fig. 8-5 Large dural tear. (From Pereira Filho Ade A, et al: Symptomatic thoracic spinal cord compression caused by postsurgical pseudomeningocele. *Arq Neuropsiquiatr* 65[2-A]:279-282, 2007.)

The treatment for dural tears occurring intraoperatively is direct repair of the dura with a thin silk or Prolene suture that nicely approximates the dura tissue edges to each other without impinging the neural elements. Wang et al[5] describe primary repair followed by short-term bed rest. This protocol led to no long-term deleterious effects or increased rates of infection, neural damage, or arachnoiditis. In addition, closed suction wound drainage does not aggravate the leak and can safely be used in the presence of a dural repair.

There are situations, however, when it may be difficult to repair a dural tear. In these cases, a thin collagen sponge can be placed over the dural leak as well as covering the rest of the exposed dura. In addition, several products can form a superficial seal over this area in conjunction with the sponge to seal off the leak. It is important to have the patient lie flat in bed for at least 48 hours after this scenario. Then the patient may gradually increase the inclination of the bed and can ambulate as long as symptoms indicative of a dural leak (e.g., headache, nausea, dizziness) do not occur.

For patients who have continued dural leakage of CSF, other options are available as well. Kitchel et al[6] describe the effectiveness and safety of a temporary subarachnoid shunt placed in the upper lumbar spine that is removed after 4 days. These patients must be

monitored very carefully. Many of these authors' patients were treated successfully in this manner with resolution of CSF drainage and symptoms and no permanent sequelae. An undetected postoperative CSF leak or cases with persistent drainage are more commonly treated with reoperation, identification, and repair of the dural leak.

Pseudoarthrosis

Lumbar spine fusion has become a widely used procedure, being performed increasingly over the past 2 decades. Initially, the surgery was only indicated for Potts disease, severe spinal deformity, unstable spine trauma, and tumor excisions leading to instability. The current indications for lumbar spine fusion have broadened and include any spinal instability and painful degenerative disc disease in carefully selected patients. Methods to achieve fusion have evolved and include new instrumentation devices, various biologics, and different approaches. A surgeon can now perform an anterior lumbar interbody fusion or posterior lumbar fusions from midline to true lateral. The lateral approach involves accessing the retroperitoneal space and traversing carefully through the psoas muscle to enter the disc space. Even though technology and biologics to achieve fusion have improved, pseudoarthrosis may still occur. *Pseudoarthrosis* is defined as an incomplete spinal fusion when a fusion is attempted. A large prospective review of revision surgeries revealed that 23.6% of these revision fusion surgeries were performed for pseudoarthrosis.[7] However, this may underestimate the true incidence of pseudoarthrosis because many patients remain asymptomatic despite the lack of a complete fusion.

Pseudoarthrosis is essentially a failed attempt at spinal fusion. Typically it manifests longer than 6 months after a spinal fusion procedure and presents with continued back pain and even recurrent radicular pain. The diagnosis is based on the clinical presentation and updated imaging studies. A pseudoarthrosis should be suspected when a patient has persistent complaints that are not relieved with physical therapy and other modalities. Flexion and extension radiographs show a continued degree of motion at the fused levels despite the instrumentation present. In addition, lucency may be seen around the pedicle screw instrumentation on the radiographs. A more precise radiographic tool to assess fusion is a thin-cut CT scan. CT scans more reliably assess fusion masses posterolaterally as well as in the interbody area.

Risk factors for nonunion include metabolic abnormalities, smoking, infection, and excessive motion at the fusion site (**Box 8-1**). Several studies have shown that not using instrumentation leads to increased pseudoarthrosis as well (**Figs. 8-6 and 8-7**). Fischgrund et al[8] published the results of a prospective, randomized trial comparing decompression and posterolateral fusion with and without instrumentation in patients with degenerative spondylolisthesis and spinal stenosis. Average patient follow up was 2 years with the fusion rate significantly better with

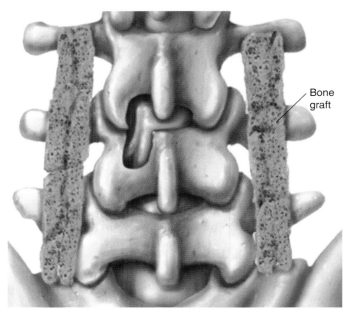

Fig. 8-6 Fusion with bone graft only (no instrumentation) increases the risk for pseudoarthrosis.

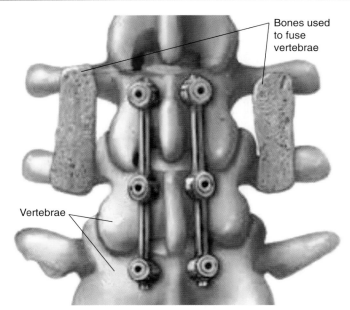

Fig. 8-8 Fusion shown with bone graft and instrumentation.

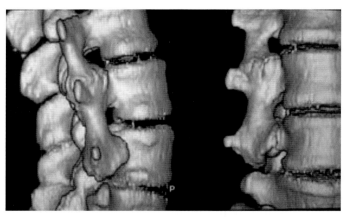

Fig. 8-7 Fusion with bone graft only (no instrumentation) increases the risk for pseudoarthrosis.

instrumentation than without (82% vs. 45%). However, they noted that good to excellent results occurred in both groups whether they fused or not. In 2004 Kornblum et al[9] reviewed the noninstrumented fusion patients from the Fischgrund trial with 5 to 14 years of follow-up. They found that there was a significant difference between the long-term results of both groups. The pseudoarthrosis patients ended up having worse clinical outcomes with many of them requiring revision operations. Thus, evidence does support the use of posterior instrumentation (**Fig. 8-8**) to achieve higher fusion rates and better clinical outcomes.

Similar to the cervical spine, longer segment fusion cases in the lumbar spine have a higher rate of pseudoarthrosis than those with fewer segments fused. Increased rates of nonunion are also seen at the thoracolumbar junction and the lumbosacral junction. Attempts to achieve higher fusion rates at the lumbopelvic junction include the use of interbody fusion at L5–S1 and iliac fixation to protect the S1 promontory screws. As previously mentioned, patients with pseudoarthrosis had significantly worse

outcomes than those who had complete fusion. Smoking, the use of allograft, extension of fusion to the sacrum, preexisting hip arthritis, and a thoracoabdominal approach may be associated with increased risk.[10]

Adjacent Segment Degeneration

After lumbar fusion is attained, an important question arises as to what the future holds at the adjacent levels that have not been operated on. It is unclear if lumbar ASD (**Fig. 8-9**) occurs as a result of lumbar spinal fusion or is part of a larger preexisting multifactorial disease process. Studies suggest an increase in risk for ASD in patients who underwent spinal fusion compared with patients who received nonfusion or no treatment. Annualized incidence rates for symptomatic ASD requiring reoperation from case series ranged from 0% to 3.9%. Approximately 26% of patients receiving lumbar fusion develop new lumbar ASD within the first 10 years after fusion based on one study.[11] The L3–L4 segment appears to be one of the most frequently involved levels, according to multiple studies. Because of this concern for ASD, many technologic advances have been made to decompress and stabilize the lumbar spine without rigid fusion. Some examples include the artificial disc replacement, pedicle-based motion-preserving devices, facet replacements, and interspinous implants. There has been much research done to validate the efficacy of many of these products. However, more time is needed to adequately assess the rates of ASD with these products versus that of lumbar spinal fusion.

Conclusion

Back pain is one of the most common causes of acute and chronic pain. When conservative care fails to relieve pain or acute neurological changes have occurred, spinal surgery must be considered. Lumbar surgery often includes decompression of the soft and bony tissues, leading to lumbar stenosis of any variety. If one presents with segmental instability or is at risk for instability, lumbar fusion is often considered. The risks of any spinal surgery are significant, but spinal fusion itself has specific risks. The most common of these risks include infection, dural tear, pseudoarthrosis, and ASD. These risks can often be reduced with careful patient selection, meticulous surgical technique, and best care practices. Despite changes in surgical technique or equipment, these risks still exist. Many emerging techniques and equipment improvements have been directed at reducing these complications, but quality evidence is still needed to prove their efficacy.

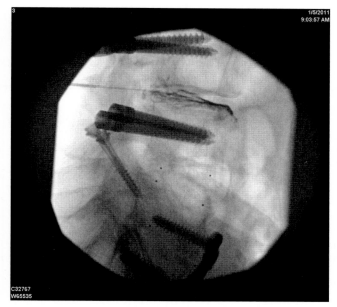

Fig. 8-9   Discogram showing adjacent level concordant pain at degenerated adjacent segment.

References

1. Weinstein MA, McCabe JP, Cammisa FP: Postoperative spinal wound infection: a review of 2,391 consecutive index procedures. *J Spinal Disord* 13(5):422-426, 2000.
2. Fang A, Hu SS, Endres N, Bradford DS: Risk factors for infection after spinal surgery. *Spine* 30(12):1460-1465, 2005.
3. Khan MH, Rihn J, Steele G, et al: Postoperative management protocol for incidental dural tears during degenerative lumbar spine surgery: a review of 3,183 consecutive degenerative lumbar cases. *Spine* 31(22):2609-2613, 2006.
4. Cammisa FP, Girardi FP, Sangani PK, et al: Incidental durotomy in spine surgery. *Spine* 25(20):2663-2667, 2000.
5. Wang JC, Bohlman HH, Riew KD: Dural tears secondary to operations on the lumbar spine. Management and results after a two year minimum follow up of eighty-eight patients. *J Bone Joint Surg Am* 80(12):1728-1732, 1998.
6. Kitchel SH, Eismont FJ, Green BA: Closed subarachnoid drainage for management of cerebrospinal fluid leakage after an operation on the spine. *J Bone Joint Surg Am* 71(7):984-987, 1989.
7. Martin BI, Mirza SK, Comstock BA, et al: Reoperation rates following lumbar spine surgery and the influence of spinal fusion procedures. *Spine* 32:382-387, 2007.
8. Fischgrund JS, Mackay M, Herkowitz HN, et al: Volvo Award winner in clinical studies: Degenerative lumbar spondylolisthesis with spinal stenosis: a prospective, randomized study comparing decompressive laminectomy and arthrodesis with and without spinal instrumentation. *Spine* 22:2807-2812, 1997.
9. Kornblum MB, Fischgrund JS, Herkowitz HN, et al: Degenerative lumbar spondylolisthesis with spinal stenosis: a prospective long term study comparing fusion and pseudoarthrosis. *Spine* 29:726-733, 2004.
10. Kim YJ, Bridwell KH, Lenke LG, et al: Pseudoarthrosis in long adult spinal deformity instrumentation and fusion to the sacrum: prevalence and risk factor analysis of 144 cases. *Spine* 31:2329-2336, 2006.
11. Park P, Garton HJ, Gala VC, et al: Adjacent segment disease after lumbar or lumbosacral fusion: review of the literature. *Spine (Phila PA 1976)* 29(17):1938-1944, 2004.

9 Complications of Nucleus Replacement and Motion-Sparing Technologies

Iain H. Kalfas

CHAPTER OVERVIEW

Chapter Synopsis: Spinal fusion surgery can provide successful outcomes in treatment of low back pain arising from disc degeneration, but the surgery can result in spinal degeneration adjacent to the fusion. So-called motion-sparing technologies present newer alternatives. Lumbar arthroplasty replaces the degenerating collagen disc with newly improved artificial materials. Similarly, nucleoplasty replaces the disc's watery center to preserve structural integrity. These technologies may provide better outcomes and prevent adjacent disc degeneration, but further long-term studies are needed before these more expensive procedures become routine. In addition, the procedures carry many of the same risks as fusion surgery, as well as other potential device-related complications.

Important Points:
- Fusion has been a long-standing strategy to treat complex degenerative disc disease, and although validated, numerous studies demonstrate increased mechanical stress on adjacent levels and may translate into increased patient morbidity and health care costs.
- Motion-sparing technologies have been developed to reduce adjacent level degeneration and include artificial discs, nucleus replacement devices, facet replacement devices, and posterior lumbar dynamic stabilization devices.
- Lumbar disc arthroplasty has strict patient selection criteria, is poorly validated, and many times these patients respond to nonsurgical management.
- Nucleoplasty implants are considered investigational and are of either injectable or preformed types, and advancement of the technology is limited by postoperative extrusion of the device and further destruction of the vertebral endplates.
- Although lumbar arthroplasty and nucleoplasty results seemed to be promising, long-term follow-up has failed to demonstrate reliable and reproducible improvement in outcomes as compared with fusion.

Introduction

Surgery for the management of degenerative disorders of the spinal column continues to evolve. Although a majority of these procedures address simple decompression of the neural elements, the use of spinal fusion has been rapidly increasing. Fusion has long been accepted as a means for managing complex spinal deformities and instability. However, the primary reason for its increasing frequency has been its application to the management of degenerative disc disease and the treatment of chronic low back pain. Although this application remains controversial among spinal surgeons, several studies have shown that fusion for degenerative disc disease at one or two levels can improve outcomes compared with the natural history of low back pain.[1,2]

Although many patients do well after lumbar fusion surgery, some patients can develop further degeneration at spinal levels adjacent to the fusion. Numerous biomechanical studies have demonstrated an increase in mechanical stresses within motion segments adjacent to fused segments.[3-5] As adjacent segment degeneration progresses, additional surgery to decompress and stabilize the involved segments may be necessary. This results in increased morbidity and expense of care and can propagate the

cycle of additional adjacent segment degeneration and the subsequent need for even more surgery.

This long-standing problem with adjacent segment degeneration has led many to investigate alternatives to spinal fusion as a means of reducing the mechanical stresses placed on these segments. In particular, the development of a variety of motion-sparing technologies has been enthusiastically embraced as the ideal technology to manage degenerative disorders of the spine while limiting the potential for adjacent segment degeneration.

Motion-sparing technology encompasses a spectrum of devices. The most common of these devices are artificial discs for both the lumbar and cervical regions. Other motion-sparing technologies include nucleus replacement devices, interspinous devices, facet replacement devices, and posterior lumbar dynamic stabilization devices.

Each of these devices allows for some motion at the operated levels, subsequently decreasing the mechanical stresses felt at adjacent levels.[6] In theory, this may reduce the incidence of degeneration at adjacent segments caused by fusion, resulting in improved long-term patient outcomes. This technology is attractive to both spinal surgeons as well as informed patients who both recognize the theoretical advantages to a spine fusion alternative. However, these devices are costly, and many lack the long-term follow-up needed to justify the added expense.

Although motion-sparing technologies have been developed to reduce the long-term complications associated with fusion procedures, they are not immune from their own set of postoperative problems. This chapter reviews the complications that can occur through the use of motion-sparing technology, specifically lumbar artificial disc replacement (arthroplasty) and lumbar nucleus replacement (nucleoplasty).

Lumbar Arthroplasty

The search for a surgical alternative to fusion and a means of treating painful lumbar discs dates back several decades. The initial efforts to design and develop an artificial lumbar disc began in the 1950s. Numerous designs were created and patented with few reaching the level of clinical study because of limitations with biomaterial design, lack of appropriate surgical approaches, and inconclusive patient selection strategies.

These early failures with artificial disc technology gradually improved aided by advancements in the design and application of artificial hip and knee joints. In the early 1980s Shellnack and Buttner-Janz[7] introduced the SB Charité lumbar artificial disc. The device used a sliding, unconstrained polyethylene core placed between two metallic endplates. When inserted into the affected disc space through an anterior surgical approach, it permitted relatively normal motion of the intervertebral segment.

After two early design changes, the SB Charité disc (DePuy Spine, Raynham, MA) eventually underwent a rigorous multicenter, prospective, randomized study with encouraging early and midterm results. It became the first lumbar disc device to receive Food and Drug Administration (FDA) approval. Widespread use of the device began in 2004. The ProDisc device (Synthes Spine, Paoli, PA) also received early FDA approval and is currently in use (**Fig. 9-1**). Several other lumbar disc replacement devices are currently in varying stages of design, development, clinical analysis, and approval.

Indications and Contraindications

Lumbar disc arthroplasty is approved for use in patients with single-level painful, degenerative disc disease. Bertagnoli[8] defined the ideal patient for disc arthroplasty as having a single level of disc disease, greater than 4 mm of retained disc height, no evidence of osteoarthritis of the facet joints, and intact posterior elements. Essentially, this type of patient is young, has an almost normal spine with only single-level disease defined by magnetic resonance imaging or discography, and has no neurologic deficits. This type of patient is relatively rare and is often successfully treated without any type of surgery.

One study evaluated 252 patients who underwent surgery for lumbar spinal disorders. Only 6.3% were deemed potential candidates for disc replacement based on the Charité exclusion criteria. Only one patient was thought by the authors to be an ideal candidate for disc replacement.[9]

Lumbar disc arthroplasty is contraindicated in patients with painful facet arthropathy, instability (i.e., spondylolisthesis), collapsed disc space, significant neural compression, or neurologic deficits. The clinical trials of the arthroplasty devices also included age older than 60 years as a contraindication to the procedure.[10]

Clinical Results

Lumbar arthroplasty has been promoted as a replacement for fusion. Preserving intersegmental motion is believed to reduce the

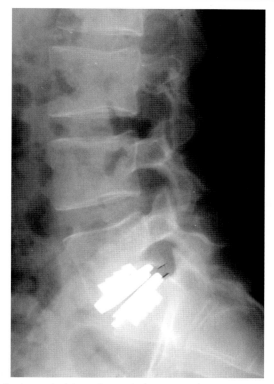

Fig. 9-1   Lateral plain radiograph demonstrating proper positioning of a ProDisc lumbar arthroplasty device within the L5–S1 disc space.

potential for the development of adjacent level degenerative changes that can be seen after fusion procedures. Several early studies were retrospective in design and demonstrated superior results for disc replacement.[8,11,12] David[13] evaluated 106 patients who had received implantation of a Charité disc with a minimum 10-year follow-up. In this study, 87 patients (82.1%) achieved excellent or good clinical outcome. Of the 96 patients working preoperatively, 86 (89.6%) returned to work. A total of 90.6% of the implanted devices were still mobile at long-term follow-up.

The first major randomized, controlled clinical study of lumbar arthroplasty evaluated the use of the Charité device. The control group selected for this study was the use of an anterior lumbar interbody fusion (ALIF) with threaded titanium cages. The selection of this control group has been criticized as an outdated technology not in current use because of relatively high failure rates and better alternatives.[14] The use of threaded cages before the study was indicated primarily in patients with a collapsed and painful disc space. However, these patients were excluded from the arthroplasty study. Only patients with preserved disc height were included, a suboptimal criterion for the use of threaded cages.

The study defined success as a 25% improvement in Oswestry Disability Index (ODI), no device failure, no major surgical complication, and no neurologic deterioration.[15] With the control group selected for this study, it could be predicted that the patients in this group would not do well. This was the case because only 46.5% of the control group patients were classified as achieving success. This is a poor result compared with other series of ALIF in properly selected patients in which success rates in the 85% to 95% range have been reported.[16,17]

The arthroplasty group did only slightly better achieving a success rate in only 57.1% of the patients. This modest success rate is further limited by the fact that at 2 years of follow-up, 72.2% of the arthroplasty patients were still on narcotic medication. However, the study did demonstrate safety and effectiveness of the device and ultimately contributed to final FDA approval.[15]

Currently, several other implant designs are in various stages of clinical investigation. The two devices approved for clinical use are gathering longer term follow-up in an effort to determine the effectiveness of arthroplasty at limiting adjacent segment degeneration. To date, little evidence exists to support a significant reduction in adjacent segment degeneration with the use of arthroplasty. Until sufficient long-term follow-up is obtained, reimbursement for the procedure will remain a challenge, further limiting the widespread application of this technology.

Complications

Surgery for lumbar arthroplasty is performed through an anterior approach. The approach-related complications for this surgery are the same as for an anterior lumbar fusion procedure. Wound infection and vascular and visceral injuries occur at the same rate with either procedure. However, selection of the appropriate implant size and the proper positioning of the device require a greater degree of technical precision than most other lumbar procedures. To adequately recreate the motion of an intact disc, the implant must be correctly centered within the disc space. Failure to precisely position and secure the implant can result in suboptimal function or extrusion of the device.

Although relatively rare, migration or extrusion of the implant is the most significant device-related complication that can occur with this procedure (**Fig. 9-2**). When present, it may result in a spinal deformity or lead to injury of major vascular structures anterior to the lumbar spine. Significant vascular complications

can also occur with any anterior revision surgery carried out through a scarred surgical field for the removal of an extruded implant. In a series of 50 patients undergoing lumbar arthroplasty, six patients required anterior revision surgery. One of these patients required three additional vascular procedures because of aortic injury that occurred with the revision surgery.[18]

Other device-related complications of lumbar arthroplasty include subsidence of the device through the vertebral endplates, loosening or fracture of the device (**Fig. 9-3**), and osteolysis of the bone surrounding the device. Malpositioning may result in suboptimal functioning of the device, which can then lead to degenerative changes in the posterior facet joints at the involved or adjacent levels. Suboptimal insertion techniques may also lead to a gradual loss of motion of the interspace or the formation of heterotopic bone bridging the disc space and essentially fusing it.[13,19] The impact of metallic and polyethylene wear debris is negligible. In the absence of device extrusion, most device-related complications can be managed by performing a posterior lumbar fusion and fixation procedure, keeping the arthroplasty device in place and avoiding higher risk anterior lumbar revision surgery.

Nucleoplasty

The intervertebral discs are designed to provide flexibility, stability, and shock absorption to the spinal column. Each disc consists of two anatomic components. The outer annulus fibrosus is composed of highly organized type I collagen fibers. The annulus forms a ring around the disc space and serves to provide tensile and torsional stability. The inner nucleus pulposus is composed of proteoglycans mixed with a randomly oriented network of type II collagen fibers. This structure provides resistance to compressive loads applied to the spinal column.

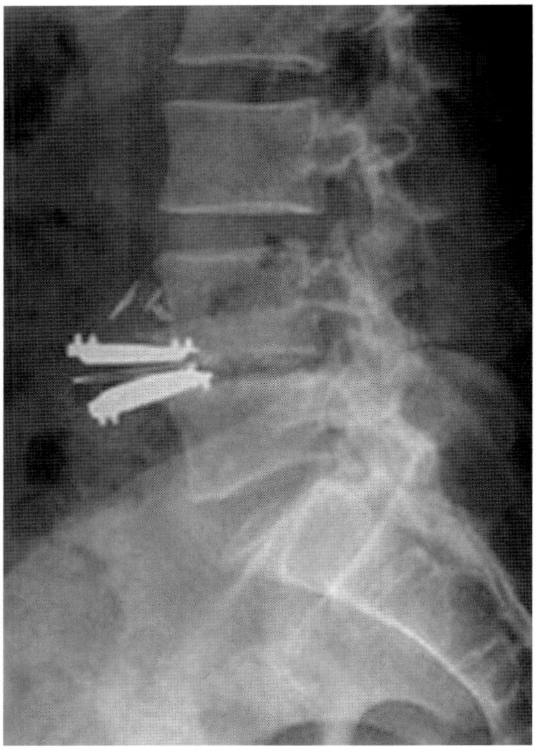

Fig. 9-2 Lateral plain radiograph demonstrating anterior extrusion of a lumbar arthroplasty device. Anterior revision surgery was needed to remove the device and to perform an interbody fusion procedure.

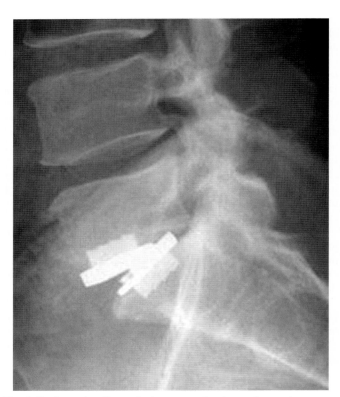

Fig. 9-3 Lateral radiograph demonstrating loosening and malalignment of a lumbar arthroplasty device.

In the first two decades of life, the nucleus pulposus has a relatively high water content, which creates positive pressure, or turgor, within the disc space. With aging, this water content begins to diminish, initiating a cascade of degenerative changes that slowly progress over several decades. The early degenerative changes include disc space narrowing as the nucleus pulposus loses its ability to resist compressive loads. These compressive loads are ultimately transmitted to the annulus and, eventually, to the facet joints. This leads to varying degrees of annular bulging, facet hypertrophy, neural compression, and motion segment instability.

The concept of nucleoplasty is predicated on the idea that limiting the early collapse of the disc space may prevent or slow down the cascade of degenerative events that typically follow this anatomic change. It represents an opportunity to intervene early and to potentially change the natural history of the degenerative process. It can be performed using minimal access techniques and does not limit the options for additional treatment as do fusion and arthroplasty.

Nucleoplasty involves the placement of a viscoelastic implant into the central portion of the disc space through either a posterior or a lateral surgical approach. This serves to restore of maintain normal disc height and provides more physiologic load transfer and shock absorption across the disc space. Restoration of disc height opens the adjacent neural foramina and provides appropriate tensioning of the annulus fibrosus. This limits the transfer of abnormal loads to the facet joints, theoretically minimizing the potential of neural compression and instability.

Types of Nucleoplasty Implants

Several nucleoplasty implants are currently in various stages of clinical investigation. These implants can be separated into two different categories: self-polymerizing injectable implants and preformed implants.

Injectable implants are designed to fill the defect left by a surgical discectomy. They consist of a synthetic monomer in liquid form that polymerizes within the disc space to form a viscoelastic polymer implant. They conform well to the shape of the discectomy void, maximizing the surface area contact with the adjacent vertebral endplates. This helps minimize the physical stress on the endplates as well as the implant itself. Unlike preformed implants, injectable implants can be placed through a relatively small annular opening and may be more resistant to postoperative extrusion.

Preformed nucleoplasty implants consist of hydrophilic hydrogels that imbibe water and enlarge within the disc space. Compared with injectable implants, they may provide superior restoration of disc turgor and height. However, because of their physical size and shape, they require a larger annular opening for insertion, increasing the potential for postoperative extrusion. Because they do not completely conform to the adjacent endplates they are in contact with, they may produce higher stress concentrations that result in remodeling of the endplates.[20]

Indications and Contraindications

Nucleoplasty implants have been used in two different patient populations. The first group consists of patients with degenerated discs and chronic low back pain. These patients have a narrowed disc space without evidence of nerve root compression. They have failed an extensive course of conservative management. Partial disc replacement allows for the removal of the presumed pain generator, the diseased nucleus, and replacement with a device that maintains relatively normal function of the disc space.[20,21]

A second group of patients presents with radiculopathy, with or without back pain, secondary to a herniated nucleus pulposus. They have failed conservative management and are candidates for a surgical discectomy procedure. Although lumbar discectomy yields consistently good results, it is well documented that a small but significant number of patients who undergo standard discectomy will develop recurrent herniations or progressive degenerative changes with symptomatic low back pain.[22-24] The loss of disc space height that frequently occurs after discectomy can promote further degenerative changes in the involved motion segment. Placement of a nucleoplasty device into the disc space may theoretically slow future degenerative changes by maintaining disc space height and normal motion.[25,26]

There are several contraindications for nucleoplasty. Placement of a nucleoplasty device into the disc space depends on a relatively competent annulus. Significant disruption of the annulus may allow for extrusion of the device. The annular opening made during a discectomy procedure needs to be kept as small as possible if nucleoplasty is planned.

Other contraindications for nucleoplasty include associated spinal pathology such as facet arthrosis, central and lateral recess stenosis, instability, deformity, and osteoporosis. Disc space height less than 5 mm has also been shown to be a relative contraindication for nucleoplasty.[20] Many of these findings are frequently present in patients with degenerative disc disease, thereby limiting the number of patients who may benefit from nucleoplasty.

Clinical Results

Clinical results of lumbar nucleoplasty remain relatively limited. One study looked at 243 patients who underwent insertion of a preformed hydrogel device for chronic discogenic low back pain. The follow-up period was 2 years, but many patients were lost to follow-up. Only 111 (46%) of the 243 patients provided 6-month follow-up data. Two-year follow-up data were provided by only 23 (9%) patients. The preoperative ODI was 52.7, dropping to 17.2 at 6 months and 9 at 24 months. The Visual Analog Scale was 7.1 preoperatively, 3.0 at 6 months, and 1.8 at 2 years. Sustained increases in disc height were observed at 2 years.[20]

Complications

The further investigation and advancement of nucleoplasty technology has been slowed by the persistence of two types of complications seen with this device. The most common complication has been postoperative extrusion of the implanted device (**Fig. 9-4**). This typically occurs through the annular defect through which the device was inserted. Several design changes have not resulted in any satisfactory reduction in the frequency of this complication.

Bertagnoli and Vazquez[27] reported that reoperation for removal of extruded implants was necessary in 12% of their study population. Risk factors for device extrusion were a disc height smaller than 5 mm, insertion of two devices into a disc space with and anteroposterior dimension of larger than 37 mm, a body mass index greater than 30, and implantation through a posterolateral annulotomy.[18] Extrusion was not seen when the device was inserted through an anterolateral transpsoas approach.

The second complication frequently seen with nucleoplasty devices is their effect on the vertebral endplates. These changes include endplate fracture, subsidence through the endplate (**Fig. 9-5**), and endplate sclerosis. A study of 46 patients demonstrated implant subsidence into the endplates in nine patients (20%) and endplate sclerosis in 28 patients (61%).[20] These changes may limit the theoretical positive effects that nucleoplasty has on the

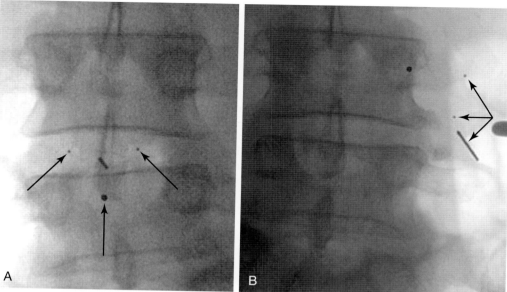

Fig. 9-4 A, Anteroposterior plain radiograph demonstrating satisfactory positioning of a preformed radiolucent nucleoplasty device within the L4–L5 disc space. Radiopaque markers outlining the device are noted by *arrows*. **B,** Anteroposterior plain radiograph demonstrating lateral extrusion of device outside of the disc space (*arrows*). This required a second surgery for removal of the implant and interbody fusion of the disc space.

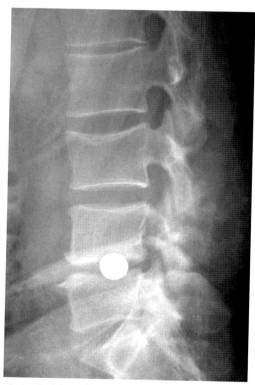

Fig. 9-5 Lateral plain radiograph demonstrating subsidence of a preformed spherical nucleoplasty device through the endplates of L4 and L5.

replacement are understood, ongoing studies will need to demonstrate long-term effectiveness. Devices and insertion techniques may need to be redesigned to limit the relatively common complications of extrusion and endplate changes before full approval is achieved.

Conclusion

Motion-sparing technology is a theoretically appealing concept for managing patients with lumbar disorders. By preserving intersegmental motion and avoiding a fusion, normal function may be better preserved and the development of adjacent segment degeneration avoided.

Both lumbar arthroplasty and nucleoplasty have undergone several years of clinical investigation and follow-up. Although early results have seemed promising, longer term follow-up has not been able to demonstrate any appreciable clinical improvement over fusion or any reliable and predictable reduction in the development of adjacent segment degenerative changes.

Device-related complications have also slowed the general acceptance of these procedures. Experience and management of these complications may facilitate improved implant designs and insertion techniques. However, longer term follow-up will be needed to fully determine the role of this technology in the management of patients with lumbar disorders.

progressive degenerative process by reducing motion or permitting a reduction in disc space height.

Currently, nucleoplasty devices are considered investigational. No device to date has received FDA approval for broad clinical use. Although the theoretical advantages of a nucleus pulposus

References

1. Fritzell P, Hagg O, Wessberg P, Nordwell A: 2001 Volvo Award Winner in Clinical Studies: lumbar fusion vs nonsurgical treatment for chronic low back pain: a multicenter randomized controlled trial from the Swedish Lumbar Study Group. *Spine* 26:2521-2532, 2001.
2. Resnick DK, Choudri TF, Dailey AT, et al: Guidelines for the performance of fusion procedures for degenerative disease of the lumbar spine: intractable pain without stenosis or spondylolisthesis. *J Neurosurg Spine* 2:670-672, 2005.

3. Kim YE, Goel VK, Weinstein JN, Lim TH: Effect of disc degeneration at one level on the adjacent level in axial mode. *Spine* 16:331-335, 1991.

4. Rao RD, David KS, Wang M: Biomechanical changes at adjacent segments following anterior lumbar interbody fusion using tapered cages. *Spine* 30:2772-2776, 2005.

5. Weinhoffer SL, Guyer RD, Herbert M, Griffith SL: Intradiscal pressure measurements above an instrumented fusion. A cadaveric study. *Spine* 20:526-531, 1995.

6. Goel VK, Grauer JN, Patel, T, et al: Effects of Charité artificial disc on the implanted and adjacent spinal segment mechanics using a hybrid testing protocol. *Spine* 30:2755-2764, 2005.

7. Buttner-Janz K, Shellnack K: Principles and initial results with the Charité modular type SB cartilage disk endoprosthesis. *Magy Traumatol Orthop Helyreallito* 31:136-140, 1988.

8. Bertagnoli R, Kumar S: Indications for full prosthetic disc arthroplasty. A correlation of clinical outcome against a variety of indications. *Eur Spine J* 11(suppl 2):131-136, 2002.

9. Simmons JW: *Inclusion criteria for disc arthroplasty*, Philadelphia, 2005, North American Spine Society.

10. Zigler JD, Lorenz MA, Bunch WH: Editorial response to the Charité Lumbar Disc Arthroplasty Study Parts 1 and 2. *Spine* 30:E388-E390, 2005.

11. Mayer HM, Wiechert K, Korge A: Minimally invasive disc replacement: surgical technique and preliminary surgical results. *Eur Spine J* 11(suppl):S124-S130, 2002.

12. Lemaire JP, Skalli W, Lavaste F: Intervertebral disc prosthesis. Results and prospects for the year 2000. *Clin Orthop* 337:64-76, 1997.

13. David T: Long-term results of one-level lumbar arthroplasty. *Spine* 32:661-666, 2007.

14. Mirza SK: Point of view: commentary on the research reports that led to Food and Drug Administration approval of an artificial disc. *Spine* 30:1561-1564, 2005.

15. Blumenthal S, McAfee PC, Guyer RD, et al: A prospective, randomized, multicenter Food and Drug Administration investigational device exemptions study of lumbar total disc replacement with the Charité artificial disc versus lumbar fusion: part I: evaluation of clinical outcomes. *Spine* 30:1565-1575, 2005.

16. Sasso RC, Kitchel SH, Dawson EG: A prospective, randomized controlled clinical trial of anterior lumbar interbody fusion using a titanium cylindrical threaded fusion device. *Spine* 29:1113-1122, 2004.

17. Burkus JK, Gornet MF, Dickman CA, Zdeblick TA: Anterior lumbar interbody fusion using rhBMP-2 with tapered interbody cages. *J Spinal Disord Tech* 15:337-349, 2002.

18. Zeegers WS, Bohnen LM, Laaper M: Artificial disc replacement with the modular type SB Charité III: 2-year results in 50 prospectively studied patients. *Eur Spine J* 8:210-217, 1999.

19. Punt IM, Visser VM, van Rhijn LW, et al: Complications and reoperations of the SB Charité lumbar disc prosthesis: experience in 75 patients. *Eur Spine J* 17:36-43, 2008.

20. Bertagnoli R, Schonmayr R: Surgical and clinical results with the PDN prosthetic disc-nucleus device. *Eur Spine J* 11(suppl 2):S143-S148, 2002.

21. Shim CS, Lee SH, Park CW: Partial disc replacement with the PDN prosthetic disc nucleus device: early clinical results. *J Spinal Disord Tech* 16: 324-330, 2003.

22. Lowell TD, Errico TJ, Fehlings MG, et al: Microdiskectomy for lumbar disc herniation: a review of 100 cases. *Orthopedics* 18:985-990, 1995.

23. Smorgick Y, Floman Y, Millgram MA, et al: Mid to long-term outcome of disc excision in adolescent disc herniations. *Spine J* 6:380-384, 2006.

24. Yorimitsu E, Chiba K, Toyama Y, Hirabayashi K: Long-term outcomes of standard discectomy for lumbar disc herniations: a follow-up of more than 10 years. *Spine* 26:652-657, 2001.

25. Jin D, Qu D, Zhao L, et al: Prosthetic disc nucleus (PDN) replacement for lumbar disc herniation: preliminary report with six month follow-up. *J Spinal Disord Tech* 16:331-337, 2003.

26. Coric D, Mummaneni PV: Nucleus replacement technologies. *J Neurosurg Spine* 8:115-120, 2008.

27. Bertagnoli R, Vazquez RJ: The anterolateral transpsoatic approach: a new technique for implanting prosthetic disc nucleus devices. *J Spinal Disord Tech* 16:398-404, 2003.

10 Complications of Spinal Injections and Surgery for Disc Herniation

William C. Thompson IV

CHAPTER OVERVIEW

Chapter Synopsis: Two of the most common interventions for chronic back pain arising from degenerative disc disease are epidural injection of steroids and surgical lumbar discectomy. The risks associated with steroid injection depend on the approach: interlaminar, transforaminal, or caudal; each presents its own anatomic challenges. Patients can also react to the corticosteroid, the local anesthetic, or the contrast agent. Discectomy carries the risks of any surgical procedure, which also vary depending on the anatomic location. Although the risks are quite low, rarely, catastrophic consequences can result from vascular or nerve damage.

Important Points:

- A detailed history and physical examination of the patient and review of pertinent diagnostic studies and laboratory values in order to identify patient-specific risk factors before intervention is critical.
- Appreciation of the inherent interindividual variability in the location of critical structures and understanding of the anatomy of the planned procedural approach to the epidural space can help limit complications.
- Use of fluoroscopic imaging (particularly with continuous fluoroscopy during the instillation of contrast) is essential unless otherwise contraindicated.
- Strict maintenance of aseptic technique, with consideration toward wearing a mask in addition to sterile gloves, will minimize the risk of infectious complication.
- Because of the importance of early detection of potentially catastrophic complications, a high index of suspicion for the occurrence of rare complications such as hematoma and abscess postprocedurally needs to be maintained.

Introduction

Back pain is among the most common pain-related complaints that lead patients to seek care from physicians. Underlying disc herniation and subsequent radicular symptoms from direct compression of nerve roots or inflammatory mediators related to disc disruption are a frequent cause of the pain leading to these physician visits. The expenditure on care for these patients has been rapidly increasing over the past several years, and one recent study estimates that total health care expenditures for adults with back and neck pain increased by 82% in the United States between 1997 and 2006.[1] These costs are attributable to a variety of diagnostic and treatment measures instituted for the alleviation of patient suffering, and a large portion of the costs is clearly related to interventional therapies for back pain such as epidural injections and surgery.

Epidural steroid injections (ESIs) are a commonly instituted therapy for degenerative disc disease with radicular symptoms. The utilization of this type of therapy has also increased substantially in recent years.[2] In the same time period, there has been a similarly substantial increase in lumbar surgeries of which lumbar discectomy is the most commonly performed for patients with disc herniation causing lumbar radicular symptoms.[3,4] With use of any medical therapy (both pharmacologic and interventional), there is always a degree of risk to the patient, and a comprehensive knowledge of the nature of that risk is paramount to minimizing complications to the greatest extent possible.

Complications of Epidural Steroid Injections

Epidural steroid injections are performed by one of three general techniques: interlaminar, transforaminal, and caudal. The interlaminar and transforaminal approaches are applied in the cervical, thoracic, and lumbar spine for radicular symptoms in the upper and lower extremities, respectively. The caudal approach is, for obvious reasons, only applicable for lumbar radicular symptoms. There is variability in which approach is used to treat cervical or lumbar radicular symptoms between the interlaminar and transforaminal route among interventional pain medicine specialists. The transforaminal approach is advocated to better direct the deposition of corticosteroids at the location of pathology, which is within the neural foramen. However, as discussed later, this anatomic location is also occupied by critical arterial vascular structures that can be inadvertently entered or injured during the injection. The interlaminar approach, on the other hand, is advocated to be safer because of the decreased risk of intraarterial injection and being more in line with the approach used to provide epidural analgesia as an established skill set of the many practitioners who enter pain medicine from anesthesiology backgrounds. Caudal access to the epidural space is among the earliest described methods of providing ESIs and is used by many practitioners as their primary method of administering ESIs for patients with lumbosacral radiculopathy.[5] It has an added advantage as well in patients with previous lumbar laminectomy that can make accessing the epidural space from other routes more challenging, particularly from an interlaminar approach.

Broadly speaking, as seen in **Table 10-1**, the potential complications of ESIs can be differentiated into the following categories: (1) medication reactions, (2) vascular injury or intravascular injection, (3) bleeding, (4) infection, (5) needle trauma (including dural puncture), and (6) miscellaneous.

Medication Reactions

During a typical ESI, three types of medications are administered: a local anesthetic, a corticosteroid preparation, and a contrast agent. Reactions to these medications can be either allergic in nature or related to the known pharmacology of the drugs themselves (**Table 10-2**).

With respect to allergic reactions, there is a known incidence of allergy to all of the aforementioned medications used in ESI. In terms of local anesthetics, the most frequently used in the context of ESI are the amide local anesthetics lidocaine and bupivacaine. Allergy to amide local anesthetics is quite rare and usually a contact dermatitis reaction, but it can occasionally be an anaphylactic-type reaction.[6] In one such case report of an anaphylactic-type reaction to amide local anesthetics, a patient without a known history of local anesthetic allergy developed an anaphylactic response to lidocaine and bupivacaine administered during a lumbar injection (presumably an ESI, although the report does not mention the exact procedure performed) after two uneventful injections with the same agents previously.[6] Corticosteroid preparations have also been reported to cause allergic reactions when administered epidurally, and although symptoms are most frequently seen

immediately after administration, they can result in a delayed onset of symptoms up to several hours later.[7] Contrast allergy, particularly to iodinated contrast agents, is also reported in the literature, although life-threatening anaphylactic reactions are rare.[8] Reported factors that increase the risk of reaction to contrast agents include a history of previous reaction to contrast agent, asthma, atopy, and advanced heart disease.[9]

Thankfully, the risk of allergic-type reactions to the medications administered during ESI is overall quite low. Key to minimizing this risk is performing a detailed history from patients of any history of allergy to the agents to be administered or history of the aforementioned risk factors, proper monitoring of patients periprocedurally, and being prepared to immediately institute appropriate therapy to patients if they have a reaction.

Toxicity associated with local anesthetic administration is exceedingly rare with doses commonly administered during ESIs and is more frequently seen with other interventional procedures used in pain medicine (e.g., sympathetic blockade). Inadvertent intravascular injection of local anesthetics into the vertebral artery during a cervical transforaminal ESI, however, has been reported to cause seizures (and even death) at lower doses of local anesthetic than those typically reported to cause seizures when administered intravenously.[10] Presumably, the direct access to the cerebral circulation increases the risk of seizure from inadvertent intravascular administration of local anesthetics in the cervical spine.

Corticosteroids have a wide range of potential physiologic effects, including when they are administered epidurally. Adverse effects associated with corticosteroids include facial erythema (flushing), dizziness, insomnia, fluid retention, hyperglycemia (which can be particularly problematic in diabetic patients), a labile mood, headache, osteoporosis, and gastritis or peptic ulcer formation, although this list is by no means all inclusive. In addition, with repeated corticosteroid administration, the cumulative effects of the administered steroid can indeed cause Cushing syndrome in patients even when the steroid administered was primarily by the epidural route. Careful monitoring of the total amount of steroid given to a patient is paramount to minimizing the severity and incidence of these complications. A comprehensive history of the patient should be obtained that includes any corticosteroid medication taken by the patient (including oral and parenterally administered), all interventional procedures performed on the patient by outside providers involving corticosteroid administration (e.g., joint injections, trigger point injections), and a complete record of the corticosteroids administered by the interventional pain physician. Patients with coexistent diabetes mellitus warrant an extra level of monitoring given the hyperglycemia associated with these medications. A history of recent blood sugar control (finger stick glucose values, recent hemoglobin A1c values, insulin administration) can give an indication as to the stability of the disease and may warrant involvement of the patient's endocrinologist or primary care physician in planning periprocedural diabetes management. The same can be said for patients with severe congestive heart failure and some cardiomyopathies. These patients could be at risk for decompensation in the event of significant fluid retention related to corticosteroid administration and may warrant periprocedural involvement of a cardiologist and possibly a reduced dosage of steroid to minimize the likelihood of cardiac decompensation.

Vascular Injury and Intravascular Injection

Depending on the approach to the epidural space, various vascular structures can inadvertently be cannulated or injured by the needles used for ESIs. A solid knowledge of the vascular anatomy of the

Table 10-1: Potential Complications of Epidural Steroid Injections

Category of Complication	Example
Medication reactions	Allergic reaction, local anesthetic toxicity, steroid effect
Vascular injury or intravascular injection	Artery of Adamkiewicz, vertebral artery
Bleeding	Epidural hematoma
Infection	Epidural abscess, meningitis
Needle trauma	Spinal cord injury, nerve root injury, dural puncture
Miscellaneous	Urinary complications, vasovagal reactions

Table 10-2: Medication Reactions in Epidural Steroid Injections

Medication	Potential Reaction	Serious Complications
Local anesthetics	Toxicity	Seizure, cardiac arrest
Corticosteroids	Physiologic effects	Hyperglycemia, fluid retention, Cushing syndrome
All medications commonly used in epidural steroid injections (local anesthetics, corticosteroids, contrast agents)	Allergic reaction	Anaphylaxis

spinal cord allows for a full understanding of the risks and consequences of injury to or injection into these vessels, but it is critical to realize that there is considerable anatomic variation among individuals in the locations of the vascular structures supplying the cord. As such, in addition to anatomic knowledge, careful and safe procedural technique will allow the practitioner to minimize complications from vascular injury.

The vascular supply to the spinal cord is commonly understood to consist of paired posterior spinal arteries and a single anterior spinal artery, the latter supplying the anterior two-thirds of the spinal cord. The anterior spinal artery has additional vascular supply from radiculomedullary arteries as it progresses caudally along the spinal cord. In the cervical spine, there is an average of three such radiculomedullary arteries that originate from branches of the vertebral arteries and occasionally have contributions from the ascending and deep cervical arteries as well.[11,12] Progressing more caudally, the supply to the anterior spinal artery is more limited, with the primary contribution arising from the artery of Adamkiewicz, a radiculomedullary artery of variable anatomic origin. Most commonly (reportedly 85% of the time), this artery arises between T9 and L2, and 80% of the time, it is located on the left.[13] See **Fig. 10-1** for a representation of this blood supply.

Because the blood supply to the anterior two-thirds of the spinal cord is dependent primarily on a few radiculomedullary arteries, with the low thoracic cord dependent on a single radiculomedullary artery (the artery of Adamkiewicz), injury to or embolization of any of these arteries can lead to a catastrophic neurologic outcome. Anatomic variation in the location of these arteries compounds the risk and should lead to vigilance in the performance of transforaminal injections. Indeed, there are reports in the literature of paraplegia and anterior spinal artery syndrome resulting from presumed embolism or injury to the artery of Adamkiewicz at almost all lumbar levels with one case as low as S1.[11,14]

In the cervical spine, as seen in **Fig. 10-2**, the vertebral artery is found anteriorly within the foramen most frequently at C6 and above.[12] Injury to this structure is also associated with catastrophic outcomes, as was reported in one case in which autopsy revealed that a puncture of the vertebral artery during a C7 transforaminal ESI led to a dissection and eventual thrombosis of the artery, causing death of the patient.[15] Multiple reports can be found in the literature of brain infarction and spinal cord infarction associated with the transforaminal approach to cervical ESIs with the postulated mechanisms being embolism of particulate steroid particles versus direct injury to the vertebral or radiculomedullary arteries supplying the anterior spinal artery, respectively.[10,15-20]

Avoiding these devastating complications is a primary procedural challenge facing interventional pain physicians. With respect to avoiding intravascular injection and subsequent embolic phenomena, it appears that the use of live fluoroscopy (with digital subtraction if available) is an essential step, particularly with the transforaminal approach, even though it may not be 100% effective. **Fig. 10-3** illustrates the benefits of digital subtraction angiography in this image that shows the artery of Adamkiewicz in a spinal angiogram at the L3-L4 level. Use of intermittent fluoroscopy (in lieu of live, continuous fluoroscopy) during contrast injection can cause the proceduralist to miss the appearance of vascular uptake.[21,22] In addition, it should be noted that a recent study showed an 8.9% incidence of simultaneous epidural and vascular patterns on injection of contrast during lumbar transforaminal injections, a finding that reinforces the critical importance of diligence during contrast injection in transforaminal ESIs, particularly when one considers that a radiculomedullary artery supplying the anterior spinal artery can occur at almost any vertebral level.[23]

The nature of the agent injected also can be a factor in the outcomes of inadvertent intravascular injection. A study by Tiso et al[24] looked at the role of particulate corticosteroids through analysis of particulate size and microscopic characteristics of the particles. In sum, they found that triamcinolone and methylprednisolone had a tendency to form aggregates in excess of 100 μm (which may increase the risk of vascular occlusion after intravascular injection) and recommend that in the case of cervical transforaminal ESIs, that only corticosteroid solutions (dexamethasone and betamethasone sodium phosphate) be used. This sentiment is further supported by review performed by Scanlon et al[10] who note that thus far all of the commonly used corticosteroids have been associated with brain or spinal cord infarction except dexamethasone.

Bleeding

Epidural hematoma is a well-known but very rare risk of neuraxial anesthesia and ESI. Estimates of its prevalence vary, but an approximate incidence is fewer than one in 150,000 epidural anesthetics, although there is suggestion that this risk has increased with the advent of newer anticoagulant medications.[25] In addition to being associated with neuraxial intervention, epidural hematoma has been reported to occur spontaneously in the general population, often in conjunction with anticoagulation, with one study reporting an incidence of 0.1 per 100,000 people.[26,27] Depending on the location, symptoms generally present with an onset of severe back or neck pain and progressive neurologic dysfunction (sensory or motor deficits and occasionally with bowel or bladder dysfunction). A high index of suspicion and rapid diagnosis are the key to better outcomes in the case of epidural hematoma as the definitive treatment of laminectomy and hematoma evacuation has been associated with better recovery of neurologic function when performed promptly within 8 hours of the onset of neurologic symptoms.[28,29]

Without question, anticoagulant therapy is the most readily identifiable risk factor for the development of epidural hematoma in conjunction with interventional techniques. With epidural hematoma being such a rare clinical entity, performance of randomized trials to elucidate the best management strategies for anticoagulant use remains a challenging prospect. As such, the large majority of recommendations in this regard are summarized treatment guidelines formulated in the context of the available literature (e.g., case reports), expert opinion, and extrapolation from other clinical knowledge of bleeding risk. The American Society of Regional Anesthesia and Pain Medicine have recently updated one such set of guidelines.[25] Although focused primarily on epidural and spinal anesthesia for surgery, they do include case reports (though rare) on epidural hematomas in the context of ESIs. In the absence of more pain medicine–specific guidelines, many practitioners apply these guidelines toward their own practice with regard to ESIs. An adaptation of these recommendations for clinical scenarios commonly encountered in an outpatient pain practice appears in **Table 10-3**. Specific note is made that this is just an adaptation and that all clinical decision making is best left to the individual practitioner, who would benefit from reading these guidelines directly.

Note should be made of the fact that the presented guidelines do not address patient-specific factors that may affect their risk of epidural hematoma after ESI. In fact, a case study cited by the authors of the guidelines represents a case of epidural hematoma after an ESI in a patient for whom bridging therapy with enoxaparin was utilized during Coumadin discontinuation for an ESI in which all of the guidelines were followed, and it was hypothesized by the authors that coexistent renal insufficiency was responsible

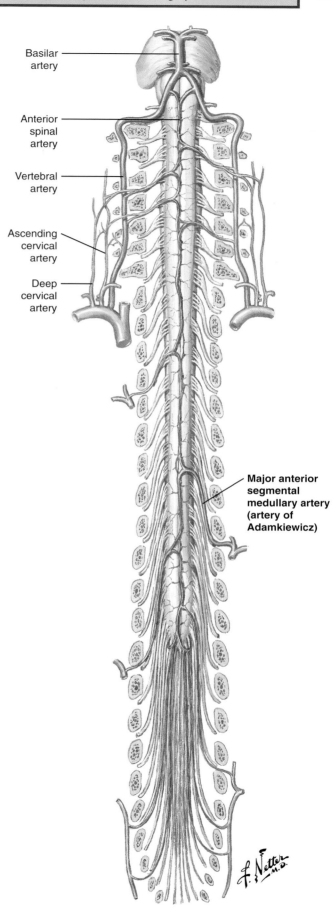

Basilar artery

Anterior spinal artery

Vertebral artery

Ascending cervical artery

Deep cervical artery

Major anterior segmental medullary artery (artery of Adamkiewicz)

Fig. 10-1   The arterial supply of the spinal cord. As described in the text, note the artery of Adamkiewicz and the relative lack of other major contributors to the arterial supply in this region. (Netter illustration from www.netterimages.com. © Elsevier, Inc. All rights reserved.)

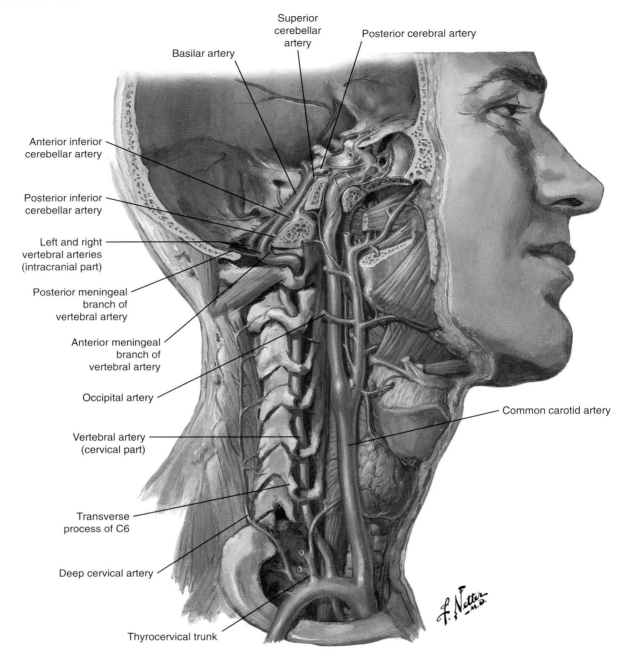

Basilar artery

Superior cerebellar artery

Posterior cerebral artery

Anterior inferior cerebellar artery

Posterior inferior cerebellar artery

Left and right vertebral arteries (intracranial part)

Posterior meningeal branch of vertebral artery

Anterior meningeal branch of vertebral artery

Occipital artery

Vertebral artery (cervical part)

Transverse process of C6

Deep cervical artery

Thyrocervical trunk

Common carotid artery

Fig. 10-2 Arteries to the brain and meninges. Note the location of the vertebral artery within the neural foramen and the downstream structures supplied by this critical artery. (Netter illustration from www.netterimages.com. © Elsevier, Inc. All rights reserved.)

for a prolonged enoxaparin effect.[30] Another report documented a similar clinical scenario, with epidural hematoma despite strict adherence to the guidelines in the absence of renal insufficiency.[27] Further emphasizing the importance of patient-specific factors is a case report of epidural hematoma resulting in paraplegia in a 67-year-old woman after an ESI with undiagnosed coagulopathy.[31] Additionally, it appears that the risk of epidural hematoma is also contributed to by the use of multiple different agents that can all affect the coagulation cascade.

Vigilance toward obtaining a complete history and evaluation of the patient, careful periprocedural management of anticoagulant medications, and prompt recognition of the clinical presentation of epidural hematoma if it occurs will minimize the incidence and morbidity of this rare complication of ESI.

Infection

Although infection is also a possible complication of ESI, serious infection such as epidural abscess is a rare event. There is no commonly agreed upon incidence for this complication in the context of ESI, but some study has been done on the incidence of spontaneous epidural abscess and found it to be 0.88 cases per 100,000 person-years using data from one county's population in the United States.[32] A recent review of the published cases of epidural abscess and meningitis associated with ESI does, however, provide some insight into the characteristics and presentation of these patients. The authors report that the mean age was 54 years and that of the 14 reported cases, nine had a condition that may be expected to decrease immune system function (diabetes mellitus, metastatic cancer, myeloproliferative disorder, oral corticosteroid

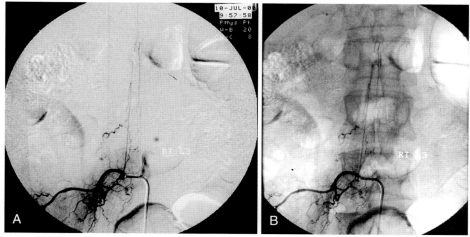

Fig. 10-3 A view of the artery of Adamkiewicz under subtraction angiography. Note the characteristic appearance of this vessel. (From Houten JK, Errico TJ: Paraplegia after lumbosacral nerve root block: report of three cases, *Spine J* 2(1):70-75, 2002.)

Table 10-3: An Adaptation of the American Society of Regional Anesthesia and Pain Medicine Guidelines on Regional Anesthesia in Patients Receiving Antithrombotic or Thrombolytic Therapy

Medication	Pre-Block Hold Recommendation	Post-Block Hold Recommendation
Heparin (subcutaneous)*	4 hr	1 hr
LMWH: prophylaxis dosing	10-12 hr	24 hr
LMWH: treatment dosing	24 hr	24 hr
Coumadin	4–5 days and normalized INR before proceeding with block	
NSAIDs (including aspirin)	No hold recommended	
Clopidogrel	7 days	
Ticlopidine	14 days	
Herbal supplements (garlic, ginseng, ginkgo)	No hold recommended	

*Recommendations are for standard dosing regimen of 5000 units twice daily. Per the American Society of Regional Anesthesia and Pain Medicine's guidelines, the safety of 10,000 units daily or more than twice-daily dosing has not been established.
INR, International Normalized Ratio; LMWH, low-molecular-weight heparin; NSAID, nonsteroidal antiinflammatory drug.
From Horlocker T, et al. Regional anesthesia in the patient receiving antithrombotic or thrombolytic therapy: American Society of Regional Anesthesia and Pain Medicine Evidence-Based Guidelines (Third Edition). *Reg Anesth Pain Med* 35(1), 2010.

use). The mean onset of symptoms was 7 days after injection and the most common causative organism was *Staphylococcus aureus*.[33]

Their observation of *S. aureus* as the most common causative organism has been reinforced by several other analyses of epidural abscess data, although gram-negative species (often arising from unintentional bowel penetration) and even fungal species have been reported.[20,33-38] The presentation is classically described as involving back pain and fever in the initial stages, with progressive neurologic deficits (motor, bowel and bladder, and sensory) developing later.[37] As with epidural hematoma, early diagnosis with advanced imaging (magnetic resonance imaging) and early intervention with antibiotics and surgery are the keys to minimizing morbidity of epidural abscess.

In addition to epidural abscess, other infectious complications of ESI are possible and have been reported. In the event of inadvertent dural puncture during the procedure, there exists the risk of postdural puncture meningitis. An interesting review of this clinical entity was performed by Baer,[35] who reported that mouth commensals (e.g., *Streptococcus viridans*) were the most frequent causative organisms of postdural puncture meningitis and that epidemiologic studies have identified the sources in some cases as being from the mouths and upper airways of medical personnel performing the procedures resulting in dural puncture. Reports also exist of cases of vertebral osteomyelitis (with soft tissue but not epidural abscess) and discitis after an ESI.[39,40]

Avoidance of infectious complications of ESIs begins with meticulous adherence to aseptic technique, including skin preparation with an appropriate antiseptic, sterile draping of the injection area, and use of sterile gloves and equipment (**Table 10-4**). Although it is controversial, many argue that wearing a mask while performing procedures that involve entry into the neuraxis is another important step to minimize infectious complications. Careful assessment of the patient for any coexistent infection at the time of the procedure will allow for identification of increased infectious risk and may lead to postponement of the procedure because of the risk of epidural abscess or infection arising from hematogenous spread. Furthermore, a history consistent with potential immunocompromise should reinforce the critical nature of aseptic technique and a risk-to-benefit analysis of the proposed injection and may lead to the decision to provide antibiotic prophylaxis as has been proposed by some interventionalists.

Needle Trauma

With any type of interventional procedure, unintended injury to adjacent anatomic structures is possible, and ESIs are no exception. The most common such complication is perhaps inadvertent dural

Table 10-4: Avoiding Infectious Complications of Epidural Steroid Injections

- Prepare the skin with an appropriate antiseptic solution.
- Perform sterile draping of the injection area.
- Ensure strict maintenance of aseptic technique with sterile gloves and equipment.
- Assess patients for any coexistent infection at time of procedure and postpone or reschedule if appropriate.
- Consider having the interventional pain physician and all assistants preparing surgical trays or drawing medications wear masks for procedures that involve entry into the neuraxis.

Table 10-5: Treatment Options for Postdural Puncture Headache

Activity Limitation	Medications	Invasive
• Bedrest	• Acetaminophen • NSAIDs • Caffeine	• Epidural blood patch

NSAID, nonsteroidal antiinflammatory drug.

puncture (or "wet tap"), which occurs at a reported frequency of approximately one in 200 epidurals.[20] Many of these patients experience postdural puncture headaches (PDPHs) as a result. PDPHs are classically reported as severe dull headaches that are positional (with decreased symptoms in the supine position). **Table 10-5** reviews some of the potential treatments for PDPH if it occurs.

Although most commonly thought of in association with the interlaminar approach to the epidural space, inadvertent dural puncture can also occur with other approaches to the epidural space and may not be associated with cerebrospinal fluid (CSF) flashback on removal of the stylet from the needle, particularly with the transforaminal approach.[41] Careful interpretation of contrast pattern will identify the subarachnoid or subdural position of the needle in these circumstances. Failure to recognize the dural puncture and administration of medications intrathecally can be problematic and lead to a potentially high spinal block from local anesthetic and even arachnoiditis (especially if methylprednisolone acetate is administered in this location).[9]

In the cervical and thoracic spine, direct injury to the spinal cord can occur during an ESI both through interlaminar and transforaminal approaches, and a number of case reports have documented this serious complication.[42-45] Too deep a level of procedural sedation has been proposed to be a contributor to this outcome with the hypothesis that the patient would have otherwise reported paresthesia or other symptom upon contact of the needle to the spinal cord. However, in one of the reported cases, the patient was not sedated and did not report any symptoms during intracord injection of steroid and local anesthetic, suggesting that reliance on patient report alone may note be sufficient to guard against this complication.[44] Caution must be exercised as well to avoid trauma to the nerve roots themselves because they are clearly not immune to inadvertent injury during an ESI either through the transforaminal or interlaminar approach.[46]

Minimization of complications resulting from needle trauma is achieved through diligent adherence to proper technique, although even with the utmost of care, these types of events can occur, albeit rarely. One factor that is unquestionably of benefit in avoiding direct injury to the spinal cord and nerve roots is the use of biplanar fluoroscopy and contrast to confirm needle location. Avoiding

deep sedation may be of benefit because the patient can report symptoms from pending neurologic injury. Reliance on loss of resistance alone may not be sufficient in the cervical spine; a recent anatomic study of cadavers revealed that there are frequently midline discontinuities in the ligamentum flavum in the cervical and high thoracic spine.[47] Obtaining fluoroscopic information of the needle tip position has the potential to prevent advancing the epidural needle too far while attempting to find the loss of resistance in this area.

Miscellaneous

Urinary complications such as urinary retention can occur with local anesthetic administration in the lumbosacral region. In many instances, this is a problem that will resolve along with resolution of the local anesthetic effect. It is reported that urinary complications are more frequently seen in elderly patients (especially men), multiparous women, and patients with a history of inguinal and perineal surgery.[20]

Vasovagal reactions in the periprocedural period are commonly reported and often resolve without sequelae. One retrospective review found that these reactions were more common in patients undergoing cervical as opposed to lumbar ESI.[48] Additionally, common minor post procedural complications include injection site soreness, increased axial neck pain (in the case of cervical ESIs), and facial flushing.[49]

Complications of Discectomy

When considering the complications of injection therapy for disc herniation, it is useful to briefly consider the complications that are possible with the alternative of surgical intervention for the treatment of disc herniation: discectomy. As with all surgical procedures, there is the minimal risk of anesthesia-related complications. Complications more specific to discectomy depend on the site of surgery (i.e., the cervical vs. lumbar spine).

Cervical Discectomy

One of the most commonly performed spinal surgical procedures is anterior cervical discectomy and fusion (ACDF), and this represents the most common approach to cervical discectomy (see **Fig. 10-4**).[50] One recent retrospective study analyzed the complication rates of this procedure in 1015 patients undergoing ACDF (note is made that only first-time operations were included in their analysis). Among their findings were that the morbidity rate was 19.3% with the most commonly observed complications being postoperative dysphagia (9.5%), hematoma (5.6%), and recurrent laryngeal nerve palsy (3.1%) (**Table 10-6**).[51] Among the most rare complications observed in their study was also the most catastrophic: esophageal perforation occurred in 0.3%, but one of these cases was fatal. Indeed, injury to adjacent structures is a risk of the ACDF procedure; vascular injury to the carotid artery and jugular vein as well as injury to the thoracic duct have also occurred, although the incidence is rare. These authors in their literature review cited an overall complication rate of ACDF as being between 0.45% and 19.6% based on published case series.[51]

Lumbar Discectomy

In the lumbar spine, lumbar discectomy is most often performed from a posterior approach (**Fig. 10-5**). Reports on the overall complication rate vary in the literature with reported values varying from 1.5% to 15.8%.[52-56] The most commonly reported complications were dural tears or CSF leak, infection, acute urinary retention, and transient or permanent radiculopathy (**Table 10-7**).

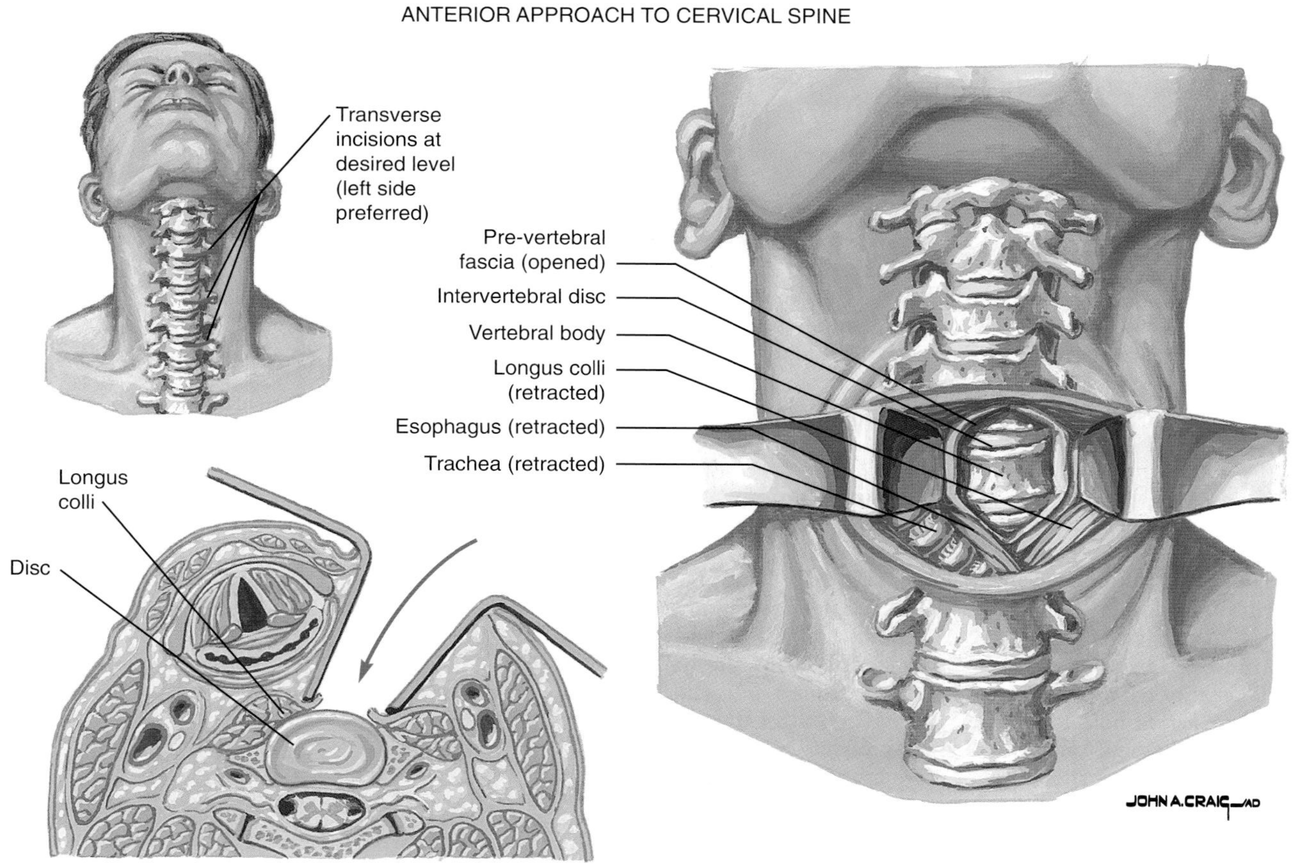

ANTERIOR APPROACH TO CERVICAL SPINE

Transverse incisions at desired level (left side preferred)

Pre-vertebral fascia (opened)
Intervertebral disc
Vertebral body
Longus colli (retracted)
Esophagus (retracted)
Trachea (retracted)

Longus colli

Disc

JOHN A. CRAIG—AD

Fig. 10-4 The most common approach to cervical disc surgery is the anterior approach. The disc of interest is visualized directly after retraction of the anterior structures of the neck. (Netter illustration from www.netterimages.com. © Elsevier, Inc. All rights reserved.)

Table 10-6: Complications of Cervical Discectomy	
More common complications	• Postoperative dysphagia • Hematoma • Recurrent laryngeal nerve palsy
Rare complications	• Esophageal perforation • Carotid injury • Jugular injury • Thoracic duct injury

From Fountas KN, Zapsalaki EZ, Nikolakakos LG, et al: Anterior cervical discectomy and fusion associated complications. *Spine* 32(21), 2007.

The most catastrophic reported complications are thankfully also among the most rare and involve injury to deep structures in the abdomen, particularly to major vessels and the bowel. With a reported incidence of 0.016% to 0.06%, the majority of intraabdominal injuries are vascular (most often involving the left common iliac artery) and can lead to acute decompensation in the perioperative period (with high mortality rate) or arteriovenous fistula formation.[53,55] Interestingly, retroperitoneal hematoma from just such a major vascular injury has even been reported in a patient undergoing the minimally invasive percutaneous endoscopic approach to discectomy, and as such, an awareness of this potential complication is critical regardless of the surgical approach.[57]

Thoracic Discectomy

Symptomatic thoracic disc herniations are a relatively rare entity, far less common than those seen in the cervical and lumbar levels. This is thought to be related to the lesser mobility of the thoracic

spinal segments given their articulation with the rib cage.[58] The surgical approaches for these herniations can involve either an anterior approach (via thoracotomy or video-assisted thoracoscopic surgery) or posterior approach (costotransversectomy, minimally invasive discectomy) with the choice often made depending on the location of the herniation (either central or lateral respectively).[59] When using the anterior approach, by nature of the surgical technique, the possible complications include those associated with all thoracic surgery (e.g., lung injury, injury to great vessels, chest tube complications). Posterior approaches can mean avoidance of intrathoracic injury but may necessitate large incisions or resection of ribs and can be associated with more manipulation of the spinal cord in order to achieve visualization of the disc material.[58]

Conclusion

Intervention for the treatment of pain resulting from disc herniation is an increasingly common scenario in modern medicine. No intervention in medicine is without some degree of risk of complication, but thankfully, the overall complication rate is quite low. Minimizing the occurrence of complications from ESIs starts and ends with diligence on the part of the interventional pain medicine specialist. Particularly important are:

■ Obtaining a detailed history and physical examination of the patient and review of pertinent diagnostic studies and laboratory values to identify patient-specific factors that affect the risks of these interventions

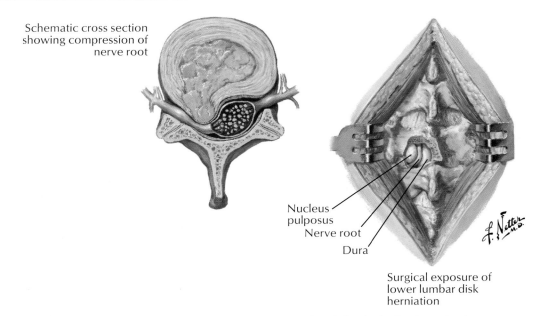

Schematic cross section showing compression of nerve root

Nucleus pulposus
Nerve root
Dura

Surgical exposure of lower lumbar disk herniation

Fig. 10-5 As opposed to the approach in the cervical spine, surgery for disc herniation in the lumbar spine is most commonly performed from the posterior approach as depicted. (Netter illustration from www.netterimages.com. © Elsevier, Inc. All rights reserved.)

Table 10-7: Complications of Lumbar Discectomy	
More common complications	• Dural tear or CSF leak • Infection • Urinary retention • Transient radiculopathy
Rare complications	• Permanent radiculopathy • Hematoma (retroperitoneal, epidural) • Injury to major vessels • Bowel injury

CSF, cerebrospinal fluid.
Data from Wu X, Zhuang S, Mao Z, Chen H: Microendoscopic discectomy for lumbar disc herniation. *Spine* 31(23), 2006; Raptis S, Quigley F, Barker S: Vascular complications of elective lower lumbar disc surgery. *Aust N Z J Surg* 64, 1994; Bell G: Implications of the spine patient outcomes research trial in the clinical management of lumber disk herniation. *Cleve Clin J Med* 74(8), 2007; Cases-Baldo MJ, Soria-Aledo V, Miguel-Perello JA, et al: Unnoticed small bowel perforation as a complication of lumbar discectomy. *Spine J* 11(1), 2011; Fallah A, Massicotte EM, Fehlings MG, et al: Admission and acute complication rate for outpatient lumbar microdiscectomy. *Can J Neurol Sci* 37(1), 2010.

- A strong foundation in the anatomy of the planned procedural approach to the epidural space with recognition of the inherent interindividual variability in the location of critical structures
- Use of fluoroscopic imaging (particularly with the transforaminal approach to the epidural space), with continuous fluoroscopy during the instillation of contrast
- Strict maintenance of aseptic technique
- A high index of suspicion for the occurrence of rare complications such as hematoma and abscess after the procedure

References

1. Martin BI, Turner JA, Mirza SK, et al: Trends in health care expenditures, utilization and health status among US Adults with spine problems, 1997-2006. *Spine* 34(19):2077-2084, 2009.
2. Friedly J, Chan L, Deyo R: Increases in lumbosacral injections in the Medicare population: 1994-2001. *Spine* 32(16):1754-1760, 2007.
3. Deyo RA, Gray DT, Kreuter W, et al: United States trends in lumbar fusion surgery for degenerative conditions. *Spine* 30:1441-1445, 2005.
4. Weinstein JN, Tosteson TD, Lurie JD, et al: Surgical vs nonoperative treatment for lumbar disk herniation. *JAMA* 296(20):2441-2450, 2006.
5. Evans W: Intrasacral epidural injection in the treatment of sciatica. *Lancet* 216(5597):1225-1229, 1930.
6. Caron AB: Allergy to multiple local anesthetics. *Allergy Asthma Proc* 28(5):600-601, 2007.
7. Simon DL, Kunz RD, German JD, Zivkovich V: Allergic or pseudoallergic reaction following epidural steroid deposition and skin testing. *Reg Anesth* 14(5):253-255, 1989.
8. Tramer MR, von Elm E, Loubeyre P, Hauser C: Pharmacologic preventions of serious anaphylactic reactions due to iodinated contrast media: systematic review. *BMJ* 333(7570):675-680, 2006.
9. Rathmell, JP. *Atlas of image-guided intervention in regional anesthesia and pain medicine*, Philadelphia, 2006, Lippincott Williams & Wilkins, pp 20-21.
10. Scanlon GC, Moeller-Bertram T, Romanowsky SM, Wallace MS: Cervical transforaminal epidural injections: more dangerous than we think. *Spine* 32(11):1249-1256, 2007.
11. Houten JK, Errico TJ: Paraplegia after lumbosacral nerve root block: report of three cases. *Spine J* 2(1):70-75, 2002.
12. Huntoon MA: Anatomy of the cervical intervertebral foramina: vulnerable arteries and ischemic neurologic injuries after transforaminal epidural injections. *Pain* 117:104-111, 2005.
13. Lo D, Vallee JN, Spelle L, et al: Unusual origin of the artery of Adamkiewicz from the fourth lumbar artery. *Neuroradiology* 44(2):153-157, 2002.
14. Lyders EM, Morris PP: A case of spinal cord infarction following lumbar transforaminal epidural steroid injection: MR imaging and angiographic findings. *Am J Neuroradiol* 30(9):1691-1693, 2009.
15. Rozin L, Rozin R, Koehler SA, et al. Death during transforaminal epidural steroid nerve root block (C7) due to perforation of the left vertebral artery. *Am J Forensic Med Pathol* 24(4):351-355, 2003.
16. Benny B, Azari P, Briones D: Complications of cervical transforaminal epidural steroid injections. *Am J Phys Med Rehabil* 89(7):601-607, 2010.
17. Brouwers PJAM, Kottnik EJBL, Simon MAM, Prevo RL: A cervical anterior spinal artery syndrome after diagnostic blockade of the right C6-nerve root. *Pain* 91:397-399, 2001.

18. Ludwig MA, Burns SP: Spinal cord infarction following cervical transforaminal epidural injection: a case report. *Spine* 30(10):E366-E368, 2005.

19. Windsor R, Overton A, Sugar R: Cervical transforaminal injection three case reports detailing complications, a review of the literature and a suggested technique. *Pain Physician* 6(4):457-465, 2003.

20. Windsor RE, Storm S, Sugar R: Prevention and management of complications from common spinal injections. *Pain Physician* 6:473-483, 2003.

21. Smuck M, Chiodo A, Tong H, et al: Accuracy of intermittent fluoroscopy to detect intravascular injection during transforaminal epidural injections. *Arch Phys Med Rehabil* 87:e38, 2006.

22. Baker R, Dreyfuss P, Mercer S, Bogduk N: Cervical transforaminal injection of corticosteroids into a radicular artery: a possible mechanism for spinal cord injury. *Pain* 103:211-215, 2003.

23. Smuck M, Fuller BJ, Yoder B, Huerta J: Incidence of simultaneous epidural and vascular injection during lumbosacral transforaminal epidural injections. *Spine J* 7(1):79-82, 2007.

24. Tiso RL, Cutler T, Catania JA, Whalen K: Adverse central nervous system sequelae after selective transforaminal block: the role of corticosteroids. *Spine J* 4(4):468-474, 2004.

25. Horlocker T, et al. Regional anesthesia in the patient receiving antithrombotic or thrombolytic therapy: American Society of Regional Anesthesia and Pain Medicine Evidence-Based Guidelines (Third Edition). *Reg Anesth Pain Med* 35(1):64-101, 2010.

26. Baek BS, Hur JW, Kwon KY, Lee HK: Spontaneous spinal epidural hematoma. *J Korean Neurosurg Soc* 44:40-42, 2008.

27. Xu R, Bydon M, Gokasian ZL, et al: Epidural steroid injection resulting in epidural hematoma in a patient despite strict adherence to anticoagulation guidelines. *J Neurosurg Spine* 11(3):358-364, 2009.

28. Vandermeulen EP, Van Aken H, Mermylen J: Anticoagulants and spinal-epidural anesthesia. *Anesth Analg* 79(6):1165-1177, 1994.

29. Stoll A, Sanchez M: Epidural hematoma after epidural block: implications for its use in pain management. *Surg Neurol* 57(4):235-240, 2002.

30. Ain RJ, Vance MB: Epidural hematoma after epidural steroid injection in a patient withholding enoxaparin per guidelines. *Anesthesiology* 102(3):701-703, 2005.

31. Yoo HS, Park SW, Han JH, et al: Paraplegia caused by an epidural hematoma in a patient with unrecognized chronic idiopathic thrombocytopenic purpura following an epidural steroid injection. *Spine* 34(10):E376-E379, 2009.

32. Ptaszynski AE, Hooten WM, Huntoon MA: The incidence of spontaneous epidural abscess in Olmsted County from 1990-2000: a rare cause of spinal pain. *Pain Med* 8:338-343, 2007.

33. Hooten WM, Kinney MO, Huntoon MA: Epidural abscess and meningitis after epidural corticosteroid injection. *Mayo Clin Proc* 79(5):682-686, 2004.

34. Knight JW, Cordingley JJ, Palazzo MG: Epidural abscess following epidural steroid and local anaesthetic injection. *Anaesthesia* 52(6):576-578, 1997.

35. Baer ET: Post-dural puncture bacterial meningitis. *Anesthesiology* 105(2):381-393, 2006.

36. Saigal G, Donovan Post MJ, Kozic D: Thoracic intradural *Aspergillus* abscess formation following epidural steroid injection. *Am J Neuroradiol* 25(4):642-644, 2004.

37. Reihsaus E, Waldbaur H, Seeling W: Spinal epidural abscess: a meta-analysis of 915 patients. *Neurosurg Rev* 23(4):175-204, 2000.

38. Gaul C, Neundorfer B, Winterholler M: Iatrogenic (para)spinal abscesses and meningitis following injection therapy for low back pain. *Pain* 116:407-410, 2005.

39. Simopoulos TT, Kraemer JJ, Glazer P, Bajwa ZH: Vertebral osteomyelitis: a potentially catastrophic outcome after lumbar epidural steroid injection. *Pain Physician* 11(5):693-697, 2008.

40. Hooten WM, Mizerak A, Carns PE, Huntoon MA: Discitis after lumbar epidural corticosteroid injection: a case report and analysis of the case report literature. *Pain Med* 7(1):46-51, 2006.

41. Goodman BS, Posecion LW, Mallempati S, Bayazitoglu M: Complications and pitfalls of lumbar interlaminar and transforaminal epidural injections. *Curr Rev Musculoskelet Med* 1(3-4):212-222, 2008.

42. Hodges SD, Castleberg RL, Miller T, et al: Cervical epidural steroid injection with intrinsic spinal cord damage. *Spine* 23:2137-2142, 1998.

43. Lee JH, Lee JK, Seo BR, et al: Spinal cord injury produced by direct damage during cervical transforaminal epidural injection. *Reg Anesth Pain Med* 33(4):377-379, 2008.

44. Tripathi M, Nath SS, Gupta RK: Paraplegia after intracord injection during attempted epidural steroid injection in an awake patient. *Anesth Analg* 101:1209-1211, 2005.

45. Khan S, Pioro EP: Cervical epidural injections complicated by syrinx formation: a case report. *Spine* 35(13):E614-E616, 2010.

46. Field J, Rathmell JP, Stephenson JH, Katz NP: Neuropathic pain following cervical epidural steroid injection. *Anesthesiology* 93:885-888, 2000.

47. Lirk P, Kolbitsch C, Putz G, et al: Cervical and high thoracic ligamentum flavum frequently fails to fuse in midline. *Anesthesiology* 99(6):1387-1390, 2003.

48. Trentman TL, Rosenfeld DM, Seamans DP, et al: Vasovagal reactions and other complications of cervical vs lumbar translaminar epidural steroid injections. *Pain Pract* 9(1):59-64, 2009.

49. Abbasi A, Malhotra G, Malanga G, et al: Complications of interlaminar cervical epidural steroid injections: a review of the literature. *Spine* 32(19):2144-2151, 2007.

50. Angevine PD, Arons RR, McCormick PC: National and regional rates and variation of cervical discectomy with and without anterior fusion, 1990-1999. *Spine* 28:931-940, 2003.

51. Fountas KN, Zapsalaki EZ, Nikolakakos LG, et al: Anterior cervical discectomy and fusion associated complications. *Spine* 32(21):2310-2317, 2007.

52. Wu X, Zhuang S, Mao Z, Chen H: Microendoscopic discectomy for lumbar disc herniation. *Spine* 31(23):2689-2694, 2006.

53. Raptis S, Quigley F, Barker S: Vascular complications of elective lower lumbar disc surgery. *Aust N Z J Surg* 64:216-219, 1994.

54. Bell G: Implications of the spine patient outcomes research trial in the clinical management of lumber disk herniation. *Cleve Clin J Med* 74(8):572-576, 2007.

55. Cases-Baldo MJ, Soria-Aledo V, Miguel-Perello JA, et al: Unnoticed small bowel perforation as a complication of lumbar discectomy. *Spine J* 11(1):e5-e8, 2011.

56. Fallah A, Massicotte EM, Fehlings MG, et al: Admission and acute complication rate for outpatient lumbar microdiscectomy. *Can J Neurol Sci* 37(1):49-53, 2010.

57. Ahn Y, Kim JU, Lee BH, et al: Postoperative retroperitoneal hematoma following transforaminal percutaneous endoscopic lumbar discectomy. *J Neurosurg Spine* 10(6):595-602, 2009.

58. Sheikh H, Samartzis P, Perez-Cruet MJ: Techniques for the operative management of thoracic disc herniation: minimally invasive thoracic microdiscectomy. *Orthop Clin North Am* 38:351-361, 2007.

59. Canale ST, Beaty JH: *Campbell's operative orthopedics*, ed 11, Philadelphia, 2008, Mosby Elsevier, pp 2195-2199.

11 Radiation Safety and Complications of Fluoroscopy, Ultrasonography, and Computed Tomography

Tristan C. Pico

CHAPTER OVERVIEW

Chapter Synopsis: Fluoroscopy and other imaging technologies have proved invaluable. The guidance they provide makes possible many interventional treatments for pain. But by its nature, fluoroscopy carries some inherent risk from radiation. An estimated 15% of the radiation we are exposed to arises from medically necessary procedures. Damage occurs either directly to the DNA or downstream, carried out by reactive oxygen species. Certain technical and precautionary measures can reduce the total radiation exposure to both patients and practitioners. Reaction to contrast media also poses a rare but severe risk. Ultrasonography is gaining ground as a guidance technique for some interventional procedures; it carries fewer risks than fluoroscopy but has not yet become commonplace.

Important Points:
- There is no accepted safe dose of radiation.
- Patient doses can be minimized by limiting the time of fluoroscopy; proper positioning of the C-arm; use of collimation; and if necessary, shielding the patient.
- Scattered radiation exposure, the major radiation risk to procedure room staff, can be reduced by use of personal protective equipment such as lead aprons, lead shielding, and maximizing the distance from the x-ray source.
- Consideration should be given to the use of protective glasses and gloves that are specially designed to reduce x-ray exposure.
- Procedure room staff should be monitored for cumulative x-ray exposure.
- Use of contrast media increases patient safety but should be used judiciously.
- Modalities such as ultrasound guidance may help reduce x-ray exposure.

Introduction

Fluoroscopy has become an invaluable tool for interventional pain procedures. Its use has allowed a significant improvement in correct needle placement. In addition, advanced procedures such as discograms and kyphoplasty would be impossible to perform effectively or safely without this imaging modality. Although fluoroscopy provides significant benefits in effectiveness and safety in performing injections, it is not without its own risks. Fluoroscopy relies on ionizing radiation, which is known to cause a number of deleterious effects. Other imaging modalities have been developed to address the shortcomings of fluoroscopy but have their own weaknesses. This chapter addresses radiation safety, the deleterious effects of radiation exposure with respect to the patient and practitioner, and alternative modalities.

Terminology

Any discussion of radiation safety requires a basic understanding of the nomenclature specific to this field. The literature is inconsistent in its use of units, with no standardization on using conventional or SI units. Fortunately, for the purposes of the clinician using fluoroscopy, many of these units can often be considered equivalent. Exposure is a quantity of radiation intensity. It is expressed in the conventional units of Roentgen (R) and the SI units of Coulomb/kg (C/kg). The energy absorbed from the exposure is described in conventional units as radiation absorbed dose (rad) and in SI units as Gray (Gy). Different types of radiation cause different biologic effects despite having similar absorbed doses. To predict the biologic effect from different types of radiation, rad is converted to radiation equivalent man (rem) or Sievert (Sv) in SI units. This conversion is accomplished by multiplying either rad or Gy by a quality factor unique to the type of radiation. As an example, whereas the quality factor for x-ray radiation is 1, it is 20 for α particle or fast neutron radiation.[1] This quality factor of 1 allows exposure, dose, and dose equivalent to be considered equal for practical purposes despite their different meanings and uses, so 1 R $\approx$ 1 rad $\approx$ 1 rem. Conversions between units are summarized in **Table 11-1**.

Radiation Physics

Radiation is energy transmitted as waves or particles. The radiation used in fluoroscopy is from a narrow band of the electromagnetic spectrum known as x-rays. X-rays are generated by passing a current (measured in milliamperes or mA) through a negatively charged heated filament (the cathode). The electrons that are produced are accelerated via high voltage (kilovolt peak or kVp) toward the positively charged anode. The energy released at the anode-electron interaction is X-radiation. The x-rays that pass through the body are captured either by film or an image intensifier to form an image that is useful for diagnostic purposes.

The image produced by the X-radiation can be altered by either modulating the current or voltage of the x-ray tube. A higher tube current (mA) will cause an increase in the number of electrons striking the anode and thus increase the number of x-rays produced. By increasing the voltage (kVp), the released electrons will have higher energy, and thus the X-radiation will have higher energy and penetrance. The amount of radiation reaching the image intensifier over a period of time is called the *radiographic density*; the higher the amount of radiation, the brighter the image appears on the fluoroscope monitor. In general, a 15% increase in kVp will have the same effect on radiographic density as doubling the mA.[2] Modern C-arms incorporate automatic brightness control (ABC) to optimize the brightness and contrast of the image. This is accomplished by automatic adjustment of mA and kVp.[1]

Background radiation is unavoidable radiation from both natural sources as well as medical procedures. The average individual receives approximately 3.6 mSv/yr with 15% of this coming from medically necessary radiation when averaged across the population.[2] The amount of background radiation from natural sources varies according to region.[3]

Basics of C-Arm Design

X-radiation is produced in the x-ray tube and directed toward the image intensifier. The image intensifier is composed of two phosphor screens. The input phosphor is spherical, and in combination with the output phosphor, the x-ray image is amplified and converted to visible light, allowing a TV camera to then transmit the image to a screen distant from the image intensifier. Collimation is the process of restricting the x-ray beam to only the clinically important anatomic area. The two types of collimators are iris and adjustable. An adjustable collimator is composed of lead shutters that can be closed to create a rectangular field. An iris variable aperture collimator creates a smaller circular field of radiation. Both collimators reduce the radiation field that reaches the image intensifier and the overall dose to the patient. A basic anatomy of a typical C-arm can be seen in **Fig. 11-1**.

Table 11-1: Units of Radiation Exposure and Dose

	Conventional Units	SI Units	Unit Conversion
Exposure	Roentgen (R)	Coulomb/kg (C/kg)	$1\ R = 2.5 \times 10^{-4}\ C/kg$
Radiation absorbed dose	rad	Gray (Gy)	100 rad = 1 Gy
Radiation equivalent man	rem	Sievert (Sv)	100 rem = 1 Sv

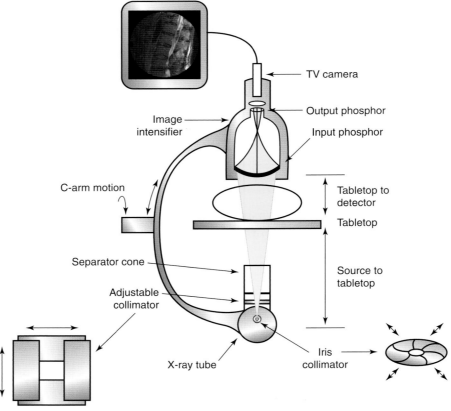

Fig. 11-1 Illustration of C-arm.

Two types of distortion can occur because of the construction of the image intensifier. Vignetting is the decreased spatial resolution and brightness at the periphery of the fluoroscopic image. The second is pincushion distortion, which is caused by the spherical construction of the input phosphor.[2] This creates a fisheye effect as signal from the spherical input phosphor is transmitted to the flat output phosphor. A visual description of this effect can be seen in **Fig. 11-2**. Both of these distortions can be avoided by placing the anatomic structure of interest in the center of the fluoroscopic image.

Radiation Biology

Damage to the body from radiation occurs from direct cellular damage and indirect damage from creation of reactive oxygen species. Direct cellular damage is most likely to occur in cells that are in the G1 or M phases of the cell cycle. In the G1 stage, proteins are synthesized that prepare the cell for replication. During the M stage, DNA is packaged tightly into chromosomes, and there is an increased risk of a lethal double-strand DNA break.[4] Not all radiation damage is lethal to the cell because complex mechanisms repair both single- and double-strand DNA breaks.[5] The repair process is usually completed in 1 to 2 hours, so an increase in time between radiation doses causes an increase in cell survival.[4]

Indirect cellular damage is the result of hydrolysis of water, resulting in production of reactive oxidative species. Two-thirds of radiation-induced DNA damage is attributable to hydroxyl radicals.[4] For example, a reactive oxygen species may combine with protein, resulting in the loss of important enzymatic activity in the cell.[6] Antioxidants that can scavenge free radicals are therefore important in minimizing this type of damage. Molecules that have sulfhydryl groups and amine groups can scavenge these destructive entities.[4]

Damage Caused by Radiation

The effects of radiation on the body are divided into deterministic (nonstochastic) and probabilistic (stochastic). Deterministic effects are directly related to the dose received and exhibit a threshold below which the effect does not normally occur and above which the effect is dose dependent. Typically, these effects are related to cell death. An example is found in skin injury from exposure to radiation. An acute dose of 2 Gy causes early transient erythema, which occurs several hours after the dose and resolves within days.[7] At an acute dose of 7 Gy, permanent epilation (loss of hair) occurs in about 3 weeks. **Table 11-2** gives a more complete enumeration of deterministic effects.[8] As described later in this chapter, many of the deterministic effects are not seen because of relatively low doses of radiation administered in the typical interventional pain fluoroscopy suite.

Probabilistic effects are attributable to mutation within the cell. There is no threshold dose below which these changes cannot occur. The severity of the effect is not dose dependent; however, the chance of the effect occurring is dose dependent. For example, if a malignant growth is induced by a 2-Gy absorbed dose and another is induced by a 0.2-Gy absorbed dose, the malignancy induced by the larger absorbed dose is not more severe than that induced by the smaller absorbed dose. The chance of induction of either malignancy by the higher dose is more likely, however.

As the probabilistic risks of radiation exposure have no threshold value, the guiding concept in radiation safety has been to keep doses "as low as reasonably achievable." This is known as the ALARA concept and is accepted by all regulatory agencies.[1] The maximum permissible dose (MPD) is the upper limit of rem one could receive without substantial risk of a clinically significant reaction. **Table 11-3** lists the annual MPDs for different anatomic structures. A dose of 25 rem can lead to measurable hematologic depression, and a whole-body total radiation dose of 100 rem can lead to radiation sickness, nausea, fatigue, hemapoietic disturbances, alopecia, and radiation dermatitis.[9] It is thought that x-rays may account for 1% of all cancers in the United States.[10]

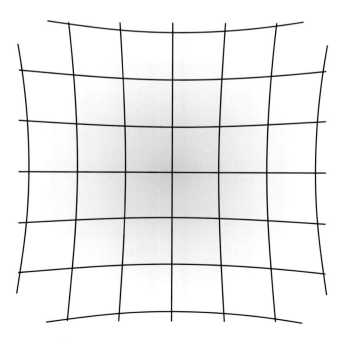

Fig. 11-2   Example of pincushion distortion.

Table 11-2: Skin Entrance Dose Thresholds for Radiation-Induced Skin Injury		
Effect	**Dose (Gy)**	**Onset**
Early transient erythema	2	Hours
Main erythema	6	10 days
Permanent epilation	7	3 weeks
Dry desquamation	14	4 weeks
Moist desquamation	18	4 weeks
Secondary ulceration	24	6 weeks
Late erythema	15	8-10 weeks
Ischemic dermal necrosis	18	>10 weeks
Dermal atrophy	10	12 weeks-1 year
Induration (invasive fibrosis)	10	>1 year
Telangiectasia	10	>1 year
Late dermal necrosis	>12	>1 year

From Brown KR, Rzucidlo ER: Acute and chronic radiation injury, *J Vasc Surg* 53(suppl):15S-21S, 2011.

Table 11-3: Annual Maximum Permissible Dose Per Target Organ or Area

Organ or Area	Annual Maximum Permissible Dose (rem)
Thyroid	50
Extremities	50
Lens of the eye	15
Gonads	50
Whole body	5
Pregnant women	0.5

From National Council on Radiation Protection and Measurements (NCRP): *Report No. 116. Limitation of exposure to ionizing radiation,* Bethesda, MD, 1993, NCRP Publications.

Patient Safety

The goal of patient safety is accomplished by reducing the radiation dose to the minimum amount needed to perform the diagnostic or interventional procedure. Certain patients are at higher risk from a given absorbed dose. Patients with connective tissue disorders such as lupus or DNA repair abnormalities such as xeroderma pigmentosum appear to have radiation hypersensitivity.[8] Obesity is also a risk factor because higher doses of x-radiation are necessary to obtain the same images as in a thin person. Lastly, different medications are known radiosensitizers. Use of chemotherapeutic agents such as doxorubicin, bleomycin, and methotrexate can increase the risk of radiation-induced injury.[8]

Several methods are used for increasing patient safety. Fractionating the dose of radiation and thus allowing time for healing between exposures is known to increase tolerance to the damaging effects of radiation. Molecular repair of the cell begins within hours of the radiation dose, and cellular repopulation of the tissue begins within days of the radiation dose.[8] Positioning of the C-arm also changes the dose of radiation. Varying the position of the beam helps protect the skin by decreasing the dose in any given area of skin. Increasing the angle of entry of the beam also puts the skin closer to the x-ray source.[11] By reducing the overall amount of tissue the beam must traverse, the total dose can be minimized while adequate image quality is maintained. This is accomplished by keeping extraneous tissue, such as arms or breast tissue, out of the path of the beam. By removing the extraneous tissue, the ABC algorithm will thus calculate a lower dose of radiation to obtain an equivalent image.

Minimizing the amount of fluoroscopy time is also crucial to reduce the dose. Continuous fluoroscopy delivers high doses of radiation. One minute of continuous or cinefluoroscopy typically delivers an exposure of 1 to 10 R/min. As a comparison, a typical single posteroanterior chest radiograph has uses an exposure of 15 mR. At a typical exposure of 2 R/min, 1 minute of continuous fluoroscopy can deliver an equivalent exposure of approximately 130 chest radiographs.[4] Using short bursts of fluoroscopy instead of continuous fluoroscopy can markedly decrease the delivered dose. Modern fluoroscopy units include a pulsed fluoroscopy mode. This mode uses frequent periodic spot images with periods between without any exposure. Using pulsed fluoroscopy instead of continuous fluoroscopy can allow up to a 40% decrease in absorbed dose.[12] This mode is usually acceptable in procedures in which continuous fluoroscopy has been typically used, such as placement of spinal cord stimulator leads. Features of the C-arm

imaging software, such as last image hold, reduce the need for repeat images and thereby reduce the radiation dose.[13]

Patient exposure can also be reduced by optimizing equipment factors. Appropriate filtration of 2.5 mm total aluminum equivalent should be in place at the x-ray source. This eliminates the low-power x-ray waves that do not contribute to creation of the image but do contribute to the total patient dose. Collimation should be used when possible to reduce radiation exposure.[14] This not only reduces the amount of x-radiation received by the patient but can also improve image quality by excluding areas of significantly different densities. Keeping the image intensifier as close to the patient as possible also helps to reduce patient radiation dose.[2]

Practitioner Safety

By putting patient safety first through adherence to the ALARA principle, practitioners also maximize the safety of the staff present in the procedure center. The main sources of radiation exposure to practitioners are from leakage from the x-ray tube and scatter from the patient and surroundings.[13] Leakage from the x-ray tube is decreased through proper shielding and maintenance of the C-arm. Scatter occurs through two different mechanisms. The Compton effect occurs when an x-ray impacts an outer shell electron and is deflected. The photoelectric effect occurs when an x-ray impacts an inner shell electron and ejects it. An outer shell electron will then occupy the vacant shell and thus emit an x-ray as secondary radiation.[1] Both of these effects cause the x-radiation to deviate or scatter from the intended path of the beam.

The patient is the major source of radiation exposure to the practitioner because of scatter. The scatter exposure level from the patient is often 0.1% of the entrance skin exposure. At a typical exposure of 2 R/min, the scatter exposure 1 m from the patient would be 2 mR/min. However, the amount of scatter is increased two to three times if the radiation source is on the same side of the table as the practitioner, as in a cross-table lateral view.[1]

Maximizing the distance from the radiation source is an effective means of decreasing the radiation exposure for practitioners. Radiation exposure falls as the square of the distance.[1] Standing away from the patient while performing spot images is useful. The use of forceps or other remote handling devices when manipulating an object in the field and the use of extension tubing while injecting under continuous fluoroscopy are ways to minimize exposure.[15,16]

Proper shielding plays in important role in reducing the radiation dose. Lead aprons absorb approximately 90% to 95% of the scattered radiation that reaches them.[17] Wrap-around aprons should be used by anyone present in the procedure room who spends a significant amount of time with their backs to the radiation source. Thyroid shields also are an important adjunct to the lead apron, and similar to lead aprons, they should be 5 mm lead equivalent at a minimum.[1] X-ray attenuating sterile surgical gloves provide extra protection but should not be considered a substitute for the practitioner keeping his or her hands out of the field. Additionally, ABC increases the output of radiation if a protective glove is in the field, overcoming any protective effects of the glove.

Radiation-induced cataracts have been described in interventional radiologists with a lens dose that approached 150 mSv/yr.[18] Protective eyeglasses can significantly attenuate scatter to the lens and should have a minimal lead equivalent of 0.35 mm.[19] These are recommended for personnel with collar badge readings of greater than 400 mrem per month.[2] Use of these glasses reduce exposure to 2% to 3% of baseline dose, resulting in a total annual dose of only a few μSv.[20]

Another major concern is overall cancer risk. In a longitudinal study of 88,766 U.S. radiation technologists by the National Cancer Institute and University of Minnesota, there was no increase in all-cause mortality, cancer, or cardiovascular disease in technologists who work with fluoroscopy compared with those who did not. The exception to this was in workers who started before 1950, when doses were higher. In this subpopulation there was some increased risk of leukemia, thyroid disease, and female breast cancer.[2] Jartti et al[21] studied physicians who worked with x-rays using exposure data from 1970 to 2001 and found a slight increase in female breast cancer but no statistically significant change in overall mortality or cancer risk from the baseline population.

Happily for patients and practitioners alike, interventional pain procedures require very little radiation exposure compared with other diagnostic studies and interventions. Botwin et al[14] performed 100 transforaminal epidural steroid injections (TFESIs) under fluoroscopic guidance using spot images. The average fluoroscopy time to perform the injections was 15.16 seconds. Cumulative radiation doses to the practitioner were measured both inside and outside the lead apron and at the hand and eye. There was a cumulative dose of 30 mrem outside the apron and 0 mrem inside. The total dose was 40 mrem at the eye and 70 mrem at the hand of the practitioner. The average dose per procedure was shown to be 0.3 mrem outside the apron, 0 mrem inside the apron, 0.4 mrem at the eye, and 0.7 mrem at the hand.[14] These doses indicate that one could perform thousands of TFESIs per year and still be within the MPD. Manchikanti et al[13] reported on the dose to the practitioner from 509 patients undergoing 800 procedures, including interlaminar epidural, transforaminal epidural, and facet joint nerve injections. They reported a mean dose of 0.629 mrem outside the apron at the chest per patient to the practitioner.[13]

Advanced interventions demand more frequent visualization of the anatomy and often require some use of continuous fluoroscopy during critical portions of the procedure. This results in a higher dose of radiation for both the patient and practitioner. Botwin et al[22] also studied the dose of radiation delivered to the practitioner during lumbar discography. A total of 37 patients underwent 106 discograms (levels). The average dose per level was determined to be 2.35 mrem outside the apron, 0.18 mrem inside the apron, 1.49 mrem at the eye, and 3.66 mrem at the hand. Fluoroscopy time per level averaged 57.77 seconds.[22] Boszczyk et al[23] reported on 15 sessions of kyphoplasty with 27 levels performed. Patients received an average total entrance skin dose of 1 Gy.

Contrast Media

One of the benefits of fluoroscopy is the ability to confirm needle placement in real time. This ability is augmented by the use of contrast media because it allows confirmation that the needle is not in the subdural or intravascular space. All of the currently used contrast media are based on the 2,4,6-triiodinated benzene ring. They have a higher viscosity and greater osmolality than blood, plasma, or cerebrospinal fluid.[24] Those most commonly used in interventional pain procedures, such as Omnipaque, Isovue, and Visipaque, are considered low-osmolality contrast media (LOCM) because their osmolality is only two to three times that of serum.[24] LOCM have a much lower incidence of mild and moderate contrast reactions (0.2% vs. 6% to 8% for high-osmolality contrast media), but the incidence of severe reactions is similar. Anaphylactoid reactions are less common with LOCM.[25]

Contrast reactions fall into two groups: anaphylactoid or idiosyncratic and nonanaphylactoid. Anaphylactoid reactions are the most serious type of reaction, are independent of dose, and occasionally lead to fatal outcomes. These reactions are more common in patients with asthma, patients with previous reactions, patients with cardiovascular disease and renal disease, and patients taking β-blockers.[24] Symptoms associated with anaphylactoid reactions range from skin rash, nausea, and itching to severe reactions such as hypotension, overt bronchospasm, laryngeal edema, seizures, and life-threatening arrhythmias. The overall risk for severe reactions from LOCM is 0.03%.[26]

Nonanaphylactoid reactions depend on the ionicity, osmolality, iodine concentration of the media, volume, and route of administration. Higher volumes and intraarterial injection are more likely to cause a reaction.[27] Reactions are believed to be caused by pertubation of homeostasis of the body, specifically blood circulation. The respiratory, gastrointestinal, and nervous systems are also commonly affected. Symptoms are typically warmth, a metallic taste, nausea, vomiting, bradycardia, hypotension, vasovagal reactions, neuropathy, and delayed reactions.[24] Pretreatment with a corticosteroid, antihistamine, or both may be considered in a patient with previous reactions or with significant risk factors for a reaction.

Computed Tomography–Guided Interventional Procedures

Fluoroscopy may be the most familiar imaging modality among interventional pain practitioners, but computed tomography (CT)–guided injections are becoming more common. These have typically been performed by interventional radiologists and deliver large doses of x-radiation.[28] CT fluoroscopy is a recently developed mode of image acquisition that allows for faster image reconstruction, near-continuous image update, and in-room table control and image viewing.[28] There is reduced spatial resolution compared with typical CT images. The rate of image acquisition is typically four to eight images per second, similar to pulsed fluoroscopy. Carlson et al[28] performed 203 CT fluoroscopy–guided procedures such as biopsies, aspirations, and catheter drainages. CT fluoroscopy times ranged anywhere from 7.5 seconds for aspirations to 13.8 seconds for catheter drainages. Patient doses ranged from a mean of 34 mGy (3400 mrad) for aspiration to 53 mGy (5200 mrad) for catheter drainages. In comparison, conventional CT guidance doses were 738 mGy for aspirations and 936 mGy for catheter drainages.[28] Silverman et al[16] performed a similar study using CT fluoroscopic guidance but reported much higher doses. The mean reported patient dose was 300 mGy (30,000 mrad) with a mean CT fluoroscopy time of 79 seconds from 107 abdominal biopsy and catheter drainage procedures.

Wagner[29] reported on the use of CT fluoroscopy for selective nerve root blocks. In a subset of 54 patients, he reported a mean CT fluoroscopy time of 2 seconds with a mean dose to the practitioner of 0.73 mrem per procedure. Compared with the study by Botwin et al,[14] this is approximately twice the dose received by the practitioner but is similar to the dose reported by Manchikanti et al.[13] Many studies referenced in this study did not use contrast media to verify placement of the needle. This is because of the improved spatial resolution of CT versus conventional fluoroscopy and thus presumed superiority in determining needle placement. One purported advantage of CT guidance is the ability to avoid contrast. However, contrast is still useful for determination of intravascular injection because negative aspiration is not a reliable indicator of proper needle placement.

Ultrasound-Guided Interventional Procedures

Ultrasound guidance for interventional pain procedures has recently been advanced as an alternative to fluoroscopic guidance in chronic pain interventions. The advantages of using ultrasound guidance are real-time visualization of the soft tissues, nerves, vessels, and injectate around the nerve.[30] Additionally, exposure to ionizing radiation is avoided. The disadvantages are the bony artifacts and limited resolution of deep tissues.[30] Although some risks, such as cavitation and an increase in temperature, are associated with ultrasonography, its widespread use in obstetrics underlies the inherent safety of this modality.[31] Successful ultrasound-guided blocks for chronic pain have been described for lumbar medial branch blocks, lumbar facet injections, lumbar selective nerve root blocks, cervical selective nerve root blocks, occipital nerve blocks, cervical medial branch blocks, cervical facet injections, stellate ganglion blocks, and transabdominal celiac plexus neurolysis.[30,32-38] Despite the significant interest in this imaging modality, most of the publications are feasibility studies, and few randomized controlled trials have been published.

Conclusion

Fluoroscopy has allowed interventional chronic pain management to be performed in a safe and efficacious manner. However, exposure to ionizing radiation remains a concern. Because no dose of x-radiation can be considered safe, exposure to the patient, staff, and pain practitioner must always be minimized. Further research into alternative imaging modalities such as ultrasound guidance may help improve patient safety.

References

1. Bushberg TB, Seibert JA, et al: *The essential physics of medical imaging*, ed 2, Philadelphia, 2002, Lippincott Williams & Wilkins.
2. Fishman SM, Smith H, Meleger A, Seibert JA: Radiation safety in pain medicine. *Reg Anesth Pain Med* 27(3):296-305, 2002.
3. Zeng W: Communicating radiation exposure; a simple approach. *J Nucl Med Technol* 29(3):156-158, 2001.
4. Brown KR, Rzucidlo ER: Acute and chronic radiation injury. *J Vasc Surg* 53(suppl):15S-21S, 2011.
5. Peterson CL, Cote J: Cellular machineries for chromosomal DNA repair. *Genes Dev* 18:602-616, 2004.
6. Dowd S, Tilson E: *Practical radiation protection and applied radiobiology*, Philadelphia, 1999, Saunders.
7. Hymes SR, Strom EA, Fife C: Radiation dermatitis: clinical presentation, pathophysiology, and treatment. *J Am Acad Dermatol* 54:23-46, 2006.
8. Koenig TR, Wolff D, Mettler FA, Wagner LK: Skin injuries from fluoroscopically guided procedures: part 1, characteristics of radiation injury. *AJR Am J Roentgenol* 177:3-11, 2001.
9. National Council on Radiation Protection and Measurements (NCRP): *Report No. 116. Limitation of exposure to ionizing radiation*, Bethesda, MD, 1993, NCRP Publications.
10. Berrington de Gozalez A, Darby S: Risk of cancer from diagnostic x-rays: estimates for the UK and 14 other countries. *Lancet* 363:345-351, 2004.
11. Koenig TR, Mettler FA, Wagner LK: Skin injuries from fluoroscopically guided procedures: Part 2, review of 73 cases and recommendations for minimizing dose delivered to patient. *AJR Am J Roentgenol* 177:13-20, 2001.
12. Wininger KL, Deshpande KK, Deshpande KK: Radiation exposure in percutaneous spinal cord stimulation mapping: a preliminary report. *Pain Physician* 13:7-18, 2010.
13. Manchikanti L, Cash KA, Moss TL, Pampati V: Effectiveness of protective measures in reducing risk of radiation exposure in interventional pain management: a prospective evaluation. *Pain Physician* 6:301-305, 2003.
14. Botwin KP, Thomas S, Gruber RD, et al: Radiation exposure of the spinal interventionalist performing fluoroscopically guided lumbar transforaminal epidural steroid injections. *Arch Phys Med Rehabil* 83(5):697-701, 2002.
15. Nawfel RD, Judy PF, Silverman SG, et al: Patient and personnel exposure during CT fluoroscopy-guided interventional procedures. *Radiology* 216:180-184, 2000.
16. Silverman SG, Tuncali K, Adams DF, et al: CT fluoroscopy-guided abdominal interventions: techniques, results, and radiation exposure. *Radiology* 212:673-681, 1999.
17. Statkiewicz-Sherer MA, Viscanti PJ, et al: *Radiation protection in medical radiography*, ed 3, St. Louis, 1998, Mosby.
18. Vañó E, González L, Beneytez F, Moreno F: Lens injuries induced by occupational exposure to non-optimized interventional radiology laboratories. *Br J Radiol* 71:728-733, 1998.
19. National Council on Radiation Protection and Measurements (NCRP): *Report No. 93 Ionizing radiation exposure of the population of the United States*, Bethesda, MD, 1987, NCRP Publications.
20. Vano E, Gonzalez L, Fernández JM, Haskal ZJ: Eye lens exposure to radiation in interventional suites: caution is warranted. *Radiology* 248:945-953, 2008.
21. Jartti P, Pukkala E, Uitti J, Auvinen A: Cancer incidence among physicians occupationally exposed to ionizing radiation in Finland. *J Work Environ Health* 32:368-373, 2006.
22. Botwin KP, Fuoco GS, Torres FM, et al: Radiation exposure to the spinal interventionalist performing lumbar discography. *Pain Physician* 6:295-300, 2003.
23. Boszczyk BM, Bierschneider M, Panzer S, et al: Fluoroscopic radiation exposure of the kyphoplasty patient. *Eur Spine J* 15:347-355, 2006.
24. Singh J, Daftary A: Iodinated contrast media and their adverse reactions. *J Nucl Med Technol* 36:69-74, 2008.
25. Cochran ST, Bomyea K, Sayre JW: Trends in adverse events after IV administration of contrast media. *AJR Am J Roentgenol* 176:1385-1388, 2001.
26. Cochran ST: Anaphylactoid reactions to radiocontrast media. *Curr Allergy Asthma Rep* 5:28-31, 2005.
27. Limbruno U, De Caterina R: Vasomotor effects of iodinated contrast media: just side effects? *Curr Vasc Pharmacol* 1:321-328, 2003.
28. Carlson SK, Bender CE, Classic KL, et al: Benefits and safety of CT fluoroscopy in interventional radiologic procedures. *Radiology* 219:515-520, 2001.
29. Wagner AL: Selective lumbar nerve root blocks with CT fluoroscopic guidance: technique, results, procedure time, and radiation dose. *Am J Neuroradiol* 25:1592-1594, 2004.
30. Narouze SN, Vydyanathan A, Kapural L, et al: Ultrasound-guided cervical selective nerve root block: a fluoroscopically-controlled feasibility study. *Reg Anesth Pain Med* 34:343-348, 2009.
31. American College of Obstetricians and Gynecologists: ACOG Practice Bulletin No. 101: ultrasonography in pregnancy. *Obstet Gynecol* 113(2 Pt 1):451-461, 2009.
32. Shim JK, Moon JC, Yoon KB, et al: Ultrasound-guided Lumbar medial-branch block: a clinical study with fluoroscopy control. *Reg Anesth Pain Med* 31:451-454, 2006.
33. Galiano K, Obwegeser AA, Bodner G, et al: Ultrasound guidance for facet joint injections in the lumbar spine: a computed tomography-controlled feasibility study. *Anesth Analg* 101:579-583, 2005.
34. Galiano K, Obwegeser AA, Bodner G, et al: Real-time sonographic imaging for periradicular injections in the lumbar spine: a sonographic anatomic study of a new technique. *J Ultrasound Med* 24:33-38, 2005.
35. Eichenberger U, Greher M, Kapral S, et al: Sonographic visualization and ultrasound-guided block of the third occipital nerve: prospective for a new method to diagnose C2-C3 zygapophysial joint pain. *Anesthesiology* 104:303-308, 2006.

36. Galiano K, Obwegeser AA, Bodner G, et al: Ultrasound-guided facet joint injections in the middle to lower cervical spine: a CT-controlled sonoanatomic study. *Clin J Pain* 22:538-543, 2006.

37. Kapral S, Krafft P, Gosch M, et al: Ultrasound imaging for stellate ganglion block: direct visualization of puncture site and local anesthetic spread. *Reg Anesth* 20:323-328, 1995.

38. Bhatnagar S, Gupta D, Mishra S, et al: Bedside ultrasound-guided celiac plexus neurolysis with bilateral paramedian needle entry technique can be an effective pain control technique in advanced upper abdominal cancer pain. *J Palliat Med* 11(9):1195-1199, 2008.

12 Complications Associated with Head and Neck Blocks, Upper Extremity Blocks, Lower Extremity Blocks, and Differential Diagnostic Blocks

Collin F. M. Clarke, Pari Azari, Chang Po Kuo, and Billy K. Huh

CHAPTER OVERVIEW

Chapter Synopsis: A diverse group of interventional techniques for chronic pain includes head and neck blocks, upper and lower extremity blocks, and differential diagnostic blocks. Although these minimally invasive procedures carry a very low risk, there are rarely catastrophic complications. The consequences vary considerably depending on the site of injection. Sites such as the trigeminal ganglion, buried inside the brain and surrounded by vasculature, pose particular anatomic challenges. Other procedures focus on sites in close anatomic proximity to structures, including nerves, brain, blood vessels, and lungs, and carry risks of particular complications depending on the affected structure.

Important Points:
- Appropriate patient selection with definitive endpoints of treatment is paramount.
- Procedures should only be performed by or under the direct supervision of those who have subspecialty training in interventional pain management.
- Development of standardized procedural approaches, including preprocedure timeouts and sterile techniques, may decrease the likelihood of adverse events.
- Thorough understanding of relevant anatomy and the ability to use imaging, whether fluoroscopy or ultrasonography, are vital to procedural success.
- Although uncommon, catastrophic complications have been reported.
- Complications related to the spine, major vessels, and airway may require emergent surgical intervention. Early recognition is imperative.

Introduction

As with any medical procedure, the physician performing the procedure should weigh the benefits versus the risks. Interventional procedures have significant potential benefit for those suffering from chronic pain. Although uncommon, complications may result in catastrophic outcomes. This chapter reviews the complications associated with a diverse group of procedures, including head and neck blocks, upper extremity blocks, lower extremity blocks, and differential diagnostic blocks. The complications associated with these can generally be divided into vascular, infectious, neural,

pharmacologic, and anatomically related to the specific sight of injection (**Table 12-1**).

Vascular

Many neural structures are intimately connected with vasculature. Overall, the likelihood of a vascular complication is rare but potentially devastating. Reported vascular complications include airway, neural, and microvascular compression related to hematoma formation.[1-3] Additionally, arterial dissection, pseudoaneurysm, and vascular insufficiency secondary to vasospasm have all been cited in the literature.[4-6]

Table 12-1: Overview of Complications Associated with Head and Neck Block, Upper Extremity Block, Lower Extremity Block, and Differential Diagnostic Block Procedures

Vascular[1-6]	• Hematoma
	  • Airway compression
	  • Neural compression
	  • Microvascular compression
	• Vascular insufficiency secondary to vasospasm
	• Artery dissection
	• Pseudoaneurysm

Infectious	• Abscess • Septic arthritis • Meningitis • Discitis

Pharmacologic	• Local anesthetic
	  • CNS toxicity
	  • Cardiovascular toxicity
	  • High or total spinal
	• Steroid
	  • Pituitary adrenal axis suppression
	  • Particulate steroid-induced vascular occlusion

Neural[2,14-16]	• Direct needle trauma • Barotrauma from high-pressure injection • Compression from hematoma • Local anesthetic neural toxicity

CNS, central nervous system.

Infection

The likelihood of infection from any single injection is extremely rare. Infection requiring intervention after an indwelling catheter has been reported as high as 0.8%.[7] With interventional procedures involving the neuraxis, terrible sequelae, including epidural abscess or meningitis, may occur. Evidence demonstrates that catheter insertion (particularly >48 hours), intensive care unit admission, male sex, lack of prophylactic antibiotics, and lack of provider experience increase the likelihood of infection.[8]

Local Anesthetic Toxicity

The proximity of many neural structures to major vessels predisposes itself to the potential for local anesthetic toxicity. Inadvertent vascular puncture is the most likely cause of toxicity, but it has been suggested that with no identifiable puncture, clinical doses may cause toxicity.[9] It appears that clinically significant local anesthetic toxicity occurs between 7.5 and 20 times per 10000 regional anesthetics.[10] Local anesthetic toxicity can be categorized by symptoms involving the central nervous system (CNS) and those related to cardiovascular toxicity (**Table 12-2**).

Neurologic

The likelihood of long-term neurologic injury is low, reported below 0.02%.[13] When these injuries do occur, the outcome is often devastating to the clinician and patient alike. Nerve injury may present in a spectrum from paresthesias to paralysis, with neuropathic pain being a dreaded outcome.

Etiologies attributed to nerve injury include direct needle trauma, barotrauma from high-pressure injection, compression from hematoma, and local anesthetic neural toxicity.[2,14-16]

Table 12-2: Signs and Symptoms Associated with Local Anesthetic Toxicity

Central nervous system[11]	• Lightheadedness • Dizziness • Blurred vision • Tinnitus • Disorientation • Muscle twitching • Tonic-clonic seizure
Cardiovascular[12]	• Initially hypertension and tachycardia caused by CNS excitation • Myocardial depression • Ventricular arrhythmias • Conduction delays • Profound contractile dysfunction • Eventual cardiovascular collapse

CNS, central nervous system.

Complications of Head and Neck Blocks

Head and neck blocks are indispensable in management of various orofacial pain and headache syndromes. However, because of the limited space and close proximity to important structures such as arteries, nerves, brain, and lungs, there is potential for significant complications. The most common complications of head and neck procedures are related to injury to blood vessels leading to bleeding and systemic toxicity from vascular or subdural injection of local anesthetics, which can cause seizure, hemodynamic instability, or even cardiac arrest. Therefore, image-guided (fluoroscopy or ultrasonography) needle placement is highly recommended when performing procedures in the head and neck area. The collateral damage to surrounding structures from needle, radiofrequency ablation (RFA), chemical ablation, or balloon compression can vary depending on the specific anatomic location of the targets.

A variety of percutaneous techniques are available for targets at head and neck, including sphenopalatine ganglion (SPG), Gasserian ganglion, atlantoaxial joint (AAJ) and atlantooccipital joint (AOJ), stellate ganglion, and C2 dorsal root ganglion. See **Table 12-3** for a description of complications associated with head and neck injections.

Gasserian Ganglion Block and Neurolysis

The Gasserian (trigeminal) ganglion lies within the Meckel cave, which contains cerebrospinal fluid (CSF), and local anesthetic deposited in this area may spread to other cranial nerves and can potentially cause brainstem anesthesia.[17] Infection, CSF leak, bleeding, and nerve damage are also likely with Gasserian ganglion block or ablation because it is located in the middle of the brain surrounded by blood vessels. Literature studies show that RFA of the Gasserian ganglion is associated with the highest incidence of complications, with nearly one-third of patients developing some form of complications.[18] Postoperative trigeminal sensory loss affects virtually all patients treated with RFA, and it is considered a side effect rather than a complication.

Sphenopalatine Ganglion Block

Epistaxis is more frequent with an intranasal approach to SPG block; intravascular injection or hematoma formation can occur after maxillary artery injury, which lies within the pterygopalatine fossa (PPF). Cheek hematoma is the most common complication. Infection is always possible especially with inadvertent needle entry into the nasal or oral cavity.[19] Reflex bradycardia is likely with RFA

Table 12-3: Common Head and Neck Blocks with Associated Complications

Gasserian ganglion block and neurolysis[17,32]	• Brainstem anesthesia • Significant bleed • CSF leak • Permanent trigeminal sensory loss
SPG block[20-24]	• Cheek hematoma (most common complication) • Epistaxis (more frequent with intranasal approach) • Intravascular injection • Hematoma formation within the PPF • Reflex bradycardia is likely with RFA because of the rich parasympathetic connections to the SPG • Permanent or temporary hyperesthesia or dysesthesia in the palate, maxilla, or posterior pharynx • Temporary diplopia
AAJ and AOJ injections[19]	• Seizure secondary to vertebral artery injection • CSF leak • High spinal • Spinal cord injury • Syringomyelia
Stellate ganglion block[1,33,34]	• Horner syndrome • Recurrent laryngeal nerve block • Vagus nerve block • Phrenic nerve block • Hematoma • Airway compromise • Disc perforation • Esophageal perforation • High spinal block
C2 dorsal root ganglion injection	• Total spinal block leading to a rapid decrease in blood pressure and difficulty breathing • Seizure • Bleeding • Infection • Increased pain • Nerve damage, paralysis, stroke, and even death

AAJ, atlantoaxial joint; AOJ, atlantooccipital joint; CSF, cerebrospinal fluid; PPF, pterygopalatine fossa; RFA, radiofrequency ablation; SPG, sphenopalatine ganglion.

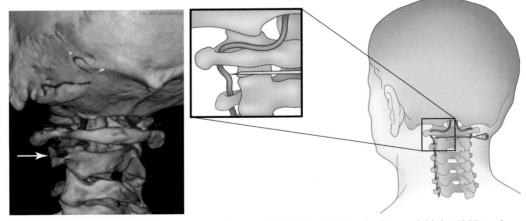

Fig. 12-1 The close proximity of the vertebral artery to the atlantooccipital joint (AOJ) and atlantoaxial joint (AAJ) to the vertebral artery results in a significant risk of intraarterial injection. (Modified from Edlow BL, Wainger BJ, Frosch MP, et al: Posterior circulation stroke after C1-C2 intraarticular facet steroid injection: evidence for diffuse microvascular injury, *Anesthesiology* 112:1532-1535, 2010.)

because of the rich parasympathetic connections to the SPG.[20] RFA of the SPG can result in permanent or temporary hyperesthesia or dysesthesia in the palate, maxilla, or posterior pharynx.[21-23] Temporary diplopia, which is more common after local anesthetic injections rather than RFA, is caused by the spread of the injectate from the PPF to the inferior orbital fissure containing the abducent nerve.[24] Temporary diplopia is likely if the needle tip is deep inside the PPF and the volume of injectate is greater than 1 to 2 mL.

Atlantoaxial Joint and Atlantooccipital Joint Injections

The AAJ and AOJ are in very close proximity to the vertebral artery (**Fig. 12-1**). Consequently, particular attention should be paid to avoid intravascular injection because vertebral artery anatomy can be unpredictable. Intraarterial injection may cause seizure or posterior circulation stroke.[25] Inadvertent puncture of the C2 dural sleeve with CSF leak or high spinal spread of the local anesthetic may occur with AAJ injection if the needle is directed too medially.

This can result in a rapid and profound decrease in blood pressure followed by apnea and death. Therefore, intravenous access should be established before the procedure. Spinal cord injury and syringomyelia are potential serious complications if the needle is directed even further medially.[19]

Stellate Ganglion Block

Many important structures lie close to the stellate ganglion. Hence, technical complications from injury to the nerves and viscera are possible during insertion of the needle.[17,26,27] This includes injury to the brachial plexus; trauma to the trachea and esophagus; injury to the pleura and lung (pneumothorax, hemothorax, which may require chest tube insertion); and bleeding and local hematoma, especially if the patient was taking anticoagulants. This can lead to airway compression (**Fig. 12-2**).[28,29] Vasovagal attacks can also occur, especially with inadvertent manipulation of carotid sinus during the block. Infectious complications are possible if there was a breach in the aseptic barrier. These can include local abscess, cellulitis, and osteitis of the vertebral body and transverse process.[30]

Complications related to the injectates include dose, volume, type of local anesthetic and site of deposition of the solution. Accidental block of the recurrent laryngeal nerve can cause hoarseness of voice while phrenic nerve paralysis can lead to respiratory depression especially if there is contralateral dysfunction of the phrenic nerve, or in patients with a preexisting respiratory problem. Therefore, bilateral stellate ganglia block is generally not recommended.[17,26] Intraarterial injection into the vertebral artery or the carotid artery can produce a high concentration of local anesthetic agent in the CNS, leading to seizures. Intravenous injection can also lead to seizure, if a high volume of local anesthetic is used.[17] Medial epidural spread and intrathecal injection of local anesthetic, producing high spinal blockade, has also been documented. Horner syndrome is often the final consequence of sympathetic blockade; although not a complication, it can be unpleasant. Air embolism

has also been reported. Loss of cardioaccelerator activity may lead to various bradyarrhythmias and hypotension.[17]

Complications from RFA are similar to the complications produced by local anesthetic sympathetic ganglia block, with the exception of a longer lasting block and potential neuritis. Because of an increased chance of injury to the surrounding structures, phenol or alcohol neurolysis is not recommended.[31]

C2 Dorsal Root Ganglion Injection

The C2 dorsal root ganglion block is an injection performed on the cervical spine to relieve headaches that originate from the C2 level. A needle is placed near the second cervical vertebral foramen at the location of the exiting C2 nerve root where the ganglion exists. Correct location of the needle tip should be always confirmed with the assistance of fluoroscopy before local anesthetic is injected or the ablation procedure is performed.

Complications of Upper Extremity Blocks

Upper extremity blockade is most commonly performed in the perioperative environment for intraoperative and postoperative analgesia. Physicians performing these procedures should consider the use of ultrasound to minimize the risks associated with peripheral nerve blocks. The majority of literature regarding this blockade comes from practitioners of regional anesthesia. However, upper extremity blockade may be a useful tool to the pain clinician for treatment and diagnosis. In the case of upper extremity neural blockade, complications can generally be divided into vascular, infectious, neural, local anesthetic toxicity, and anatomically related to the specific site of injection (**Table 12-4**). A large French study has reported that the overall incidence of serious complication from peripheral nerve block is 0.04%.[13]

The brachial plexus is intimately connected with a variety of vascular structures. Overall, the likelihood of a vascular complication is rare but potentially devastating. Reported vascular complications include hematoma, resulting in airway, neural, and microvascular compression.[1-3] Arterial dissection,

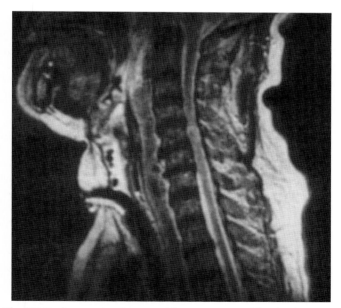

Fig. 12-2 Large retropharyngeal hematoma resulting in airway obstruction extending into the mediastinum after stellate ganglion block. Demonstrated on T2-weighted magnetic resonance image. (From Mishio M, Matsumoto T, Okuda Y, Kitajima T: Delayed severe airway obstruction due to hematoma following stellate ganglion block, *Reg Anesth Pain Med* 23:516-519, 1998.)

Table 12-4: Upper Extremity Blocks and Their Site-Specific Advantages and Complications	
Interscalene block[44-49]	• Pneumothoraces • Prolonged phrenic nerve palsy • Recurrent laryngeal nerve palsy • Prolonged Horner syndrome • Intrathecal block • Epidural block
Supraclavicular block[37-40]	• Transient phrenic nerve paresis (≈50% of patients) • Transient Horner syndrome • Recurrent laryngeal involvement • Pneumothorax
Infraclavicular block[38,39]	• Distanced from central and neuraxial structures • Pneumothoraces have been reported[42,43]
Axillary block[37]	• Distanced from the centroneuraxis structures • Increased potential for vascular uptake secondary to technique for injection

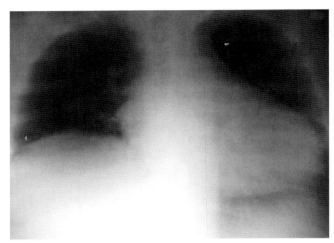

Fig. 12-3 Chest radiograph typical of a right phrenic nerve palsy after interscalene block. (From Cangiani L, Rezende L, Neto A: Phrenic nerve block after interscalene brachial plexus block. Case report, *Rev Bras Anestesiol* 58:7, 2008.)

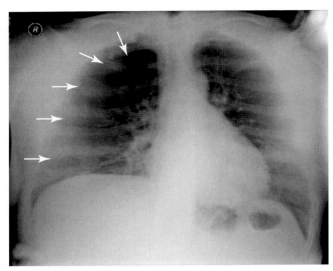

Fig. 12-4 Right pneumothorax (*arrows*) after a right supraclavicular block. (From Bhatia A, Lai J, Chan VW, Brull R: Case report: pneumothorax as a complication of the ultrasound-guided supraclavicular approach for brachial plexus block, *Anesth Analg* 111:817-819, 2010.)

pseudoaneurysm, and vascular insufficiency secondary to vasospasm have also been reported.[4-6]

The likelihood of long-term neural injury is low, reported below 0.02%.[13] When these injuries do occur, the outcome is often devastating to the clinician and patient alike. Nerve injury may present in a spectrum of paresthesias, paralysis, and neuropathic pain.

The proximity of the brachial plexus to major vascular structures predisposes itself to the potential for local anesthetic toxicity. Inadvertent vascular puncture is the most likely cause of toxicity, but it has been suggested that even with no identifiable puncture clinical doses may cause toxicity.[9] Clinically significant local anesthetic toxicity occurs between 7.5 and 20 times per 10,000 regional anesthetics.[10]

Interscalene Block

The approach at the interscalene level carries the greatest anatomic risk because it is adjacent to many central structures. Some reports state a complication rate as high as 1.1%[35] This approach yields an almost 100% incidence of unilateral phrenic nerve palsy (**Fig. 12-3**) and should be used with caution in those with respiratory insufficiency.[36]

Supraclavicular Block

The supraclavicular nerve block has the advantage of being slightly farther away from the central and neuraxial structures but does consistently miss the long thoracic and dorsal scapular nerves and may miss the subclavius and suprascapular nerves, all of which may be important to complete shoulder blockade.[3] It does, however, remain close enough that local anesthesia spread involves the phrenic nerve in about 50% of patients.[37] Additionally, reports have shown transient Horner syndrome and recurrent laryngeal involvement with this approach.[38,39] It has been suggested that there is an increased likelihood of pneumothorax with this approach compared with the infraclavicular approach (**Fig. 12-4**).[40,41]

Infraclavicular Block

Similarly to the axillary block, the infraclavicular approach is some distance from central and neuraxial structures. This provides some decreased risk of anatomically related complications. It must be

kept in mind that the pleural space is close to the neurovascular bundle at this level, and pneumothoraces have been reported.[42,43]

Axillary Block

The axillary injection site for brachial plexus blockade carries the least risk for structural injury and complication because of its distance from centroneuraxis structures. The one potential complication that some authors suggest is an increased potential for vascular uptake of the medication because of an increase in distance between intended neural structures, with most providers using a "fanlike" needle technique for injection.[37]

Complications of Lower Extremity Blocks

The incidence of nerve injury after neural block is very low.[50] An observational study demonstrated a 1.7% incidence of postoperative neurologic dysfunction after 3996 nerve blocks performed with multiple injection techniques.[51] Complications of lower extremity blocks share many characteristics that are similar from one to another (**Table 12-5**). The complications could be simply separated as local complications and systemic complications.

Local complications include nerve damage and injury to surrounding anatomic structures. Nerve puncture by the block needle and intraneural injection of local anesthetic is a feared complication and is thought to be a major contributor to neurologic injury after peripheral nerve blocks.[52] High injection pressure has also been postulated as a cause of neural injury.[15] Fortunately, it has been shown that injection of local anesthetics beyond the epineurium does not result in nerve damage.[52,53] Paresthesia or dysesthesia without motor deficit may be attributable to injury of the nervi nervorum, which innervate the epineurium and mesoneurium.[52] Leakage around the puncture site, especially when a catheter has been introduced, may favor bacterial contamination. Furthermore, infection may be a result of inadequate sterilization and might result in sepsis or CNS infection. The local complications are avoidable with adequate imaging modalities and applying standard operating procedures. Leakage around the catheter can be reduced

Table 12-5: Specific Complications Following Lower Limb Nerve Block

Psoas compartment block[57-60]	• Intrathecal (total spinal anesthesia) • Epidural spread • Intravascular injection • Peripheral nerve damage • Sympathetic block

Lumbar sympathetic block[62-65]	• Nerve damage
	  • Lumbar nerve root injury
	  • Genitofemoral neuralgia
	• Puncture of major vessel
	• Renal trauma
	• Ureteral trauma
	• Local anesthesia toxicity
	• Intrathecal block
	• Infectious
	  • Abscess
	  • Cellulitis
	  • Osteitis

Three-in-one (femoral) nerve block	• Intravascular injection • Hematoma • Nerve damage
Lateral femoral cutaneous nerve block	• Neuritis by needle trauma (unlikely) • Drug toxicity (unlikely) • Intravascular injection (rare)
Sciatic nerve block[51,68]	• Muscle trauma • Vascular puncture • Low risk of significant hypotension • Neuropathy or nerve damage
Nerve blocks at the ankle	• Multiple injections result in discomfort for the patient • Persisting paresthesias may occur but are usually self-limited • Intravascular injection is possible but unlikely • Low incidence of local anesthetic toxicity

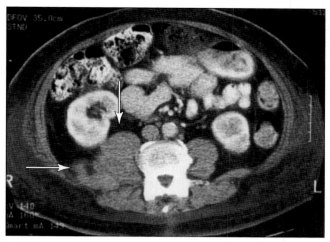

Fig. 12-5 A computed tomographic image demonstrating a large retroperitoneal hematoma (*arrows*) distorting the right psoas muscle.

by tunneling the catheter and applying a slightly compressive dressing.

Systemic complications usually result from accidental intravascular injection of local anesthetics; less frequently, overzealous administration has been implicated.[54,55] These complications can be life threatening, and both adults and children should be managed in the same way. The major difference between adults and children is that cardiovascular complications are often not preceded by neurologic signs but are concomitant with cerebral toxicity.[56] The incidence of systemic reactions to local anesthetics ranges between 3.9 and 11 in 10,000.[50]

As with upper extremity blockade, the vast majority of adverse event literature is generated from regional anesthesia. Lower extremity blocks do play a significant role for pain practitioners in regards to diagnosis and treatment of chronic pain conditions.

Psoas Compartment Block (Posterior Approach to the Lumbar Plexus)
Because of the anatomic location, blind technique in this region carries the potential for intrathecal injection with resulting total spinal anesthesia, large-volume injections are commonly associated with epidural spread with volumes greater than 20 mL.[57-60]

Peripheral nerve damage and sympathetic block from extravasation of local anesthetic are also reported with the paravertebral approach. Furthermore, case reports exist of retroperitoneal hematomas with associated lumbar plexopathies (**Fig. 12-5**).[61]

Lumbar Sympathetic Block
The lumbar sympathetic block is used for a variety of lower extremity sympathetically mediated disorders. Similar to the stellate ganglion block, complications related to this procedure are best characterized as anatomic, drug-related, or infectious. Traversing the lumbar roots for this procedure increases the likelihood of lumbar root injury. Furthermore, the close proximity of the lumbar plexus to major vessels increases the likelihood of vascular puncture.[62] Anatomic knowledge in combination with image guidance in this region is paramount because injury to vital structures, including renal and ureteral trauma, have been reported.[63,64] Furthermore, local anesthetic toxicity and intrathecal blocks have been reported.[65]

Perivascular Three-in-One (Femoral) Nerve Block
Femoral nerve block is frequently used in the perioperative period by regional anesthesiologists for analgesia with total knee replacements.[66] Complications related to this procedure include intravascular injection, hematoma, and nerve damage, all being reported infrequently.[13]

Lateral Femoral Cutaneous Nerve Block
Meralgia paresthetica is a neurologic disorder of the lateral femoral cutaneous nerve characterized by pain and paresthesia of the anterior lateral thigh. Blockade of the lateral femoral cutaneous nerve is often used more for diagnostic purposes rather than treatment. Complications of this block are rarely reported. It is recommended that ultrasonography be used for this procedure not only to minimize complication but also because of the high incidence of anatomic variation(≤25%).[67]

Sciatic Nerve Block
Again, the sciatic nerve block is more commonly used by regional anesthesiologists than chronic pain practitioners. It is most commonly used for major foot and ankle surgery. It can also be helpful

in diagnosis and treatment. Serious complications are rare but include muscle trauma and vascular puncture. Residual dysesthesias are frequently reported and usually last for 1 to 3 days with the remainder usually resolving within several months.[51,68] Blockade of the sciatic nerve most commonly occurs in the subgluteal region (Labat approach) or within the popliteal fossa. It is advisable to use ultrasonography to decrease the chance of needle puncture of adjacent vital structures.

Nerve Blocks at the Ankle

Multiple injections may result in discomfort for the patient. Persisting paresthesias may occur but are usually self-limited. Intravascular injection is possible but unlikely if aspiration for blood is negative. There is a low incidence of local anesthetic toxicity with this technique. Because of the small caliber of nerves at this level, blind techniques are most commonly used.

Differential Diagnostic Blocks

Differential diagnostic blocks are used to identify patients' varying pain complaints and to differentiate among placebo-responsive pain, sympathetic pain, somatic pain, and central pain. The two main approaches to doing a diagnostic differential nerve block are intrathecal and epidural. There are also two techniques, the anatomic approach and the pharmacologic approach. The anatomic approach uses the anatomic separation of somatic and sympathetic nervous system fibers, and the pharmacologic approach uses different concentrations of local anesthetic to affect different types of fibers.[64]

Doing a differential diagnostic block through the epidural approach is generally more time consuming because it takes longer for the blocks to occur and may provide confounding results; however, risks are thought to be decreased with the epidural approach. The complications of performing epidural and spinal differential diagnostic blocks can be related (**Box 12-1**), the most dreaded being an epidural abscess (**Fig. 12-6**).[64,65]

Summary

As with any procedure performed by a pain physician, the goal is to provide prolonged analgesia or assist in confirming a diagnosis. The procedures highlighted in this chapter do carry a specific burden of risk, being concurrently in close proximity to neural and vascular structures. Although the risk of developing a serious complication is rare, the risk, nonetheless, is ever present. Development of standardized procedural approaches, including preprocedure timeouts and sterile techniques in conjunction with a thorough understanding of relevant anatomy and appropriately chosen image guidance, is imperative to increasing procedural success while minimizing the likelihood of adverse events.

Box 12-1: Complications of Differential Diagnostic Block

Direct neural injury
Spinal cord puncture (reports only in sedated or anesthetic patients)
Dural puncture headache
Vasospastic or vasoocclusive (e.g., anterior spinal artery syndrome)
Epidural abscess
Meningitis
Discitis

Data from Hodges SD, Castleberg RL, Miller T, et al: Cervical epidural steroid injection with intrinsic spinal cord damage. Two case reports. *Spine (Phila Pa 1976)* 23: 1998; Benzon HT: Diagnostic nerve blocks. In Benzon HT, editor: *Essentials of pain medicine and regional anesthesia*, ed 2, Philadelphia, 2005, Elsevier-Churchill Livingstone; Bromage PR, Benumof JL: Paraplegia following intracord injection during attempted epidural anesthesia under general anesthesia. *Reg Anesth Pain Med* 23: 1998.

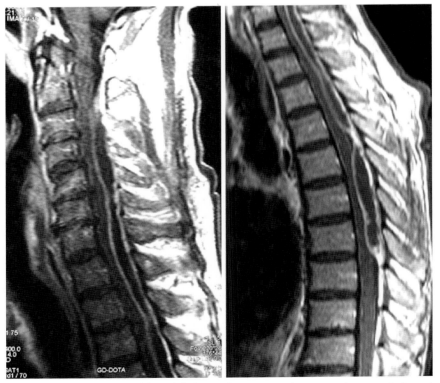

Fig. 12-6 T1-weighted magnetic resonance image with gadolinium enhancement demonstrating a posterior spinal epidural abscess from C2 to T8 after thoracic epidural catheter insertion. (From Payer M, Walser H: Evacuation of a 14-vertebral-level cervico-thoracic epidural abscess and review of surgical options for extensive spinal epidural abscesses, *J Clin Neurosci* 15:483-486, 2008.)

References

1. Higa K, Hirata K, Hirota K, et al: Retropharyngeal hematoma after stellate ganglion block: Analysis of 27 patients reported in the literature. *Anesthesiology* 105:1238-1245; discussion 5A-6A, 2006.

2. Ben-David B, Stahl S: Axillary block complicated by hematoma and radial nerve injury. *Reg Anesth Pain Med* 24:264-266, 1999.

3. Neal JM, Gerancher JC, Hebl JR, et al: Upper extremity regional anesthesia: essentials of our current understanding, 2008. *Reg Anesth Pain Med* 34:134-170, 2009.

4. Bhat R: Transient vascular insufficiency after axillary brachial plexus block in a child. *Anesth Analg* 98:1284-1285, table of contents, 2004.

5. Ott B, Neuberger L, Frey HP: Obliteration of the axillary artery after axillary block. *Anaesthesia* 44:773-774, 1989.

6. Flowers GA, Meyers JF: Pseudoaneurysm after interscalene block for a rotator cuff repair. *Arthroscopy* 20(suppl 2):67-69, 2004.

7. Neuburger M, Breitbarth J, Reisig F, et al: [Complications and adverse events in continuous peripheral regional anesthesia: results of investigations on 3,491 catheters]. *Anaesthesist* 55:33-40, 2006.

8. Capdevila X, Pirat P, Bringuier S, et al: Continuous peripheral nerve blocks in hospital wards after orthopedic surgery: a multicenter prospective analysis of the quality of postoperative analgesia and complications in 1,416 patients. *Anesthesiology* 103:1035-1045, 2005.

9. Dhir S, Ganapathy S, Lindsay P, Athwal GS: Case report: ropivacaine neurotoxicity at clinical doses in interscalene brachial plexus block. *Can J Anaesth* 54:912-916, 2007.

10. Mulroy MF: Systemic toxicity and cardiotoxicity from local anesthetics: incidence and preventive measures. *Reg Anesth Pain Med* 27:556-561, 2002.

11. Dillane D, Finucane BT: Local anesthetic systemic toxicity. *Can J Anaesth* 57:368-380, 2010.

12. Finucane BT: *Complications of regional anesthesia*, ed 2, New York, NY, 2007, Springer.

13. Auroy Y, Benhamou D, Bargues L, et al: Major complications of regional anesthesia in France. The SOS Regional Anesthesia Hotline Service. *Anesthesiology* 97:6, 2002.

14. Rice AS, McMahon SB: Peripheral nerve injury caused by injection needles used in regional anaesthesia: influence of bevel configuration, studied in a rat model. *Br J Anaesth* 69:433-438, 1992.

15. Hadzic A, Dilberovic F, Shah S, et al: Combination of intraneural injection and high injection pressure leads to fascicular injury and neurologic deficits in dogs. *Reg Anesth Pain Med* 29:417-423, 2004.

16. Hogan QH: Pathophysiology of peripheral nerve injury during regional anesthesia. *Reg Anesth Pain Med* 33:435-441, 2008.

17. Bridenbaugh PO, Cousins MJ: *Neural blockade in clinical anesthesia and management of pain*, ed 3, Philadelphia, 1998, Lippincott-Raven.

18. Lopez BC, Hamlyn PJ, Zakrzewska JM: Systematic review of ablative neurosurgical techniques for the treatment of trigeminal neuralgia. *Neurosurgery* 54:973-982; discussion 982-983, 2004.

19. Narouze S: Complications of head and neck procedures. *Tech Reg Anesth Pain Manage* 11:6, 2007.

20. Konen A: Unexpected effects due to radiofrequency thermocoagulation of the sphenopalatine ganglion: two case reports. *Pain Digest* 10:3, 2000.

21. Salar G, Ori C, Iob I, Fiore D: Percutaneous thermocoagulation for sphenopalatine ganglion neuralgia. *Acta Neurochir (Wien)* 84:24-28, 1987.

22. Sanders M, Zuurmond WW: Efficacy of sphenopalatine ganglion blockade in 66 patients suffering from cluster headache: a 12- to 70-month follow-up evaluation. *J Neurosurg* 87:876-880, 1997.

23. Narouze S, Kapural L, Casanova J, Mekhail N: Sphenopalatine ganglion radiofrequency ablation for the management of chronic cluster headache. *Headache* 49:571-577, 2009.

24. Narouze SN: Role of sphenopalatine ganglion neuroablation in the management of cluster headache. *Curr Pain Headache Rep* 14:160-163, 2010.

25. Edlow BL, Wainger BJ, Frosch MP, et al: Posterior circulation stroke after C1-C2 intraarticular facet steroid injection: evidence for diffuse microvascular injury. *Anesthesiology* 112:1532-1535, 2010.

26. Bonica JJ: *The management of pain*, ed 2, Philadelphia, 1990, Lea & Febiger.

27. Hogan QH, Abram SE: Neural blockade for diagnosis and prognosis. A review. *Anesthesiology* 86:216-241, 1997.

28. Elias M, Chakerian M: Repeated stellate ganglion blockade using a catheter for pediatric herpes zoster ophthalmicus. *Anesthesiology* 80:2, 1994.

29. Mishio M, Matsumoto T, Okuda Y, Kitajima T: Delayed severe airway obstruction due to hematoma following stellate ganglion block. *Reg Anesth Pain Med* 23:516-519, 1998.

30. Hartzler GO, Osborn MJ: Invasive electrophysiological study in the Jervell and Lange-Nielsen syndrome. *Br Heart J* 45:225-229, 1981.

31. Elias M: Cervical sympathetic and stellate ganglion blocks. *Pain Physician* 3:294-304, 2000.

32. Zakrzewska JM, Jassim S, Bulman JS: A prospective, longitudinal study on patients with trigeminal neuralgia who underwent radiofrequency thermocoagulation of the Gasserian ganglion. *Pain* 79:51-58, 1999.

33. Narouze S, Vydyanathan A, Patel N: Ultrasound-guided stellate ganglion block successfully prevented esophageal puncture. *Pain Physician* 10:747-752, 2007.

34. Whitehurst L, Harrelson JM: Brain-stem anesthesia. An unusual complication of stellate ganglion block. *J Bone Joint Surg Am* 59:541-542, 1977.

35. Lenters TR, Davies J, Matsen FA, 3rd: The types and severity of complications associated with interscalene brachial plexus block anesthesia: local and national evidence. *J Shoulder Elbow Surg* 16:379-387, 2007.

36. Cangiani L, Rezende L, Neto A: Phrenic Nerve block after interscalene brachial plexus block. Case report. *Rev Bras Anestesiol* 58:7, 2008.

37. Brown DL: Brachial plexus anesthesia: an analysis of options. *Yale J Biol Med* 66:415-431, 1993.

38. Solanki SL, Jain A, Makkar JK, Nikhar SA: Severe stridor and marked respiratory difficulty after right-sided supraclavicular brachial plexus block. *J Anesth* 25(2):305-307, 2011.

39. Perlas A, Lobo G, Lo N, et al: Ultrasound-guided supraclavicular block: outcome of 510 consecutive cases. *Reg Anesth Pain Med* 34:171-176, 2009.

40. Yang CW, Kwon HU, Cho CK, et al: A comparison of infraclavicular and supraclavicular approaches to the brachial plexus using neurostimulation. *Korean J Anesthesiol* 58:260-266, 2010.

41. Bhatia A, Lai J, Chan VW, Brull R: Case report: pneumothorax as a complication of the ultrasound-guided supraclavicular approach for brachial plexus block. *Anesth Analg* 111:817-819, 2010.

42. Sanchez HB, Mariano ER, Abrams R, Meunier M: Pneumothorax following infraclavicular brachial plexus block for hand surgery. *Orthopedics* 31:709, 2008.

43. Crews JC, Gerancher JC, Weller RS: Pneumothorax after coracoid infraclavicular brachial plexus block. *Anesth Analg* 105:275-277, 2007.

44. Borgeat A, Ekatodramis G, Kalberer F, Benz C: Acute and nonacute complications associated with interscalene block and shoulder surgery: a prospective study. *Anesthesiology* 95:875-880, 2001.

45. Urmey WF, Talts KH, Sharrock NE: One hundred percent incidence of hemidiaphragmatic paresis associated with interscalene brachial plexus anesthesia as diagnosed by ultrasonography. *Anesth Analg* 72:498-503, 1991.

46. Seltzer JL: Hoarseness and Horner's syndrome after interscalene brachial plexus block. *Anesth Analg* 56:585-586, 1977.

47. Sukhani R, Barclay J, Aasen M: Prolonged Horner's syndrome after interscalene block: a management dilemma. *Anesth Analg* 79:601-603, 1994.

48. Walter M, Rogalla P, Spies C, et al: [Intrathecal misplacement of an interscalene plexus catheter]. *Anaesthesist* 54:215-219, 2005.

49. Faust A, Fournier R, Hagon O, et al: Partial sensory and motor deficit of ipsilateral lower limb after continuous interscalene brachial plexus block. *Anesth Analg* 102:288-290, 2006.

50. Auroy Y, Narchi P, Messiah A, et al: Serious complications related to regional anesthesia: results of a prospective survey in France. *Anesthesiology* 87:479-486, 1997.

51. Fanelli G, Casati A, Garancini P, Torri G: Nerve stimulator and multiple injection technique for upper and lower limb blockade: failure rate, patient acceptance, and neurologic complications. Study Group on Regional Anesthesia. *Anesth Analg* 88:847-852, 1999.

52. Bigeleisen PE: Nerve puncture and apparent intraneural injection during ultrasound-guided axillary block does not invariably result in neurologic injury. *Anesthesiology* 105:779-783, 2006.

53. Sala-Blanch X, Pomes J, Matute P, et al: Intraneural injection during anterior approach for sciatic nerve block. *Anesthesiology* 101:1027-1030, 2004.

54. Mazoit JX, Dalens BJ: Pharmacokinetics of local anaesthetics in infants and children. *Clin Pharmacokinet* 43:17-32, 2004.

55. D'Andrea P, Calabrese A, Grandolfo M: Intercellular calcium signalling between chondrocytes and synovial cells in co-culture. *Biochem J* 329(Pt 3):681-687, 1998.

56. Maxwell LG, Martin LD, Yaster M: Bupivacaine-induced cardiac toxicity in neonates: successful treatment with intravenous phenytoin. *Anesthesiology* 80:682-686, 1994.

57. Awad IT, Duggan EM: Posterior lumbar plexus block: anatomy, approaches, and techniques. *Reg Anesth Pain Med* 30:143-149, 2005.

58. Capdevila X, Coimbra C, Choquet O: Approaches to the lumbar plexus: success, risks, and outcome. *Reg Anesth Pain Med* 30:150-162, 2005.

59. Capdevila X, Macaire P, Dadure C, et al: Continuous psoas compartment block for postoperative analgesia after total hip arthroplasty: new landmarks, technical guidelines, and clinical evaluation. *Anesth Analg* 94:1606-1613, table of contents, 2002.

60. Enneking FK, Chan V, Greger J, et al: Lower-extremity peripheral nerve blockade: essentials of our current understanding. *Reg Anesth Pain Med* 30:4-35, 2005.

61. Klein SM, D'Ercole F, Greengrass RA, Warner DS: Enoxaparin associated with psoas hematoma and lumbar plexopathy after lumbar plexus block. *Anesthesiology* 87:1576-1579, 1997.

62. Haynsworth RF, Jr, Noe CE, Fassy LR: Intralymphatic injection: another complication of lumbar sympathetic block. *Anesthesiology* 80:460-462, 1994.

63. Wheatley JK, Motamedi F, Hammonds WD: Page kidney resulting from massive subcapsular hematoma. Complication of lumbar sympathetic nerve block. *Urology* 24:361-363, 1984.

64. Dirim A, Kumsar S: Iatrogenic ureteral injury due to lumbar sympathetic block. *Scand J Urol Nephrol* 42:395-396, 2008.

65. Gay GR, Evans JA: Total spinal anesthesia following lumbar paravertebral block: a potentially lethal complication. *Anesth Analg* 50:344-348, 1971.

66. Sharma S, Iorio R, Specht LM, et al: Complications of femoral nerve block for total knee arthroplasty. *Clin Orthop Relat Res* 468:135-140, 2010.

67. Patijn J, Mekhail N, Hayek S, et al: Meralgia paresthetica. *Pain Pract* 11(3):302-308, 2011.

68. Auroy Y, Benhamou D, Bargues L, et al: Major complications of regional anesthesia in France: the SOS Regional Anesthesia Hotline Service. *Anesthesiology* 97:1274-1280, 2002.

13 Complications of Epidural Injections

Matthew T. Ranson

CHAPTER OVERVIEW

Chapter Synopsis: Epidural steroid injection (ESI) for the treatment of chronic pain requires physician expertise not only in the injection procedure itself but also in the technique of using fluoroscopic guidance. ESI carries risks associated with the injection as well as with the injected steroid. The lowest possible steroid dose should always be used to avoid drug effects. One possible complication of ESI is suppression of the hypothalamic–pituitary–adrenal axis. Transforaminal injections to the cervical spine should be carefully considered because they carry a greater risk of catastrophic complications.

Important Points:

- Epidural injections for the treatment of chronic pain should only be performed by well-trained physicians under fluoroscopic guidance.
- American Society of Regional Anesthesia guidelines should be consulted before neuraxial interventions on patients receiving anticoagulants. However, it is important to recognize these guidelines do not specifically address interventional pain procedures.
- The lowest dose of steroid that could be expected to have a clinical response should be used in the epidural space.
- No prospective data have shown that a large dose of steroid is superior to low doses.
- Cervical transforaminal injections should be approached with great caution and should only be performed when clinical issues suggest a specific nerve involved in the pain pattern.

Introduction

Epidural steroid injections (ESIs) have been associated with a myriad of complications and side effects. Although the overall incidence of complications from ESIs appears to be low,[1] there are some potentially catastrophic complications that should be considered by all physicians performing these procedures. There are two general categories of complications associated with ESIs: exogenous steroid side effects and complications associated with the actual placement of the needle by the physician performing the procedure. Complications associated with ESIs are discussed in this chapter and are organized into medication-associated complications and those complications that may result from the procedure.

Complications of Steroid Administration

Complications that may result from corticosteroid injections include hyperglycemia, Cushing syndrome, hypertension, deep venous thrombosis (DVT), secondary infections, psychological disorders, lipid accumulation (epidural lipomatosis), osteoporosis, vertebral compression fractures, avascular necrosis of joints, and numerous other endocrine and dermatologic manifestations.[2] Epidural steroid administration has been demonstrated to adversely affect native cortisol concentrations for up to 30 days from a single injection.[3] It is likely that suppression of the hypothalamic–pituitary–adrenal (HPA) axis is variable among individuals, but there is evidence that a series of three epidural injections with 40 mg of triamcinolone may suppress the HPA axis for up to 3 months.[2] Serious side effects such as steroid myopathy and Cushing syndrome have been reported after a single epidural dose of

triamcinolone.[4] Although the risk of complications from ESIs theoretically should increase with increasing frequency of injections, it appears that total dose of steroids given during a specific time may be more important in determining steroid complications.[5,6]

Particulate steroids have been under increasing scrutiny because of the theoretical risk of high particulate steroid preparations causing vascular events.

Recommendations for Avoiding Steroid Complications

The total annual dose of steroid should be limited to the smallest efficacious dose. Although there is insufficient evidence to determine the risks of epidural steroid administration, evidence suggests that large annual doses of steroids may lead to serious complications. There is no evidence that large doses of steroids are superior to low doses. Recommendations have been made to limit the amount of annual steroid dose to 3 mg/kg of triamcinolone or equivalent.[7] See **Tables 13-1** and **13-2** for commercially available steroid preparations and their relative potencies.

Transforaminal ESIs, especially in the cervical spine, have been reported to result in catastrophic complications, including stroke, paralysis, and death.[8] Although there are more case reports of complications with transforaminal injections in the cervical spine, there are some reports of neurologic injury in the lumbar spine.[9] Several mechanisms have been proposed for the development of anterior spinal artery syndrome, including mechanical trauma to a radicular artery supplying the anterior or posterior spinal arteries, vasospasm, and embolism resulting from particulate-containing steroids (**Figs. 13-1** and **13-2**).[10,11] The use of nonparticulate steroids has been suggested to be safer than particulate steroids when performing cervical transforaminal injections.[12] Cervical transforaminal injections should be approached with caution,[7] and prudent physicians should consider using nonparticulate steroid solutions such as dexamethasone when performing transforaminal epidural injections in the thoracic and upper lumbar spine.

Complications Associated with Needle Placement and Injection

Numerous complications are associated with needle placement during epidural steroid administration. Pneumocephalus, pneumothorax, vascular injection, epidural hematoma, subdural injection, infection (localized skin, meningitis, and epidural abscess formation), nerve damage, spinal cord trauma, cerebrovascular infarction, DVT, vasovagal episodes, and increased pain have all been reported during both interlaminar and transforaminal approaches to the neuraxis.[1] As with any invasive procedure, strict aseptic technique is mandatory. It has been reported that DuraPrep and alcohol-containing preparations are superior to iodine-containing antiseptic solutions in preventing infections.[13] Although ChloraPrep and DuraPrep solutions are not approved for epidural and intrathecal use, iodine has never received Food and Drug Administration approval for epidural injections.

Several studies have reported that between 25% and 40% of epidural injections performed without fluoroscopy are not delivered to the intended target.[14,15] Without the aid of fluoroscopy, the risk of intramuscular and inadvertent intrathecal injection may be substantially increased. Intrathecal injection can result in severe complications, including possible nerve injury from preservative-containing solutions, arachnoiditis, aseptic meningitis, cerebral vein thrombosis, adhesive arachnoiditis, and pneumocephaly.[16,17]

Transforaminal epidural injections are usually indicated in the treatment of radicular pain confined to one or two dermatomes.[7] There have been numerous reports of catastrophic complications associated with the transforaminal approach with most of the case reports involving the cervical region.[8,11] Most of the complications associated with the transforaminal approach have resulted in paralysis, presumably from anterior spinal syndrome, although smaller vessels and feeder arteries may also play a role. Although several mechanisms have been proposed for the development of anterior spinal artery syndrome, it is likely that the syndrome results from direct injury to a radicular artery or from embolism resulting from injection of high-particulate steroid into a radicular artery supplying the anterior spinal cord. Another proposed mechanism may be vasospasm without true embolism.[10] Epidural hematoma formation is a significant but uncommon complication in patients receiving anticoagulation therapies (**Fig. 13-3**). Epidural hematoma formation has been estimated to occur in one in 150,000 to one in 220,000 patients undergoing neuraxial procedures.[18] Although the risk of epidural hematoma in patients taking agents such as clopidogrel and warfarin seems well established, it is unclear when it is safe to perform ESIs in many of these patients. Discontinuing antifibrinolytic medications for 7 to 10 days has previously been recommended, but there are no data to establish when it is safe to perform neuraxial procedures in patients treated with these medications.[19] Additionally, there has never been a clear relationship established between aspirin administration and epidural hematoma formation. Recommendations published by the American Society of Regional Anesthesia and Pain Management (ASRA) attempt to provide guidelines for discontinuing anticoagulation in patients who are to undergo neuraxial procedures. These guidelines are based on the current scientific literature, but we will see many new drugs that impact clotting arising over the next few years, and these guidelines may not cover the new drugs appropriately.[19] It is

Table 13-1: Commercially Available Steroids

Steroid	Available Concentrations (mg/mL)	Typical Doses (mg)
Depo-Medrol (methylprednisolone)	40, 80	40-80
Celestone (betamethasone)	6	6-12
Kenalog (triamcinolone)	25, 40	40-80
Decadron (dexamethasone)	4, 8	4-10

Adapted from Deer T, Ranson M, Kappural L, Diwan SA: Guidelines for the proper use of epidural steroid injections for the chronic pain patient, *Tech Reg Anesth Pain Manage* 13(4):288-295, 2009.

Table 13-2: Relative Potencies of Steroids

Steroid	Half-Life (hr)	Relative Glucocorticoid Activity	Relative Mineralocorticoid Activity	Glucocorticoid Dose Equivalency (mg)	Relative Antiinflammatory Activity
Hydrocortisone	8-12	1	1	20	NAE
Cortisone	8-12	0.8	0.6	25	1
Prednisone	8-36	4	0.8	5	NAE
Prednisolone	8-36	4	0.8	5	3
Methylprednisone	18-36	5	0.5	4	6.2
Triamcinolone	18-36	5	0	4	5
Dexamethasone	36-54	20-30	0	0.75	26
Betamethasone	36-54	20-30	0	0.6	NAE

NAE, no available equivalency.
Adapted from Harris E: *Kelley's textbook of rheumatology*, 7th ed, Philadelphia, 2005, Saunders.

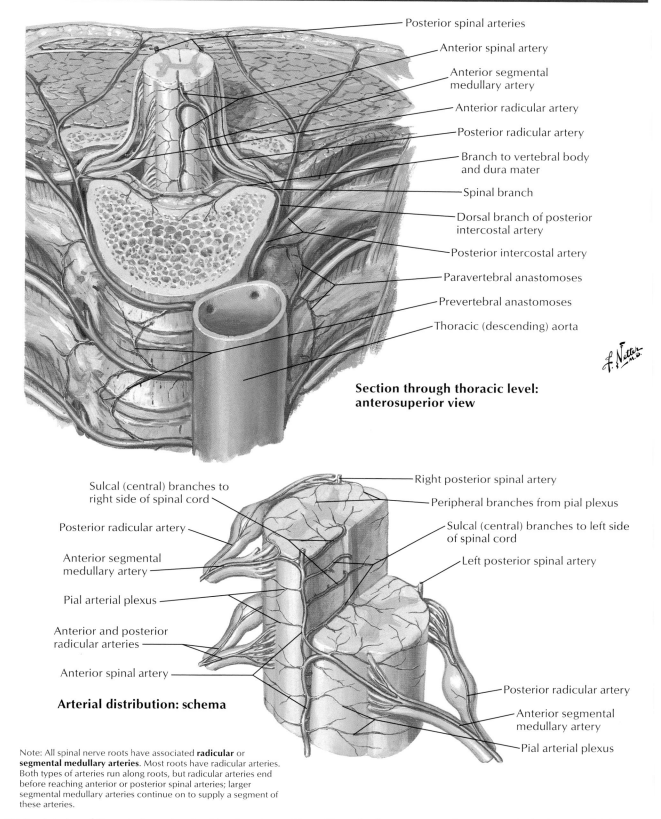

Posterior spinal arteries

Anterior spinal artery

Anterior segmental medullary artery

Anterior radicular artery

Posterior radicular artery

Branch to vertebral body and dura mater

Spinal branch

Dorsal branch of posterior intercostal artery

Posterior intercostal artery

Paravertebral anastomoses

Prevertebral anastomoses

Thoracic (descending) aorta

Section through thoracic level: anterosuperior view

Sulcal (central) branches to right side of spinal cord

Posterior radicular artery

Anterior segmental medullary artery

Pial arterial plexus

Anterior and posterior radicular arteries

Anterior spinal artery

Arterial distribution: schema

Right posterior spinal artery

Peripheral branches from pial plexus

Sulcal (central) branches to left side of spinal cord

Left posterior spinal artery

Posterior radicular artery

Anterior segmental medullary artery

Pial arterial plexus

Note: All spinal nerve roots have associated **radicular** or **segmental medullary arteries**. Most roots have radicular arteries. Both types of arteries run along roots, but radicular arteries end before reaching anterior or posterior spinal arteries; larger segmental medullary arteries continue on to supply a segment of these arteries.

Fig. 13-1 Arteries of the spinal canal and epidural anatomy. (Netter illustration from www.netterimages.com. © Elsevier, Inc. All rights reserved.)

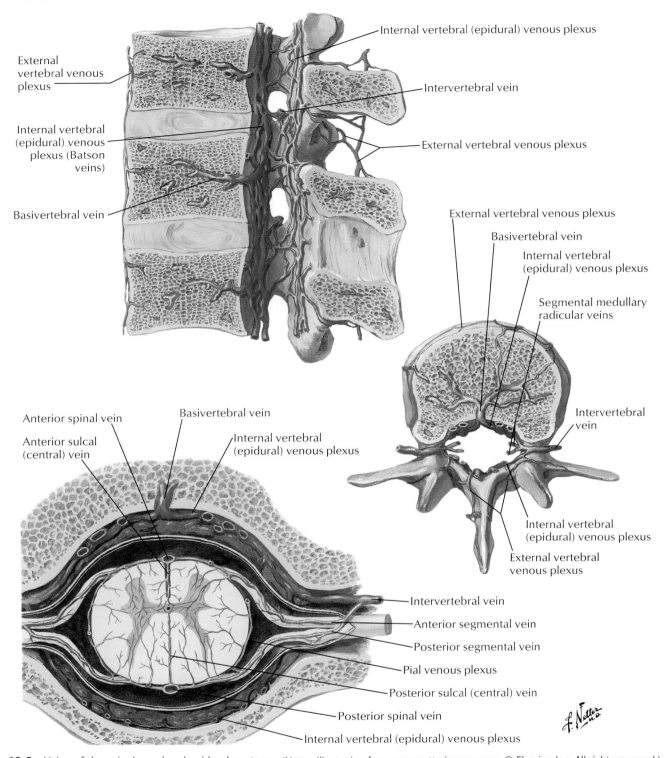

Fig. 13-2 Veins of the spinal canal and epidural anatomy. (Netter illustration from www.netterimages.com. © Elsevier, Inc. All rights reserved.)

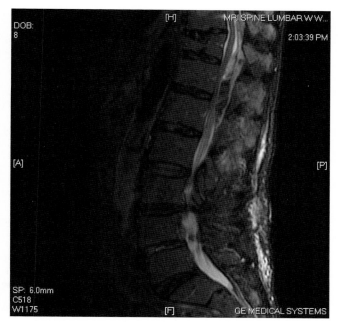

Fig. 13-3 Magnetic resonance image of epidural hematoma. (Courtesy of Timothy Deer, MD.)

Table 13-3: Complications Reported from Epidural Steroid Administration

Epidural hematoma	Cushing syndrome
Epidural abscess	Hypertension
Paralysis and quadriplegia	Deep vein thrombosis
Death	Secondary infections
Steroid induce mania	Psychological manifestations
Osteoporosis and vertebral compression fractures	Epidural lipomatosis
Suppression of the hypothalamic–pituitary–adrenal axis	Avascular necrosis of joints
Hyperglycemia	

important to consult with the treating cardiologist or neurologist when these guidelines are not inclusive of the issue in question.

Recommendations for Avoiding Complications Associated with Needle Placement

All physicians performing epidural injections should receive adequate training in the use of fluoroscopy as well as techniques of epidural needle placement by experienced physicians. Weekend courses, such as those presented at national meetings, are not sufficient to provide the training and expertise necessary for physicians to safely perform epidural injections. Additionally, although some physicians have traditionally allowed physician extenders to place epidural catheters for parturients under their supervision, given the risks of catastrophic complications that can arise from epidural needle placement, these procedures should be limited only to physicians who have received extensive training in such procedures.

Traditional injection techniques and targets to transforaminally access the epidural space have recently been challenged because injury to the artery of Adamkiewicz can be described as a "black swan" event. Furthermore, traditional needle trajectory and a target in the superior anterior portion of the foramen, directed to the "safe triangle," places the needle tip anatomically where the vasculature resides, increasing the chance of vascular injury. To avoid potential vascular injury, some physicians recommend an inferior approach to the foramen, targeting the Kambin triangle.[20]

All epidural injections should be performed with fluoroscopy. Although there is no clear consensus regarding the use of contrast and digital subtraction fluoroscopy, it seems prudent to use contrast in all transforaminal procedures. Cervical transforaminal epidural injections have not been demonstrated to be more efficacious than the interlaminar approach and have resulted in significant injuries; therefore they should be used only in cases in which the risk is believed to be outweighed by the benefit. Low-particulate steroid compounds such as dexamethasone should be considered when entering the cervical, thoracic, or upper lumbar spine. No large prospective studies have compared nonparticulate steroids with particulate steroids in the treatment of patients with chronic pain, however, some are worth mentioning. A recent prospective, blinded study examined 61 patients randomly assigned to either particulate or nonparticulate steroids of equipotent doses to treat lumbar radicular pain, examining VAS, complications, medication adjustments, and additional therapeutic interventions. The investigators concluded that nonparticulate steroid is very comparable to safety and effectiveness as particulate steroid for the treatment of lumbar radicular pain, with a statistically nonsignificant trend of less lengthy pain relief and magnitude.[21] Similarly, another prospective randomized study compared equipotent particulate versus nonparticulate steroid injections in 106 patients with lumbar radiculopathy, concluding that nonstatistically significant differences were determined for McGill Pain Questionnaire, or the Oswestry Disability Index, where a statistically significant difference was apparent for the VAS (visual analog scale) in favor of particulate steroid injections.[22]

Given the superior antiseptic properties of ChloraPrep compared with iodine, it is recommended that physicians use alcohol-containing solutions such as ChloraPrep when performing epidural injections. ASRA consensus guidelines should be consulted regarding anticoagulation medications before performing epidural procedures in anticoagulated patients. Although aspirin poses a theoretical risk of epidural hematoma formation in patients undergoing ESIs, discontinuing aspirin in a patient with significant cardiovascular disease should be contemplated with caution because of the lack of evidence implicating aspirin in epidural hematoma formation. When possible, the treating cardiologist should be consulted regarding issues of anticoagulants.

Conclusion

Conscientious physicians perform ESIs only on patients who have been thoroughly evaluated and have undergone all appropriate laboratory evaluations, including coagulation studies if indicated. ESIs should only be performed by qualified physicians who have the proper training to perform these procedures safely and properly with fluoroscopic guidance. Ultrasonography is emerging and may be an alternative to fluoroscopy in the future. Serious complications and death have been reported from epidural steroid administration (**Table 13-3**). Physicians who have not completed residency or fellowship training that included interventional pain management training are strongly encouraged to pursue postgraduate training in an accredited fellowship program in interventional pain management before performing ESIs.

References

1. Abdi S, Datta S, Lucas LF: Role of epidural steroids in the management of chronic spinal pain: a systematic review of effectiveness and complications. *Pain Physician* 8(1):127-143, 2005.
2. Manchikanti L: Role of neuraxial steroids in interventional pain management. *Pain Physician* 5(2):182-199, 2002.
3. Dubois EF, Wagemans MF, Verdouw BC, et al: Lack of relationships between cumulative methylprednisolone dose and bone mineral density in healthy men and postmenopausal women with chronic low back pain. *Clin Rheumatol* 22(1):12-17, 2003.
4. Boonen S, Van Distel G, Westhovens R, Dequeker J: Steroid myopathy induced by epidural triamcinolone injection. *Br J Rheumatol* 34(4): 385-386, 1995.
5. Knight CL, Burnell JC: Systemic side-effects of extradural steroids. *Anaesthesia* 35(6):593-594, 1980.
6. Kay J, Findling JW, Raff H: Epidural triamcinolone suppresses the pituitary-adrenal axis in human subjects. *Anesth Analg* 79(3):501-505, 1994.
7. Deer T, Ranson M, Kappural L, Diwan SA: Guidelines for the proper use of epidural steroid injections for the chronic pain patient. *Tech Reg Anesth Pain Manage* 13(4):288-295, 2009.
8. Scanlon GC, Moeller-Bertram T, Romanowsky SM, Wallace MS: Cervical transforaminal epidural steroid injections: more dangerous than we think? *Spine (Phila Pa 1976)* 32(11):1249-1256, 2007.
9. Huntoon MA Martin DP: Paralysis after transforaminal epidural injection and previous spinal surgery. *Reg Anesth Pain Med* 29(5):494-495, 2004.
10. Baker R, Dreyfuss P, Mercer S, Bogduk N: Cervical transforaminal injection of corticosteroids into a radicular artery: a possible mechanism for spinal cord injury. *Pain* 103(1-2):211-215, 2003.
11. Rathmell JP, Aprill C, Bogduk N: Cervical transforaminal injection of steroids. *Anesthesiology* 100(6):1595-1600, 2004.
12. Anwar A, Zaidah I, Rozita R: Prospective randomized single blind study of epidural steroid injection comparing triamcinolone acetonide with methylprednisolone acetate. *APLAR J Rheumatol* 8:1-53, 2005.
13. Birnbach DJ, Meadows W, Stein DJ, et al: Comparison of povidone iodine and DuraPrep, an iodophor-in-isopropyl alcohol solution, for skin disinfection prior to epidural catheter insertion in parturients. *Anesthesiology* 98(1):164-169, 2003.
14. White AH, Derby R, Wynne G: Epidural injections for the diagnosis and treatment of low-back pain. *Spine (Phila Pa 1976)* 5(1):78-86, 1980.
15. White AH: Injection techniques for the diagnosis and treatment of low back pain. *Orthop Clin North Am* 14(3):553-567, 1983.
16. Abram SE: Intrathecal steroid injection for postherpetic neuralgia: what are the risks? *Reg Anesth Pain Med* 24(4):283-285, 1999.
17. Mateo E, López-Alarcón MD, Moliner S, et al: Epidural and subarachnoidal pneumocephalus after epidural technique. *Eur J Anaesthesiol* 16(6):413-417, 1999.
18. Tryba M: [Epidural regional anesthesia and low molecular heparin: Pro]. *Anasthesiol Intensivmed Notfallmed Schmerzther* 28(3):179-181, 1993.
19. Horlocker TT, Wedel DJ, Benzon H, et al: Regional anesthesia in the anticoagulated patient: defining the risks (the second ASRA Consensus Conference on Neuraxial Anesthesia and Anticoagulation). *Reg Anesth Pain Med* 28(3):172-197, 2003.
20. Glaser SE, Shah RV: Root cause analysis of paraplegia following transforaminal epidural injections: the unsafe triangle. *Pain Physician* 13:237-244, 2010.
21. Kim D, Brown J. Efficacy and safety of lumbar epidural dexamethasone versus methylprednisolone in the treatment of lumbar radiculopathy: A comparison of soluble versus particulate steroids. *Clin J Pain* 27:518-522, 2011.
22. Park CH, Lee SH, Kim, BI. Comparison of effectiveness of lumbar transforaminal epidural injection with particulate and nonparticulate corticosteroids in lumbar radiating pain. *Pain Medicine* 11: 1654-1658, 2010.

14 Complications of Facet Joint Injections and Medial Branch Blocks

Jason E. Pope

CHAPTER OVERVIEW

Chapter Synopsis: Facet joint injections and medial branch blocks present highly effective treatments for facetogenic chronic pain arising from facet arthropathy. Most serious complications can be avoided with the usual precautions including careful patient selection and guidance using either fluoroscopy or ultrasonography. Intimate knowledge of spinal cord anatomy and interventional techniques by the physician also ensures a safe procedure. Uncommon but severe complications can arise, most commonly procedure-related nerve damage and infections. Disastrous consequences may be prevented by careful attention to any postinjection signs of complications.

Important Points:

- Appropriate Accreditation Council for Graduate Medical Education mentored subspecialty training in interventional pain management is vital to ensure patient-centered care.
- A thorough understanding of the spinal anatomy is vital to procedural success. Extrapolation of three-dimensional needle placement using two-dimensional ultrasound and fluoroscopic guidance is crucial for accurate needle placement.
- Although uncommon, devastating complications from facetogenic intraarticular or median branch injections have been reported.
- Infectious complications can be severe, and diagnosis centers on a high index of suspicion, initiation of intravenous antibiotic therapy, and prompt neurosurgical consultation for neurologic deterioration for decompression.
- Injection under live fluoroscopy with digital subtraction may help elucidate intravascular needle placement.

Introduction

Facetogenic sources of pain are common, accounting for approximately 40% of thoracic and cervical complaints and 30% of lumbar pain.[1-7] These are disorders of older adults; 89.2% of people 60 to 69 years of age have facet joint arthropathy,[8] but there is little correlation in the cervical and thoracic regions. Predicatively, facetogenic interventions are the second most commonly used and gratifying procedures performed by pain management physicians in the United States because they are relatively easy to perform with reliable radiographic landmarks, very good outcomes, and reported complications described to occur very rarely.

In a recent guideline statement, the American Society of Interventional Pain Physicians did not recommend intraarticular injections for either diagnostic or therapeutic benefit (level III evidence).[9] The International Spine Intervention Society described thoracic intraarticular injections as emerging procedures and did not provide any comments on the cervical or lumbar level.[10] The American Society of Anesthesiologists Task Force on Chronic Pain Management and the American Society of Regional Anesthesia (ASRA) and Pain Medicine reported that randomized placebo controlled trials demonstrated equivocal evidence supporting intraarticular injections, and although observational studies provided evidence for short-term pain relief, they summarily described the evidence as "may be used for symptomatic relief of facet-mediated pain."[11] Both guidelines suggest better evidence (level I or II) with median branch injections for diagnostic and therapeutic benefit using 80% pain reduction with two

comparative controlled diagnostic blocks, and based on Guyatt et al's[12] criteria, IB recommendations for radiofrequency (RF) neurotomy.[9]

By definition, facet arthropathy is diagnosed by a positive response to an intervention (i.e., controlled diagnostic injections). Commonly, this is performed with local anesthetic in combination with steroid or alone. The response is gauged by pain relief concordance and is very dependent on technique; specificity depends on the quantity of injectate. Therapeutically, facetogenic interventions center on intraarticular steroid injections; median branch steroid injections; or RF treatment using traditional (thermal), pulsed, or cooled modalities.

Complication avoidance begins with patient selection because treatment of patients with local infection near the injection site, coagulopathy, allergy to injectate, or comorbidities or conditions that preclude fluoroscopic guidance should be avoided. Appreciation and clear understanding of spinal anatomy and utilization of image guidance during needle placement are vital to ensure both quality treatment and reduced patient morbidity and mortality. Furthermore, it should be understood that appropriate training within Accreditation Council for Graduate Medical Education accredited programs and mentorship is vital to ensure treatment success; interventional hobbyists only serve to undermine accessibility of these valuable therapies to patients.

Despite appropriate care, significant and devastating complications have been described as scattered case reports, including radicular artery injury and epidural abscesses (**Box 14-1**).

Box 14-1: Complication Classification

Procedural
Vascular injury
Hematoma or bleeding
Disc injury
Postdural puncture headache
Spinal anesthesia
Neuritis
Radiofrequency treatment complications
Nerve root injury
Pneumothorax
Local postprocedural pain

Infectious
Discitis
Epidural abscess
Septic arthritis
Meningitis
Intraspinal abscess
Paraspinal abscess

Pharmacologic
Pituitary adrenal axis suppression
Local anesthetic epidural or spinal spread

Selected Complications

Vascular Injury

Briefly, the perfusion of the spinal cord depends on one anterior and two posterior vascular supplies. Paired posterior spinal arteries, arising from the posterior inferior cerebellar arteries, perfuse the posterior third of the spinal cord. The anterior spinal artery, which is a branch of the vertebral artery after it ascends through the foramen transversarium, perfuses the anterior two-thirds of the spinal cord. Unlike the posterior blood supply, the solitary anterior spinal artery requires staggered reinforcement by anterior segmental medullary arteries, and consequently, perfusion is more tenuous, and the anterior spinal cord is more susceptible to injury.

Huntoon[13] investigated cervical blood flow in a cadaveric study and noted that the ascending and deep cervical arterial branches may contribute significantly to the anterior segmental arteries, and anterior spinal artery flow may be susceptible to injury during interventional procedures (**Fig. 14-1**). There have been unpublished reports of quadriplegia from vascular occlusion by particulate steroid after attempted cervical zygapophyseal interventions. Despite well-described lateral and prone approaches for cervical median branch blocks and rhizotomies, the prone technique hypothetically may be safer because there are more reliable osteal landmarks during needle placement; however, comparative studies are lacking.

Image guidance is required. Tetraplegia was reported in a case using only landmarks to guide needle placement[14] and is not advocated. Image guidance, by either ultrasound or fluoroscopic means, is essential.

The most publicized and largest segmental spinal artery is the artery of Adamkiewicz. It is vitally important to reinforce the American Society of Anesthesiologists in the thoracolumbar region. It has a variable anatomic course. The Adamkiewicz artery is typically located between T8 and L3, but it is at T9 or T10 in 50% of people and comes from the left side in 75% of cases. Additional radiculomedullary arteries were found in 43% of patients.[15,16]

These important reinforcing segmental spinal arteries have variable location segmentally (**Fig. 14-2**) but consistent intraforaminal anatomy as they course in the superior anterior location of the

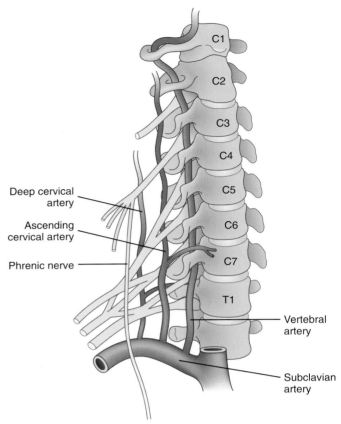

Fig. 14-1 Ascending and deep cervical arterial branches may contribute significantly to the anterior segmental and anterior spinal arterial flow.

foramen beneath the pedicle.[17] Obviously, inadvertent needle placement can result in injury. Despite well-described lateral and prone approaches for cervical median branch blocks and rhizotomies, the prone technique hypothetically may be safer because there are more reliable osteal landmarks during needle placement; however, comparative studies are lacking.

Huntoon[13] investigated cervical blood flow in a cadaveric study and noted that the ascending and deep cervical arterial branches may contribute significantly to the anterior segmental arteries. Consequently, the anterior spinal artery flow may be susceptible to injury during interventional procedures. Steroids for spinal interventional procedures are not created equal because homogenicity and potency are variable. Derby et al[18] investigated particle size and aggregation frequency of commonly used spinal corticosteroids (**Table 14-1**). The larger the particle size and the higher the aggregation, the more likely ischemic injury can result from embolic phenomena.

Inadvertent vascular ischemic injury after steroid particulate injection or vascular injury during cervical transforaminal injections.[19,20] has become increasingly common, and corollaries should be drawn to facetogenic interventions. There have been unpublished reports of quadriplegia from vascular occlusion by particulate steroid after attempted cervical zygapophyseal interventions.

Furthermore, studies for facet and epidural interventions comparing particulate versus nonparticulate steroids found no statistical difference in efficacy.[21] Injection under live fluoroscopy with or without digital subtraction may help elucidate intravascular needle placement.

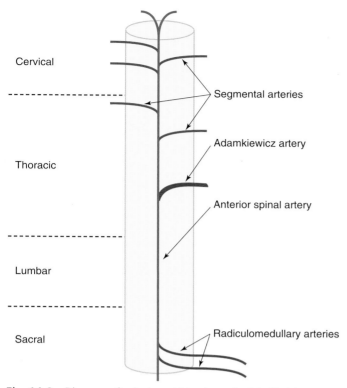

Fig. 14-2 Diagram of spinal cord blood supply. (Modified from Charles YP, Barbe B Beaujeux R, et al: Relevance of the anatomical location of the Adamkiewicz artery in the spine, *Surg Radiol Anat* 33(1):3-9, 2010.)

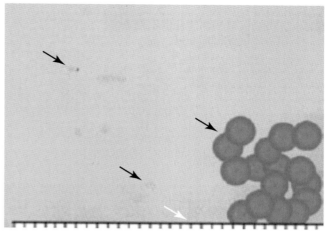

Fig. 14-3 Dexamethasone compared to red blood cells. (From Derby R, Lee SH, Date ES, et al: Size and aggregation of corticosteroids used for epidural injections, *Pain Med* 9(2):227-234, 2008.)

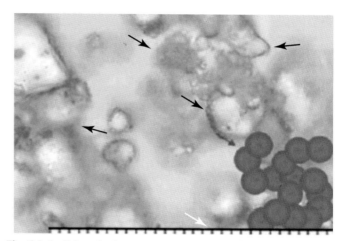

Fig. 14-4 Triamcinolone aggregates compared to red blood cells. (From Derby R, Lee SH, Date ES, et al: Size and aggregation of corticosteroids used for epidural injections, *Pain Med* 9(2):227-234, 2008.)

Table 14-1: Particle Size and Aggregation Potential for Commonly Used Corticosteroids for Spinal Injections		
Steroid	**Particle Size**	**Aggregation**
Dexamethasone	5–10× smaller than RBCs (**Fig. 14-3**)	None
Triamcinolone	Varied in size, often >RBCs (**Fig. 14-4**)	High aggregation
Betamethasone	Varied in size, often >RBCs	High aggregation
Methylprednisolone	Uniform size, smaller than RBC	Few aggregations

RBC, red blood cell.

Local tenderness has been reported in many investigations. Dobrogowsi et al[22] investigated strategies to reduce the inflammatory pain associated with the lesioning. In a randomized prospective trial, patients were randomized to intraoperative methylprednisolone (10 mg), pentoxifylline (10 mg), or saline (1 mL). No "severe local tenderness" was reported in either the methylprednisolone group or the pentoxifylline group, with minor tenderness resolving within 1 month, as compared with the saline group, which had four of 15 patients with severe pain at 1 week and one patient for longer than 1 month. Other authors report a 3-day dosage of diclofenac to be effective in reducing procedural pain after conventional RF neurotomy of lumbar median branches.[23]

Infection

Although there have been several case reports of infectious complications, appreciating the scope of facetogenic interventions, these complications continue to be very rare. Some authors contend that the immunosuppressive effects of steroids contribute to the infectious complication potential (**Table 14-2**). A consistent theme in successful treatment is prompt diagnosis and a high index of suspicion.

Epidural Abscess

Epidural abscess (**Fig. 14-5, A**) can occur spontaneously, with a reported incidence of 0.2 to 1.2 per 10,000 hospital admissions.[24] Early diagnosis is important for reduced morbidity.[25] It is very infrequently associated with facetogenic interventions (only one reported case). Commonly, nonspecific inflammatory markers, including C-reactive protein and erythrocyte sedimentation rate (ESR), are elevated. Patients may also develop leukocytosis, fever, and commonly complain of back pain. Progressive clinical phases have been described for epidural infection leading to epidural abscess, described by van Zundert.[26] Phase I involves backache and local tenderness; phase II is associated with radicular pain, fever, neck stiffness, and rigidity and commonly occurs 2 to 3 days later; phase III presents with sensory, motor, or reflex depression (often 3 to 4 days later); and phase IV is associated with paralysis.[26]

Magnetic resonance imaging (MRI) with gadolinium contrast is a very sensitive diagnostic tool, in that 80% to 90% of cases were correctly diagnosed.[24] When neurologic deterioration occurs, decompression via laminectomy is warranted and should be used within 36 hours, although neurologic sequela can still be significant.[27]

Staphylococci are the most common species identified (57% to 73% in epidural abscesses), although other gram-positive, negative,

anaerobic mycobacteria and fungi have been implicated.[28,29] The most common source of infection is a hematogenous source, typically from furunculosis.[30] Spread from adjacent paraspinal structures has also been implicated, and in a review by Darouiche et al,[31] 44% of 43 patients had vertebral body osteomyelitis (**Fig. 14-5, B**). Intravenous (IV) bacteriocidal antibiotics should be started as early as possible and continued for 4 weeks, and enteral or parenteral therapy continued for 8 to 12 weeks is typically advocated.[31] Therapy should be modified according to speciation and antibiotic resistance profile if isolation is achievable.

Septic Facet Joint Arthritis

Septic arthritis has been described secondary to zygapophyseal joint injections, both in the cervical and lumbar arena, although similar to epidural abscesses, it is more common via hematogenous spread.[32,33] The causative organisms are most commonly staphylococci. Again, a high level of suspicion is required to make a prompt diagnosis because early treatment with IV antibiotics is necessary. The presentation is similar to that of epidural abscess, and it is often difficult to differentiate it from spondylodiscitis, although typically septic arthritis is more painful.[28,34]

Lumbar facet septic arthritis typically occurs unilaterally and rarely occurs bilaterally, although it has been reported.[34] Radiographic evidence includes widening of the facet joint on plain radiographs, ultra-high signal intensity on T2-weighted images, and ring enhancement on gadolinium enhanced T1-weighted images (**Fig. 14-6**).[28,35,36]

Similar to epidural abscess treatment, IV antibiotics are given for 4 to 6 weeks to follow objective functional endpoints for treatment, such as reduction in ESR or normalization of leukocytosis. In cases without epidural extension, percutaneous drainage was successful in treatment approximately 85% of the time.[37] Surgical decompression is required if antibiotics fail or neurologic deterioration occurs. Muffoletto et al[37] suggest that patients with septic facet arthritis from iatrogenic causes were more

Table 14-2: Reported Infectious Complications After Zygapophyseal Interventions

Author, Year	Complication Reported
Heenan et al,[35] 1995	Septic arthritis
Cook et al,[39] 1999	Paraspinal abscess
Magee et al,[57] 2000	Paraspinal abscess
Rombauts et al,[58] 2000	Septic arthritis
Alcock et al,[24] 2003	Epidural abscess
Doita et al,[34] 2003	Septic arthritis
Orpen et al,[59] 2003	Septic arthritis
Gaul et al,[38] 2005	Iatrogenic paraspinal abscess and meningitis
Weingarten et al,[60] 2006	Septic arthritis
Falagas et al,[43] 2006	Spondylodiscitis
Park et al,[40] 2007	Paraspinal communicated with epidural abscess
Hoelzer et al,[41] 2008	Endocarditis after paraspinal abscess

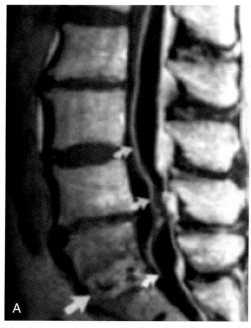
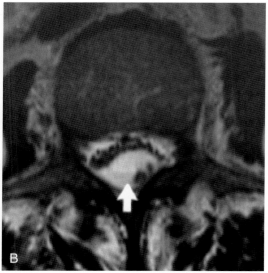

Fig. 14-5 T1-weighted magnetic resonance image of an epidural abscess L4-5 (**A**) and associated osteomyelitis L5 (**B**). (From Darouiche RO, Hamil RJ, Greenberg, et al: Bacterial spinal epidural abscess: review of 43 cases and literature survey, *Medicine* 71:369-385, 1992.)

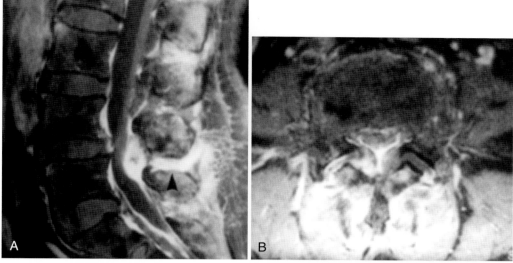

Fig. 14-6   Gadolinium-enhanced magnetic resonance image demonstrating an L4–L5 inflammatory process in the sagittal (**A**) and axial (**B**) planes. (From Doita M, Nishida K, Miyamoto H, et al: Septic arthritis of bilateral lumbar facet joints: report of a case with MRI findings in the early stage, *Spine* 28:198-202, 2003.)

likely to require surgical intervention than those with hematogenous causes.

Paraspinal Abscess

Gaul et al estimated the risk of central nervous system infectious complications after paraspinal pain intervention to be approximately one in 1000.[38] There have been numerous case reports with significant morbidity, including endocarditis.[39-41]

Paraspinal abscess presentation, onset, and treatment are similar to the aforementioned infectious complications (**Fig. 14-7**).[42] As with other therapies, prompt diagnosis and institution of bactericidal therapy are paramount.

Spondylodiscitis

Spondylodiscitis incidence from iatrogenic facetogenic interventional sources is rare,[43] and the incidence from all causes is 2.4 in 100,000.[44] The typical presentation is vague dull back pain that increases in character with continued progression of clinical signs, including fever, leukocytosis, and ESR. The aforementioned radiographic investigations, including MRI, and serologic and tissue assessment, including blood cultures biopsy, are suggested (**Fig. 14-8**).

Organisms again implicated most commonly include staphylococci. Treatment again centers on IV antibiotic therapy tailored to specific speciation and sensitivity.

Epidural Hematoma

Although the incidence of epidural hematoma formation associated with spinal procedures approximates one in 150,000 epidural procedures and one in 222,000 for spinal anesthetics, the incidence after facet interventions is largely unknown.[45] The AASRA developed guidelines to avoid the risk of bleeding complicating neuraxial procedures, and although largely for epidural and spinal perioperative anesthesia or analgesia, they can be used in the chronic pain realm. Obviously, if anatomic vascular variation is present, a predisposition to bleeding complications may be increased. The epidural space is an area surrounded by a plexus of epidural veins, commonly implicated in hematoma formation.

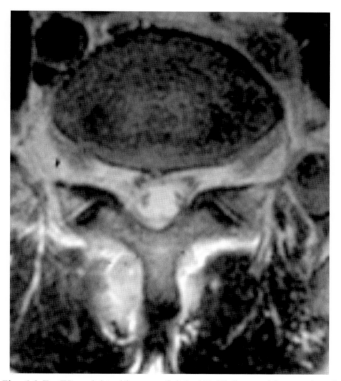

Fig. 14-7   T2-weighted image of right L5–S1 facet with associated paraspinal abscess. (From Park MS, Moon SH, Hahn SB, Lee HM: Paraspinal abscess communicated with epidural abscess after extra-articular facet joint injection, *Yonsei Med J* 48:711-714, 2007.)

Nam et al[46] reported two cases of epidural hematoma after facet block (**Fig. 14-9** and **Table 14-3**). Both patients presented with back pain and radicular pain, but no systemic disorders or coagulopathies were identified. Subsequently, both resolved with appropriate treatment, one requiring a multilevel laminectomy.

Treatment and prognosis depend on early accurate diagnosis. Commonly, the presenting complaint is severe axial back

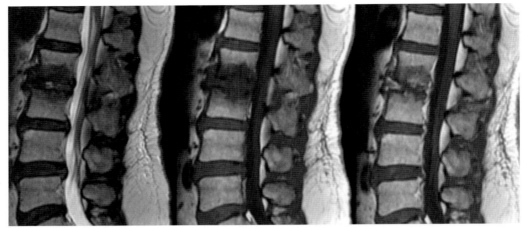

Fig. 14-8 T2, T1, with and without contrast of spondylodiscitis at the L2–L3 disc. (From Kaplan P, Helms CA, Dussault R et al: Musculoskeletal MRI: In *Spine*. Philadelphia, 2001, WB Saunders.)

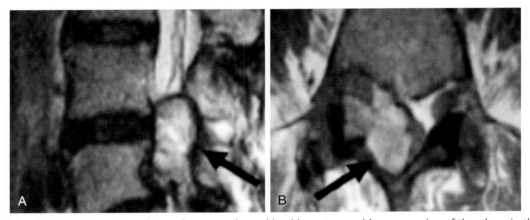

Fig. 14-9 T1-weighted magnetic resonance image demonstrating epidural hematoma with compression of thecal sac in the sagittal (**A**) and axial (**B**) plane at the L4 and L5 levels. (From Nam KH, Choi CH, Yang MS, Kang DW: Spinal epidural hematoma after pain control procedure, *J Korean Neurosurg Soc* 48: 281-284, 2010.)

Table 14-3: Pharmacologic and Bleeding Complications	
Author, Year	**Complication Reported**
Goldstone et al,[49] 1987	Spinal anesthesia
Cohen,[50] 1994	Postdural puncture headache
Heckmann et al,[14] 2006	Transient tetraplegia
Nam et al,[46] 2010	Epidural hematoma
Kay et al,[51] 1994	Pituitary–adrenal axis suppression*

*Extrapolated from epidural steroid injections.

or radicular pain, usually temporally associated with the pain procedures, usually preceded by hours to days. Complete or partial weakness leading to quadriplegia or paraplegia can occur within hours of symptom onset.

Treatment should not be delayed until radiographic confirmation. MRI with low signal intensity on T1 and high signal intensity on T2 is suggestive of an acute bleed. Slightly high signal on T1 and T2 is suggestive of an subacute bleed. Early neurosurgical consultation is paramount because the absence of neurologic sequelae is contingent on hematoma evacuation within 8 hours of neurologic deficit.[47]

Spinal Anesthesia and Post-Dural Puncture Headache

The anatomy of the spinal elements predisposes to potential dural puncture. As described in the chapter on intraarticular injection (see Chapter 12), the architecture and orientation of the facet joint vary with function and position within the vertebral column. The cervical facet joints are between the articular pillars of the vertebrae and are oriented approximately 45 degrees from the transverse plain and 80 degrees from the sagittal. The cervical facet joint can accommodate approximately 0.5 to 1.0 mL of fluid. The thoracic facet joint can accommodate no more than 0.75 mL of fluid and is more vertically oriented than the lumbar or cervical facet joints. On average, they are approximately 75 degrees from the sagittal and transverse planes. The lumbar facet joint is oriented approximately 78.5 degrees from the transverse and 122 degrees from the sagittal planes, accommodating an average of 1.0 to 1.5 mL of fluid (**Fig. 14-10**).[48]

The dural sleeve of the exiting nerve root extends laterally and is caudal to the ipsilateral pedicle. Spinal anesthesia after lumbar facet intraarticular injection has been described.[49] The authors postulated inadvertent needle placement and trajectory, potential dural cuff penetration, or intraneural injection as potential explanations.

After dural puncture, postdural puncture headache can occur, and after isolated penetration, it is largely contingent on needle

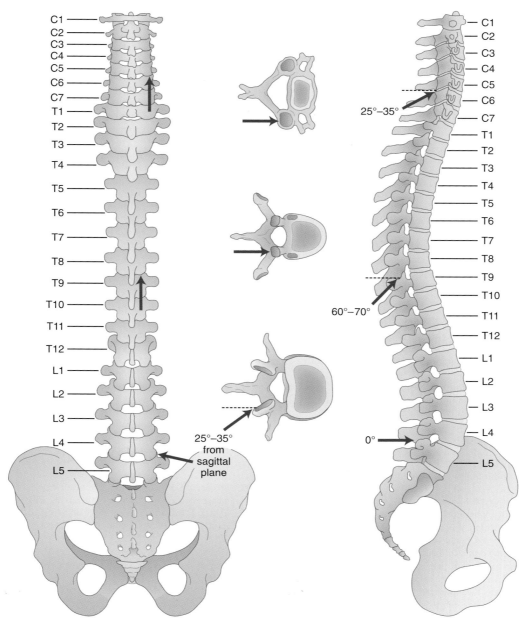

Fig. 14-10 Entry into the cervical, thoracic, and lumbar facet joints has predictable differences in the sagittal, axial, and coronal planes. (Modified from Rathmell JP: *Atlas of image-guided intervention in regional anesthesia and pain medicine*. Philadelphia, 2006, Lippincott.)

gauge and bevel shape. Typical needle gauges (22 or 25 gauge) for intraarticular or median branch procedures lessen the chance of dural puncture. Given this, Cohen[50] described this complication after successful lumbar facet block.

Even after successful, appropriate lumbar facet procedures, complications arise. It is vital that the interventionalist is familiar with neuraxial crisis management and readily has the necessary life-sustaining and supportive equipment and knowledge available. These include supplemental oxygen via ambulation bag, laryngoscope with appropriate endotracheal tube and induction medications, and suction, along with vasoactive medications for blood pressure and perfusion support. High spinals are commonly managed symptomatically, with Trendelenburg position to increase cerebral perfusion after control of the airway is achieved.

Pituitary–Adrenal Axis Suppression

Although numerous studies have demonstrated pituitary–adrenal suppression with epidural or intraarticular administration of glucocorticoids,[51-53] none has investigated axis depression from zygapophyseal interventions. From the available data, hypothalamic–pituitary–adrenal axis suppression could be assumed to be depressed for 4 weeks, and insulin sensitivity may be adversely affected for approximately 1 week. Cushing syndrome, steroid myopathy, aseptic meningitis, and anaphylactoid reactions have been reported after single epidural steroid injections.[54,55] Other glucocorticoid side effects, including musculoskeletal, ophthalmologic, gastrointestinal, cardiovascular, secondary cortisol deficiency, gynecologic, neurologic, hematologic, gynecologic, psychiatric, and dermatologic, have been described.[56]

Summary

Facetogenic interventions, either for diagnostic or therapeutic purposes, greatly serve many patients with chronic pain. Although reported complications are rare, catastrophic iatrogenic events have occurred. As with any interventional procedure, respect for the neural elements and perfected procedural technique is crucial for successful patient outcomes and reduction in morbidity and mortality.

References

1. Datta S, Lee M, Falco FJ, et al: Systematic assessment of diagnostic accuracy and therapeutic utility of lumbar facet joint interventions. *Pain Physician* 12:437-460, 2009.
2. Alturi S, Datta S, Falco FJE, Lee M: Systematic review of diagnostic utility and therapeutic effectiveness of thoracic facet joint interventions. *Pain Physician* 11:611-629, 2008.
3. Schwarzer AC, Wang S, Bogduk N, et al: Prevalence and clinical features of lumbar zygapophysial joint pain: a study in an Australian population with chronic low back pain. *Ann Rheum Dis* 54:100-106, 1995.
4. Manchikanti L, Manchikanti KN, Pampati V, et al: The prevalence of facet-joint-related chronic neck pain in postsurgical and nonpostsurgical patients: a comparative evaluation. *Pain Practice* 8:5-10, 2008.
5. Lord SM, Barnsley L, Wallis BJ, Bogduk N: Chronic zygapophysial joint pain after whiplash: A placebo-controlled prevalence study. *Spine* 21:1737-1744, 1996.
6. Manchukonda R, Manchikanti KN, Cash KA, et al: Facet joint pain in chronic spinal pain: an evaluation of prevalence and false-positive rate of diagnostic blocks. *J Spinal Disord Tech* 20:539-545, 2007.
7. Kalichman L, Li L, Kim DH, et al: Facet joint osteoarthritis and low back pain in the community-based population. *Spine* 33:2560-2565, 2008.
8. Kalichman L, Li L, Kim DH, et al: Facet joint osteoarthritis and low back pain in the community- based population. *Spine* 33:2560-2565, 2008.
9. Manchikanti L, Boswell MV, Singh V, et al: Comprehensive evidence-based guidelines for interventional techniques in the management of chronic spinal pain. *Pain Physician* 12:699-802, 2009.
10. Bogduk N, International Spine Intervention Society: *Practice guidelines spinal diagnostics and treatment procedures*, San Francisco, 2004.
11. Practice guidelines for chronic pain management: An updated report by the American Society of Anesthesiologists Task Force on Chronic Pain Management and the American Society of Regional Anesthesia and Pain Medicine. *Anesthesiology* 112:810-833, 2010.
12. Guyatt G, Gutterman D, Baumann MH, et al: Grading strength of recommendations and quality of evidence in clinical guidelines: report from an American College of Chest Physicians task force. *Chest* 129:174-181, 2006.
13. Huntoon MA: Anatomy of the cervical intervertebral foramina: vulnerable arteries and ischemic neurologic injuries after transforaminal epidural injections. *Pain* 117(1-2):104-111, 2005.
14. Heckmann JG, Maihofner C, Lanz S, et al: Transient tetraplegia after cervical facet joint injection for chronic neck pain administered without imaging guidance. *Clin Neurol Neurosurg* 108:709-711, 2006.
15. Lazorthes G, Gouaze A, Zadeh JO, et al: Arterial vascularization of the spinal cord. *J Neurosurg* 35:253-262, 1971.
16. Charles YP, Barbe B Beaujeux R, et al: Relevance of the anatomical location of the Adamkiewicz artery in the spine. *Surg Radiol Anat* 33(1):3-9, 2010.
17. Glaser SE, Shah RV: Root cause analysis of paraplegia following transforaminal epidural steroid injections: the "unsafe triangle." *Pain Physician* 13:237-244, 2010.
18. Derby R, Lee SH, Date ES, et al: Size and aggregation of corticosteroids used for epidural injections. *Pain Med* 9(2):227-234, 2008.
19. Rathmell JP, Aprill C, Bogduk N: Cervical transforaminal injection of steroids. *Anesthesiology* 100:1595-1600, 2004.
20. Rozin L, Rozin R, Koehler SA, et al: Death during transforaminal epidural steroid nerve root block (C7) due to perforation of the left vertebral artery. *Am J Forensic Med Pathol* 24:351-355, 2003.
21. Lee JW, Park KW, Chung SK, et al: Cervical transforaminal epidural steroid injection for the management of cervical radiculopathy: a comparative study of particulate versus non-particulate steroids. *Skeletal Radiol* 38(11):1077-1082, 2009.
22. Dobrogowski J, Wrzosek A, Wordliczek J: Radiofrequency denervation with or without addition of pentoxifylline or methylprednisolone for chronic lumbar zygapophysial joint pain. *Pharmacol Rep* 57:475-480, 2005.
23. Ma K, Yiqun M, Wang W, et al: Efficacy of diclofenac sodium in pain relief after conventional radiofrequency denervation for chronic facet joint pain: a double blind randomized controlled trial. *Pain Med* 12(1):27-35, 2010.
24. Alcock E, Regaard A, Browne J: Facet joint injection: a rare form cause of epidural abscess formation. *Pain* 103:209-210, 2003.
25. Mackenzie AR, Laing RBS, Kaar GF, Smith FW: Spinal epidural abscess: the importance of early diagnosis and treatment. *J Neurol Neurosurg Psychiatry* 65:209-212, 1998.
26. Van Zundert A: The epidural abscess: diagnosis and treatment. In *Highlights in regional anaesthesia and pain therapy IX*, Rome, 2000, Italy Cyprint Ltd, pp 159-162.
27. Danner RL, Hartman BJ: Update of spinal epidural abscess: 35 cases and review of literature. *Rev Infect Dis* 9:265-274, 1987.
28. Ergan M, Macro M, Benhamou CL, et al: Septic arthritis of lumbar facet joints: a review of six cases. *Rev Rheum Engl Ed* 64:386-395, 1997.
29. Bruma OJ, Craane H, Kunst MW: Vertebral osteomyelitis and epidural abscess due to mucormycosis, a case report. *Clin Neurol Neurosurg* 81(1):39-44, 1979.
30. Gouche CR, Graziotti P: Extradural abscess following local anaesthetic and steroid injection for chronic low back pain. *Br J Anaesth* 65:427-429, 1990.
31. Darouiche RO, Hamil RJ, Greenberg, et al: Bacterial spinal epidural abscess: review of 43 cases and literature survey. *Medicine* 71:369-385, 1992.
32. Stecher JM, El-Khoury GY, Hitchon PW: Cervical facet joint arthritis: a case report. *Iowa Orthop J* 30:182-187, 2010.
33. Ogura T, Mikami Y, Hase H, et al: Septic arthritis of a lumbar facet joint associated with epidural and paraspinal abscess. *Orthopedics* 28(2):173-175, 2005.
34. Doita M, Nishida K, Miyamoto H, et al: Septic arthritis of bilateral lumbar facet joints: report of a case with MRI findings in the early stage. *Spine* 28:198-202, 2003.
35. Heenan SP, Britton J: Septic arthritis in a lumbar facet joint: a rare cause of epidural abscess. *Neuroradiology* 37:109-112, 1995.
36. Fujiwara A, Tamai K, Yamato M, et al: Septic arthritis of a lumbar facet joint: report of a case with early MRI findings. *J Spinal Disord* 11:452-453, 1998.
37. Muffoletto AJ, Ketonen LM, Mader JT, et al: Hematogenous pyogenic facet joint infection. *Spine* 26:1570-1576, 2001.
38. Gaul C, Neundorfer B, Winterholler M: Iatrogenic (para-) spinal abscesses and meningitis following injection therapy for low back pain. *Pain* 116:407-410, 2005.
39. Cook NJ, Hanrahan P, Song S: Paraspinal abscess following facet joint injection. *Clin Rheumatol* 18:52-53, 1999.
40. Park MS, Moon SH, Hahn SB, Lee HM: Paraspinal abscess communicated with epidural abscess after extra-articular facet joint injection. *Yonsei Med J* 48:711-714, 2007.
41. Hoelzer BC, Weingarten TN, Hooten WM, et al: Paraspinal abscess complicated by endocarditis following a facet joint injection. *Eur J Pain* 12:261-265, 2008.
42. Puehler W, Brack A, Kopf A: Extensive abscess formation after repeated paravertebral injections for the treatment of chronic back pain. *Pain* 113:427-429, 2005.
43. Falagas ME, Bliziotis IA, Mavrogenis AF, Papagelopoulos PJ: Spondylodiscitis after facet joint injection: a case report and a review of literature. *Scand J Infect Dis* 38(4):295-299, 2006.

44. Titlic M, Josipovic-Jelic Z: Spondylodiscitis. *Bratisl Lek Listy* 109(8): 345-347, 2008.

45. Horlocker TT, Rowlingson JC, Enneking FK, et al: Regional anesthesia in the patient receiving antithrombotic or thrombolytic therapy: American Society of Regional Anesthesia and Pain Medicine Evidence-Based Guidelines (Third Edition). *Reg Anesth Pain Med* 35(1):64-101, 2010.

46. Nam KH, Choi CH, Yang MS, Kang DW: Spinal epidural hematoma after pain control procedure. *J Korean Neurosurg Soc* 48: 281-284, 2010.

47. Vandermeulen EP, Van Aken H, Vermylen J: Anticoagulants and spinal-epidural anesthesia. *Anesth Analg* 79:1165-1177, 1994.

48. Punjabi MM, Oxland T, Takata K, et al: Articular facets of the human spine. Quantitative three-dimensional anatomy. *Spine* 18:1298-1310, 1993.

49. Goldstone JC, Pennant JH: Spinal anaesthesia following facet joint injection. A report of two cases. *Anaesthesia* 42:754-756, 1987.

50. Cohen SP: Postdural puncture headache and treatment following successful lumbar facet block. *Pain Digest* 4:283-284, 1994.

51. Kay J, Findling JW, Raff H: Epidural triamcinolone suppresses the pituitary-adrenal axis in human subjects. *Anesth Analg* 79:501-505, 1994.

52. Ward A, Watson J, Wood P, et al: Glucocorticoid epidural for sciatica: Metabolic and endocrine sequelae. *Rheumatology (Oxford)* 41:68-71, 2002.

53. Cook DM, Meikle AW, Bowman R: Systemic absorption of triamcinolone after a single intraarticular injections suppresses the pituitary-adrenal axis [abstract]. *Clin Res* 36:121A, 1988.

54. Knight CL, Burnell JC: Systemic side effects of extradural steroids. *Anaesthesia* 35:593-594, 1980.

55. Boonen S, Van Distel G, Westhovens R, et al: Steroid myopathy induced by epidural triamcinolone injection. *Br J Rheumatol* 34:385-386, 1995.

56. Nesbit LT: Minimizing complications from systemic glucocorticosteroid use. *Dermatol Clin* 13:925-939, 1995.

57. Magee M, Kannangara S, Dennien B: Paraspinal abscess complicating facet joint injection. *Clin Nucl Med* 25:71-77, 2000.

58. Rombauts PA, Linden PM, Buyse AJ, et al: Septic arthritis of a lumbar facet joint caused by *Staphylococcus aureus. Spine* 25:1736-1738, 2000.

59. Orpen NM, Birch NC: Delayed presentation of septic arthritis of a lumbar facet joint after diagnostic facet joint injection. *J Spinal Disord Tech* 16:285-287, 2003.

60. Weingarten TN, Hooten WM, Huntoon MA: Septic facet joint arthritis after a corticosteroid facet injection. *Pain Med* 7(1):52-56, 2006.

15 Complications of Radiofrequency Rhizotomy for Facet Syndrome

Jason E. Pope

CHAPTER OVERVIEW

Chapter Synopsis: Radiofrequency (RF) rhizotomy can provide relief for zygapophyseal joint pain arising from facet syndrome. Careful patient selection and consideration of the available techniques can reduce the risk of complications and improve success. Diagnostic injection can also increase the ultimate effectiveness of rhizotomy. Physicians may choose thermal, pulsed, or cooling RF to ablate nerve tissue; each technique carries its own possible benefits and risks. Vascular and nerve injury account for most complications, but rhizotomy can also carry infection risks.

Important Points:
- Appropriate Accreditation Council for Graduate Medical Education mentored subspecialty training in interventional pain management is vital to ensure patient-centered care.
- Accurate and expertly placed RF needles are essential to ensure median branch neurotomy.
- RF treatments are not created equal, and an appreciation for each underscores their differences.
- Common complications, regardless of the RF modality used, include transient increased localized pain and usually self-limiting neuritis.
- Infectious complications are less common than in the diagnostic or therapeutic steroid injections, potentially related to the thermal injury created.
- Only one retrospective review has investigated complications associated with RF treatments.
- Injection of steroid or enteral antiinflammatory medications may help with postprocedural pain and neuritis.
- Burn injuries can be avoided by careful equipment interrogation and correct electrosurgical unit return plate positioning.

Introduction

Rhizotomy techniques have revolutionized treatment for many pain states and are commonly used to treat facetogenic pain after appropriate controlled diagnostic injections. Relatively recent reviews approximated lumbar, thoracic, and cervical zygapophyseal pain to be 31%, 40%, and 39%, respectively, using dual controlled diagnostic injections (**Table 15-1**).[1-3]

As with any intervention, complication avoidance begins with patient selection. Patients with local infection near the injection site, coagulopathy, allergy to injectate, or comorbidities or conditions that prevent fluoroscopic needle guidance or consent should be avoided. A clear understanding of spinal anatomy and utilization of image guidance is vital to ensure both quality treatment and reduced patient morbidity and mortality. Furthermore, it should be understood that appropriate training within Accreditation Council for Graduate Medical Education accredited programs and mentorship is pivotal to ensure treatment success; interventional hobbyists only serve to undermine accessibility of these valuable therapies to patients.

Facetogenic injections are required to make diagnosis because no physical, historical, or radiographic examination feature are unreliable,[4] but attempts at noninvasive diagnostic strategies

are ongoing.[5] Interestingly, later Cohen et al[6] looked at the cost effectiveness of one, two, or no controlled diagnostic injection before facet radiofrequency (RF) treatment and summarized that from a cost analysis perspective, proceeding to RF denervation before diagnostic injection was superior, and although efficacy determination was not a study endpoint, the treatment outcome related to duration and magnitude of pain relief was greater for the dual diagnostic blockade group.

Regardless of the diagnostic treatment algorithm used, RF techniques are a safe and effective means to treat zygapophyseal pain.[7] However, RF techniques are not created equal, and an understanding of the different modalities is crucial to understand the potential pitfalls and safety concerns.

Background

Thermal (Traditional, Conventional, or Continuous) Radiofrequency

Thermal RF was first introduced in the 1930s. The thermal lesion is created by the introduction of an insulated electrode with an active tip of (2 to 10 mm), a dispersal plate, and a power source to complete the circuit (**Fig. 15-1**).

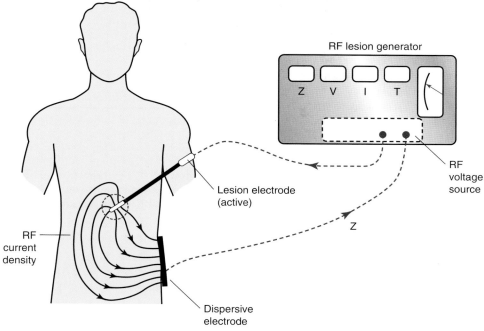

Fig. 15-1   The radiofrequency circuit.

Table 15-1: Prevalence and Diagnostic Accuracy of Zygapophyseal Joint Pain		
	Prevalence (%)*	**Diagnostic Accuracy: False Positive Rate* (%)**
Cervical	39 (23–45)	45 (37–52)
Thoracic	40 (33–48)	42 (33–51)
Lumbar	31 (28–33)	30 (27–33)

*95% confidence interval using 80% pain reduction.
Data from Manchukonda R, Manchikanti KN, Cash KA, et al: Facet joint pain in chronic spinal pain: An evaluation of prevalence and false-positive rate of diagnostic blocks, *J Spinal Disord Tech* 20:539-545, 2007.

High-frequency electrical current is then applied adjacent to the structure of the nerve that is intended to ablate; such current leads to ionic oscillation and frictional dissipation of the ions and electrolytes, which produce heat. The heat produced is directly related to the amplitude of the applied current and electrode size and indirectly related to distance from the electrode. The tip of the electrode measures the tissue temperature. Larger lesions are created by increased temperature, size of the electrode, and duration of applied current. Monopolar lesioning is performed when one electrode is used. Bipolar lesioning occurs when two electrodes are used in close proximity to one another. Laboratory evidence suggests that cellular damage occurs at temperatures of 60° to 65°C. As suggested by the aforementioned isotherm mapping from the electrode tip, 80° to 85°C is required at the needle tip, where the desired 60° to 65°C is achieved in the surrounding tissue, producing a prolate ovoid-shaped lesion (**Fig. 15-2**). Therefore, because the lesion created does not extend distal to the electrode, proper electrode position is parallel to the target nerve.

The neurotomy created by the thermal technique is dependent on proximity to the targeted nerve, size of electrode, the temperature (or amplitude of current) applied, and the duration of lesioning. When applied immediately adjacent to the dorsal root ganglion, temperatures of 45°, 55°, 65°, 75°, and 85°C produce complete

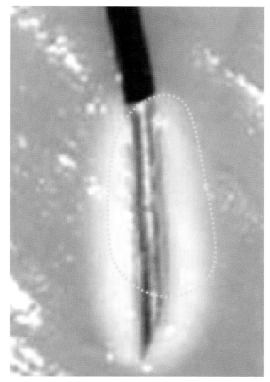

Fig. 15-2   Traditional thermal radiofrequency lesion. (Courtesy of Dr. Nagy Mekhail, MD, PhD, Cleveland Clinic.)

destruction of unmyelinated and near complete destruction of myelinated fibers.[8]

Pulsed Radiofrequency

Pulsed RF was first introduced in 1998, and the aforementioned circuit is used. Interestingly, there is no creation of a histologic lesion, and no nerve degeneration occurs (no Wallerian degeneration). The treatment is produced by providing current of 50,000 Hz in 20-msec pulses at a frequency of 2 per second. The temperature is maintained to be below 42°C or 45 V (**Fig. 15-3**). The greatest current density delivered is at the tip of the electrode; so ideal placement is perpendicular to the target nerve.

The mechanism of the therapeutic treatment is less clear compared with thermal RF and is surrounded by controversy. The mechanism appears to be independent of temperature and is neuromodulatory in nature,[9-12] and one resounding conclusion can be made: There is no histologically detected cellular destruction.

Cooled Radiofrequency

Cooled RF is a misnomer. The neurotomy produced is secondary to thermal destruction; however, the cooled RF uses a lower temperature than traditional thermal RF lesioning (**Fig. 15-4**). The traditional RF lesion size is limited by the charring of tissues around the electrode as the temperature of tissues rises. On the other hand, cooled RF maintains the temperature adjacent to the electrode at a desired lower level to prevent tissue charring, hence allowing the lesion to expand and increase in size.[13]

The resultant lesion is spherical in shape (**Fig. 15-5**). The radius of the spherical lesion equals the length of the active tip of the electrode. Simply, the tip of the electrode is the center of the spherical lesion. Therefore, the cooled RF lesion is eight times by volume the thermal RF lesion for the same length electrode tip.[13] Whereas the spherical lesion projects distally from the electrode, conventional thermal RF produces a prolate ovoid parallel to the active tip of the needle (see **Fig. 15-2**) with little or no projection distally. Consequently, unlike thermal RF, which requires parallel electrode placement adjacent to the target nerve, cooled RF lesions are independent of electrode orientation.[14]

Summarily, and as described, important differences regarding lesion size, electrode placement, and neural destruction need to be noted (**Table 15-2**).

Selected Complications

Despite routine use, complications, similar to those associated with the diagnostic or therapeutic zygapophyseal injections, are rare. See Chapter 14 for further details. Other modalities to produce lesions to treat facetogenic pain include alcohol, phenol, laser, and kryoneurolysis.[15-19] This chapter focuses on complications specific to RF neurotomy, and none will be discussed further. Theoretical risks regarding RF neurotomy are listed in **Box 15-1**.

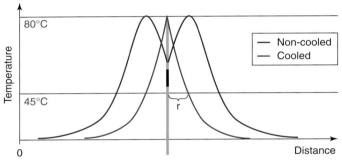

Fig. 15-4 Temperature distance comparison for cooled and thermal radiofrequency.

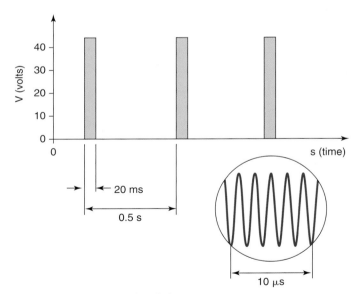

Fig. 15-3 Pulsed radiofrequency current parameters.

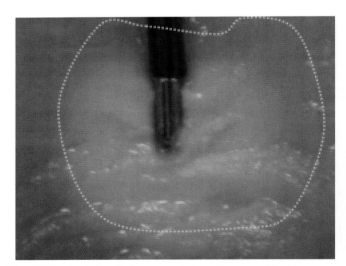

Fig. 15-5 Cooled radiofrequency lesion. (Courtesy of Dr. Nagy Mekhail, MD, PhD, Cleveland Clinic.)

Table 15-2: Radiofrequency Summary						
	Lesion Shape	**Lesion Diameter (mm)**	**Needle Orientation**	**Temperature (°C)**	**Time of Lesion (sec)**	**Neurodestruction**
Pulsed	None	None	Perpendicular	42	120	No
Conventional	Prolate spheroid	4	Parallel	80–90	90–105	Yes
Cooled	Spherical	8	Independent	60	230	Yes

Postprocedure Pain and Neuritis

There is sparse literature describing the complications associated with RF treatments (pulsed, conventional, or cooled) for facetogenic pain.[7,20-29] No cooled RF of the lumbar median branches has been formally reported, although some advocate its use. Kornick et al[30] performed a retrospective review over a 5-year period at the Mayo Clinic in Jacksonville, Florida, in a total of 92 patients receiving 616 RF lesions (80°C for 90 seconds) during 116 separate procedures. Of the 616 lesions, six complications were noted—three cases of localized pain at the RF sites lasting more than 2 weeks and three cases of neuritic pain lasting less than 2 weeks (**Table 15-3**). No motor, sensory, vascular, or infectious complications were noted.[30] A case report of neuroma formation after multiple RF ablation procedures has been described. It was successfully treated with an open minimally invasive medial branch neurectomy.[31]

Frequently, steroids are injected after denervation, which seems counterintuitive because the goal in thermal rhizotomy is to create a histologically detectable lesion, and although anecdotal evidence suggests postoperative neuritis reduction, studies are lacking. No studies to date have compared efficacy with long-term follow-up of steroid application after conventional or cooled neurotomy.

Dobrogowsi et al[32] investigated strategies to reduce the inflammatory pain associated with the lesioning. In a randomized prospective trial, patients were randomized to intraoperative methylprednisolone (10 mg), pentoxifylline (10 mg), or saline (1 mL). No "severe local tenderness" was reported in either the methylprednisolone group or pentoxifylline group, with minor tenderness resolving within 1 month, compared with the saline group, which had four of 15 patients with severe pain at 1 week and one patient for longer than 1 month. Other authors[33] report that 3-day dosage of diclofenac to be effective in reducing procedural pain after conventional RF neurotomy of lumbar median branches (**Fig. 15-6**).

Box 15-1: Theoretical Complications Associated with Radiofrequency

Procedural
Vascular injury
Hematoma or bleeding
Disc injury
Postdural puncture headache
Spinal anesthesia
Neuritis
Radiofrequency treatment complications
Nerve root injury
Pneumothorax
Burn injury
Neuroma formation

Infectious
Discitis
Epidural abscess
Septic arthritis
Meningitis
Intraspinal abscess
Paraspinal abscess

Table 15-3: Complications Reported with Radiofrequency Treatments

Author, Year	Site	Type of Lesioning	Complication Reported	Duration of Complaint	Prevalence
Kornick et al,[30] 2004	Lumbar	Conventional	Neuritis Dysesthesia	>2 weeks <2 weeks	0.5% 0.5%
Gekht et al,[31] 2010	Lumbar	Conventional	Neuroma, deafferentation injury	≈9 months	?
Cohen et al,[6] 2010	Lumbar	Conventional	Increased pain, dysesthesia	<3 months	3 of 150 patients
Tzaan et al,[39] 2000	Lumbar (n = 88); thoracic (n = 17); cervical (n = 13)	Conventional	Increased pain Neuropathic pain Leg pain or weakness	NA <3 months NA	4 of 118 patients 12 of 118 patients 3 of 118
Barnsley et al,[37] 2005	Cervical	Conventional	Superficial infection Postprocedural pain Pain exacerbation	NA ≈1 week 3 months	1 of 47 patients Most of 47 patients 1 of 47 patient
Lang et al,[38] 2010*	Cervical	Conventional	Burning dysesthesia Numbness	? "Longer period of time"	1 of 31 patients (61 procedures) 4 of 31 patients
Liliang et al,[40] 2008	Cervical	Pulsed	Postprocedural pain	≈1 week	1 of 14 patients
Kapural et al,[14] 2010	Sacroiliac, L5 dorsal ramus	Cooled	Increased pain numbness itching	<6 weeks	8 of 100 patients

*All patients received 100 mg of indomethacin on the day of the procedure.
NA, not applicable.

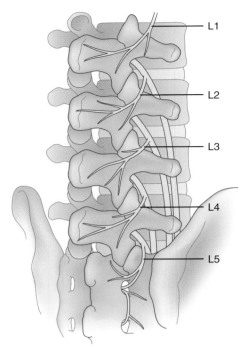

Fig. 15-6 Lumbar median branches and dorsal ramus of L5.

Burn Injuries

Burn injuries have been reported early in literature and were the result of equipment malfunction, insulation breaks within the electrodes, a unipolar electrosurgical unit return plate, or unknown causes.[34-36] Whereas operating room power supplies are ungrounded systems, office buildings are typically grounded systems. This difference dramatically impacts the chance of burn injury (or macroshock) to the patient because isolated systems are more difficult to deliver aberrant current. Furthermore, burn severity is related to current density, either greater the current or the smaller the area applied.

Infectious Complications

There very few reported infectious complications. Barnsley[37] reported a superficial infection after cervical conventional RF that resolved after enteral antibiotics were administered.[38] Furthermore, some contend that the inherent heating of the tissue during the thermal lesioning may provide some means of bacteriocidal effect.[6]

Needle Placement

Proper needle placement during RF denervation is essential, as described in Chapter 7. Improper placement can lead to thermal destruction of nontargeted tissues, including the ventral rami. Although a serious concern, with proper motor testing before lesioning with an increase of stimulation to at least 2 V at 2 Hz, this complication should be avoided.

Summary

Facet pain is a common source of low back pain, and diagnosis and successful treatment hinge on appropriate patient selection and technique. Definitive osteal landmarks demarcate needle targets, excluding the middle thoracic medial branches. With vigilance, strict sterile technique, and motor testing before RF neurotomy, complications are likely to remain low.

References

1. Datta S, Lee M, Falco FJ, et al: Systematic assessment of diagnostic accuracy and therapeutic utility of lumbar facet joint interventions. *Pain Physician* 12:437-460, 2009.
2. Alturi S, Datta S, Falco FJE, Lee M: Systematic review of diagnostic utility and therapeutic effectiveness of thoracic facet joint interventions. *Pain Physician* 11:611-629, 2008.
3. Manchukonda R, Manchikanti KN, Cash KA, et al: Facet joint pain in chronic spinal pain: An evaluation of prevalence and false-positive rate of diagnostic blocks. *J Spinal Disord Tech* 20:539-545, 2007.
4. Cohen SP, Raja SN: Pathogenesis, diagnosis, and treatment of Lumbar zygapophysial (facet) joint pain. *Anesthesiology* 106:591-614, 2007.
5. McDonald M, Cooper R, Wang MY: Use of Computed tomography-single-photon emission computed tomography fusion for diagnosing painful facet arthropathy. Technical note. *Neurosurg Focus* 22(1):E2, 2007.
6. Cohen SP, Williams KA, Kurihara C, et al: Multicenter, randomized comparative cost-effectiveness study comparing 0, 1 and 2 diagnostic medial branch (facet joint nerve) block treatment paradigms before lumbar facet radiofrequency denervation. *Anesthesiology* 113:395-405, 2010.
7. Dreyfuss P, Halbrook B, Pauza K, et al: Efficacy and validity of radiofrequency neurotomy for chronic lumbar zygapophysial joint pain. *Spine* 25:1270-1277, 2000.
8. Van Boxen K, van Eerd M, Brinkhuize T, et al: Radiofrequency and pulsed radiofrequency treatment of chronic pain syndromes: the available evidence. *Pain Med* 8: 385-393, 2008.
9. Tun K, Cemil B, Gurcay AG, et al: Ultrastructural evaluation of pulsed radiofrequency and conventional radiofrequency in rat sciatic nerve. *Surg Neuro* 72:496-501, 2009.
10. Molina JAL, Rivera MJ, Trujillo M, Berjano EJ: Thermal modeling for pulsed radiofrequency ablation: analytical study based on hyperbolic heat conduction. *Med Phys* 36:1112, 2009.
11. Cahana A, Van Zundert J, Macrea L, et al: Pulsed radiofrequency: current clinical and biological literature available. *Pain Med* 7:411-423, 2006.
12. Bogduck N: Position papers: pulsed radiofrequency. *Pain Med* 7:396-407, 2008.
13. Kapural L, Mekhail N, Hick D, et al: Histological changes and temperature distribution studies of a novel bipolar radiofrequency heating system in degenerated and nondegenerated human cadaver lumbar discs. *Pain Med* 9:68-75, 2008.
14. Kapural L, Stojanovic M, Bensitel T, Zovkic P: Cooled radiofrequency of L5 dorsal ramus for RF denervation of the sacroiliac joint: technical report. *Pain Med* 11:53-57, 2010.
15. Andres RH, Graupner T, Barlocher CB, et al: Laser guided lumbar medial branch kryorhizotomy. *J Neurosurg Spine* 13:341-345, 2010.
16. Li G, Patil C, Adler JR, et al: CyberKnife rhizotomy for facetogenic back pain: a pilot study. *Neurosurg Focus* 23(6):E2, 2007.
17. Iwatsuki K, Yoshimine T, Awazu K: Alternative denervation using laser irradiation in lumbar facet syndrome. *Lasers Surg Med* 39:225-229, 2007.
18. Barlocher CB, Krauss JK, Seiler RW: Kryorhizotomy: an alternative technique for lumbar medial branch rhizotomy in lumbar facet syndrome. *J Neurosurg* 98:14-20, 2003.
19. Staender M, Maerz U, Tonn JC, Steude U: Computerized tomography-guided kryorhizotomy in 76 patients with lumbar facet joint syndrome. *J Neurosurg Spine* 3:444-449, 2005.
20. North RB, Han M, Zahurak M, et al: Radiofrequency lumbar facet denervation: analysis of prognostic factors. *Pain* 57:77-83, 1994.
21. Gallagher J, Petriccione Di Vadi PL, Wedley JR, et al: Radiofrequency facet joint denervation in the treatment of low back pain: a prospective controlled double-blind study to assess its efficacy. *Pain Clin* 7:193-198, 1994.
22. Leclaire R, Fortin L, Lambert R, et al: Radiofrequency facet joint denervation in the treatment of low back pain. *Spine* 26:1411-1417, 2001.

23. Slappendel R, Crul BJ, Braak GJ, et al: The efficacy of radiofrequency lesioning of the cervical spinal dorsal root ganglion in a double blinded randomized study: no difference between 40 degrees C and 67 degrees C treatments. *Pain* 73:159-163, 1997.

24. Lord S, Barnsley L, Wallis B, et al: Percutaneous radio-frequency neurotomy for chronic cervical zygapophyseal-joint pain. *N Engl J Med* 335:1721-1726, 1996.

25. Mikeladze G, Espinal R, Finnegan R, et al: Pulsed radiofrequency application in treatment of chronic zygapophyseal joint pain. *Spine J* 3:360-362, 2003.

26. Cho J, Park YG, Chung SS: Percutaneous radiofrequency lumbar facet rhizotomy in mechanical low back pain syndrome. *Stereotact Funct Neurosurg* 68:212-217, 1997.

27. Royal MA, Bhakta B, Gunyea I, et al: Radiofrequency neurolysis for facet arthropathy: a retrospective case series and review of the literature. *Pain Pract* 2(1):47-52, 2002.

28. Kroll HR, Kim D, Danic MJ, et al: A randomized, double-blind, prospective study comparing the efficacy of continuous versus pulsed radiofrequency in the treatment of lumbar facet syndrome. *J Clin Anesth* 20:534-537, 2008.

29. Mancikanti L, Singh V, Falco FJE, et al: Comparative effectiveness of a one-year follow-up of thoracic medial branch blocks in management of chronic thoracic pain: a randomized, double-blind active controlled trial. *Pain Physician* 13:535-548, 2010.

30. Kornick C, Kramarich SS, Lamer TJ, Todd Sitzman B: Complications of lumbar facet radiofrequency denervation. *Spine* 29:1352-1354, 2004.

31. Gehkt G, Nottmeier EW, Lamer TJ: Painful medial branch neuroma treated with minimally invasive median branch neurectomy. *Pain Med* 11:1179-1182, 2010.

32. Dobrogowski J, Wrzosek A, Wordliczek J: Radiofrequency denervation with or without addition of pentoxifylline or methylprednisolone for chronic lumbar zygapophysial joint pain. *Pharmacol Rep* 57:475-480, 2005.

33. Ma K, Yiqun M, Wang W, et al: Efficacy of diclofenac sodium in pain relief after conventional radiofrequency denervation for chronic facet joint pain: a double blind randomized controlled trial. *Pain Med* 12(1):27-35, 2010.

34. Shealy CN: Percutaneous radiofrequency denervation for spinal facets: treatment for chronic back pain and sciatica. *J Neurosurg* 43:448-451, 1975.

35. Katz SS, Savitz MH: Percutaneous radiofrequency rhizotomy of the lumbar facets. *Mount Sinai J Med* 53:523-525, 1986.

36. Ogsbury JS, Simon RH, Lehman RAW: Facet "denervation" in the treatment of low back pain. *Pain* 3:257-263, 1977.

37. Barnsley L: Percutaneous radiofrequency neurotomy for chronic neck pain: outcomes in a series of consecutive patients. *Pain Med* 6(4):282-286, 2005.

38. Lang JK, Buchfelder M: Radiofrequency Neurotomy for headache stemming from the zygapophysial joints C2/3 and C3/4. *Cen Eur Neurosurg* 71:75-79, 2010.

39. Tzaan WC, Tasker RR: Percutaneous radiofrequency facet rhizotomy-experience with 118 procedures and reappraisal of its value. *Can J Neurol Sci* 27:125-130, 2000.

40. Liliang PC, Lu K, Hsieh CH, et al: Pulsed radiofrequency of cervical medial branches for treatment of whiplash-related cervical zygapophyseal joint pain. *Surg Neurol* 70(suppl 1):50-55, 2008.

16 Complications of Sacroiliac Joint Injection and Lateral Branch Blocks, Including Water-Cooled Rhizotomy

Jason E. Pope

CHAPTER OVERVIEW

Chapter Synopsis: Sacroiliac pain affects diverse patient populations and can be difficult to accurately diagnose. One line of treatment for sacroiliac pain in carefully selected patients can be joint injection or lateral branch block, including cooled radiofrequency (RF) rhizotomy. The most common complications arising from sacroiliac joint injections include local pain and self-resolving neuritis. Infectious risks, including viral infection, can arise but are not common. A possible complication specialized to sacroiliac interventions is suppression of the pituitary–adrenal axis.

Important Points:

- Appropriate Accreditation Council for Graduate Medical Education mentored subspecialty training in interventional pain management is vital to ensure patient-centered care.
- Accurate and expertly placed needles in appropriately selected patients are essential to ensure accurate diagnosis and successful treatment.
- The sacroiliac joint is a large structure with rich, variable innervation. Numerous techniques have been described for intraarticular, extraarticular, lateral branch, and RF treatments.
- RF treatments are not created equal, and an appreciation for each underscores their different applications and associated risks.
- Common complications, regardless of RF modality used, include transient increased localized pain and usually self-limiting neuritis.
- Infectious complications are uncommon if appropriate sterile technique and avoidance of multidosing from single-dose vials are used.
- Injection of steroids or enteral antiinflammatory medications may help with postprocedural pain and neuritis.
- Burn injuries can be avoided by understanding basic circuitry systems, careful equipment use, and correct electrosurgical unit return plate positioning.

Introduction

Estimates of sacroiliac joint sources of back and leg pain have been estimated to be between 10% and 38% using compared diagnostic injections, with a false-positive rate estimated between 0% and 53.8%.[1-3] Not only have diagnostic provocative tests failed to be accurate,[4,5] but there have been numerous efforts to treat sacroiliac joint pain, including intraarticular injections, extraarticular injections, radiofrequency (RF) treatments, fusion, and prolotherapy[6-9] with level II-3 evidence for both short- and long-term relief.[2]

Sacroiliac pain or dysfunction has been implicated in diverse patient populations and associated morbidities, including pediatric low back pain, pregnancy, cancer, infection, ankylosing spondylitis, and inflammatory bowel disease.[10-13] Controversy surrounds diagnostic accuracy and technique[14-21] because some advocate intraarticular injections but others advocate extraarticular injections or lateral branch blocks before RF treatment. Summarily, interventions are directed to either the afferent nociceptive nerves supplying the joint or the actual joint itself. A corollary can be drawn to zygapophyseal treatments because intraarticular or median branch blocks are used before RF treatment, just as sacroiliac intraarticular injection or lateral branch blocks are performed before using RF. Although widely accepted clinically, this treatment algorithm has recently been questioned.[3]

As with any treatment plan, complication avoidance begins with patient selection. Treatment of patients with local infection near the injection site, coagulopathy, allergy to injectate, or comorbidities or conditions that prevent fluoroscopic needle guidance or consent should be avoided. A clear understanding of spinal anatomy and utilization of image guidance is vital to ensure both quality treatment and reduced patient morbidity and mortality.

Table 16-1: Radiofrequency Summary

	Lesion Shape	Lesion Diameter (mm)	Needle Orientation	Temperature (°C)	Time of Lesion (sec)	Neurodestruction
Pulsed	None	None	Perpendicular	42	120	No
Conventional	Prolate spheroid	4	Parallel	80-90	90-105	Yes
Cooled[55]	Spherical	8	Independent	60	230	Yes

Box 16-1: Theoretical Complication Classification

Procedural
Vascular injury
Hematoma or bleeding
Spinal anesthesia
Neuritis
Local postprocedural pain
Burn injury
Neuroma formation
Peripheral nerve injury

Infectious
Epidural abscess
Septic arthritis
Meningitis
Herpes simplex virus

Pharmacologic
Pituitary-adrenal axis suppression
Local anesthetic epidural or spinal spread

Furthermore, it should be understood that appropriate training within Accreditation Council for Graduate Medical Education accredited programs and mentorship is pivotal to ensure treatment success; interventional hobbyists only serve to undermine accessibility of these valuable therapies to patients.

Before proceeding, readers are directed to the chapters that correspond to sacroiliac joint injections; lateral branch blocks; and traditional (see Fig. 15-2), pulsed, and cooled RF treatments (see Fig. 15-5). A brief review of the differences in RF modalities are listed in **Table 16-1**, and reviewed elsewhere in the text (see Chapter 7). Other modalities to treat sacroiliac joint pain include fusion and prolotherapy,[22] this chapter focuses on complications specific to RF neurotomy.

Even after appropriate safeguards and training, significant complications have been described in scattered case reports. Theoretical risks are listed in **Box 16-1**, and they are typically localized or systemic in nature.

Selected Complications

Meta-analysis of treatment outcomes is difficult because the treatment arm is highly variable regarding RF technique, inconsistent patient selection, outcome endpoints, and definitions of success. Although there is a plethora of literature describing sacroiliac joint interventions, few describe complications.[2-4,9,10,13,23-29]

Postprocedure Pain or Neuritis
Transient postprocedural pain often follows RF treatments and has been described in numerous studies for lumbar facetogenic interventions; however, few describe sacroiliac lateral branch

denervation. Cooled RF and traditional thermal RF have been accompanied by postprocedure local pain (**Table 16-2**), typically of a transient nature,[6,30,31] and Vallejo et al[9] reported that no complications arose from pulsed RF treatments of the lateral branches.

No published study has compared the efficacy and complications of cooled versus traditional RF. In an unpublished retrospective analysis of 88 patients at the Cleveland Clinic, there was no statistically significant difference in duration of pain relief, and anecdotally, more patients who underwent cooled RF reported transient postprocedure localized back pain. Kapural et al[6] described transient itching, numbness, and pain.

Steroids are injected after denervation to lessen postprocedural pain. This may seem counterintuitive because the goal in thermal rhizotomy is to create a histologically detectable lesion, blocking neural afferent nociception. Dobrogowsi et al[32] investigated strategies to reduce the inflammatory pain associated with the lesioning using pentoxifylline or methylprednisolone. In a randomized prospective trial, patients were randomized to 1 mL of intraoperative methylprednisolone, pentoxifylline, or saline. No "severe local tenderness" was reported in either the methylprednisolone group or the pentoxifylline group.[32] Other authors[33] contend that 3-day dosage of enteral diclofenac is effective in reducing procedural pain after conventional RF neurotomy of lumbar median branches.

False-Positive Results
False-positive results have been reported to be 0% to 53% using controlled diagnostic injections or post-block provocative sacroiliac maneuvers.[2,4-6,34] These problems may result from numerous factors, including oversedation, large-volume injectate, inaccurate needle placement, or anatomic innate defects in sacroiliac ventral or dorsal capsule. Similarly, false-negative results or treatment failures can result if interosseous or dorsal sacroiliac joint ligaments are not anesthetized because they are known to contribute to these pain complaints. Furthermore, anterior sacroiliac joint innervation is largely ignored as a significant contribution to sacroiliac joint pain.

There have been numerous techniques suggested to enter the sacroiliac joint for arthrography,[14-19] to perform lateral branch blocks,[5,8,34,35] and for denervation.[6,9,11,27,31,36-40] Whatever the method of diagnosing sacroiliac joint pain, accuracy hinges on small-volume injectate and controlled diagnostic comparative blocks, although cost effectiveness has recently come into question.[3] Cohen et al[3] suggested that the cost of RF treatment without diagnostic injection was almost $9000 cheaper, although indirect results suggest a better treatment outcome with dual diagnostic injections before neurotomy, keeping a keen eye on potential placebo cofounders.

Infections
There are scattered reports of infection for both sacroiliac injection and RF therapy. Some suggest that the thermal nature of RF treatment may decrease the chance of infection.[3] Others suggest that

Table 16-2: Reported Sacroiliac Radiofrequency Complications

Author, Year	Type of Lesioning and Location	Complication Reported	Duration of Complaint	Prevalence
Burnham et al,[56] 2007	Radiofrequency strip lesions	Not described	Transient and "mild"	NA
Yin et al,[57] 2003	Thermal, L5 DR, lateral cutaneous branch L5, S1-S3	Persistent cutaneous numbness Transient dysesthesia or hypoesthesia	>6 months 3 weeks-3 months	1 of 14 patients "Most" of 14 patients
Cohen et al,[30] 2008	Traditional L4-L5, cooled S1-S3	Postprocedure localized pain Nonpainful paresthesia	5-10 days	"Majority" of 28 patients
Kapural et al,[6] 2010	Cooled L5, S1-S3	Increased pain Numbness Itching	<6 weeks	8 of 100 patients
Cohen et al,[31] 2009	Traditional L4, DR L5, cooled S1-S3	Temporary anesthesia Superficial skin infection Hyperglycemia	<14 days Course of antibiotics 3 days	5 of 77 patients

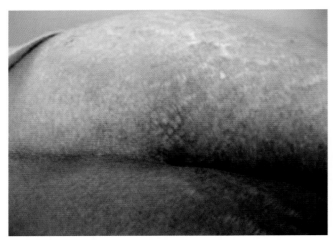

Fig. 16-1 Herpetic outbreak. (From Meydani A, Schwartz A, Foye PM, Patel AD: Herpes simplex following intra-articular sacroiliac corticosteroid injection, *Acta Dermatoven APA* 16(3):135-137, 2009.)

Table 16-3: Reported Sacroiliac Joint Block Lateral Branch Block Complications

Author	Complication Reported	Duration of Complaint	Prevalence
Wong et al,[42] 2010	*Klebsiella pneumoniae* infection *Enterobacter aerogenes* infection	NA	9 of 45 retrospective (3 *Klebsiella* and 1 *Enterobacter* infections)
Meydani et al,[41] 2009	Herpes simplex virus infection	NA	NA
Fortin et al,[58] 1999; Rupert et al,[2] 2009	Inaccurate intraarticular sacroiliac joint injection	NA	20%–54% false-positive rate
Dreyfuss et al,[8] 2009	Inaccurate block of lateral branches	NA	30% false-negative rate
Maugars et al,[59] 1996	Transient perineal anesthesia Sciatica	Few hours 3 weeks	Unknown

NA, not applicable.

steroids may innately increase the infectious potential because they are immunosuppressive.[38] Interestingly, only one report of infectious complication after block therapy was found after an exhaustive Medline search with search terms "sacroiliac and infection." Meydani et al[41] report a herpes simplex virus type II outbreak (**Fig. 16-1**) after sacroiliac injection therapy (**Table 16-3**), confirmed by unroofing vesicle and DNA analysis.

Cohen et al[31] described one superficial infection after RF treatment of 77 patients that resolved after a course of oral antibiotics. Single-use vials should always be used for individual patients because this was a major source of contamination in an *Enterobacter aerogenes* and *Klebsiella pneumoniae* bacteremia outbreak after sacroiliac joint injection reported in 2008.[42]

There have been no reported cases of epidural or paraspinal abscess after sacroiliac joint interventions. The only serious infections described in the literature are those of hematogenic septic arthritis remote from sacroiliac joint interventions.[43]

Bleeding
The incidence of hematoma after sacroiliac joint injection is unknown but is likely less than for spinal or epidural anesthetic procedures, estimated to be one in 222,000 and one in 150,000, respectively.[28] In fact, no cases have been reported. However, if epidural hematoma is suspected, it should be promptly investigated and treated. Symptom and sign presentation is dependent on the anatomic location of the bleed, and a high index of suspicion is needed for diagnosis. Early neurosurgical consultation is essential because prognosis requires expeditious evacuation within 8 hours of neurologic deficit presentation.[29]

Burn Injuries

No burn injuries have been reported with sacroiliac joint denervation; however, the potential can be extrapolated from the facetogenic literature. Burn injuries were the result of equipment malfunction, insulation breaks within the electrodes, unipolar electrosurgical unit return plate, or unknown causes.[44-46] Appreciation of circuit differences between grounded and ungrounded systems is encouraged as operating room power supplies are typically isolated, ungrounded systems, where office buildings are typically grounded systems. By design, isolated systems are more difficult to deliver aberrant current. Furthermore, burn severity is related to current density, either greater the current or the smaller the area applied.

Pituitary–Adrenal Axis Suppression

Although numerous studies have demonstrated pituitary–adrenal suppression with epidural or intraarticular administration of glucocorticoids,[47-51] none has investigated axis depression from sacroiliac interventions. From the available data, hypothalamic pituitary adrenal axis suppression could be assumed to be depressed for 4 weeks, and insulin sensitivity may be adversely affected for 1 week. Cushing syndrome, steroid myopathy, aseptic meningitis, and anaphylactoid reactions have been reported after single epidural steroid injections.[52,53] Other glucocorticoid side effects, including musculoskeletal, ophthalmologic, gastrointestinal, cardiovascular, secondary cortisol deficiency, gynecologic, neurologic, hematologic, psychiatric, and dermatologic, have been described.[54]

Summary

The sacroiliac joint is recognized as a major contributor for low back and leg pain. It has a highly variable and rich anterior and posterior innervation, with contributions from various adjacent structures. This variability permits interventional targets to be widely distributed, and subsequent meta-analysis on complications difficult. What can be taken from analysis is that careful attention to patient selection and expertly conducted interventions are vital to provide patients with the best opportunity for success while mitigating side effects and complications.

References

1. Manchikanti L, Singh V, Pampati V, et al: Evaluation of the relative contributions of various structures in chronic low back pain. *Pain Physician* 4:308-316, 2001.
2. Rupert MP, Lee M, Machikanti L, et al: Evaluation of sacroiliac joint interventions: a systemic appraisal of the literature. *Pain Physician* 12:399-418, 2009.
3. Cohen SP, Williams KA, Kurihara C, et al: Multicenter, randomized comparative cost-effectiveness study comparing 0, 1 and 2 diagnostic medial branch (facet joint nerve) block treatment paradigms before lumbar facet radiofrequency denervation. *Anesthesiology* 113:395-405, 2010.
4. Laslett M, Young SB, Aprill CN, McDonald B: Diagnosing painful sacroiliac joints: a validity study of a McKenzie evaluation and sacroiliac provocation tests. *Aust J Physiother* 49:89-97, 2003.
5. van der Wurff P, Buijs EJ, Groen GJ: A multitest regimen of pain provocation tests as an aid to reduce unnecessary minimally invasive sacroiliac joint procedures. *Arch Phys Med Rehabil* 87:10-14, 2006.
6. Kapural L, Stojanovic M, Bensitel T, Zovkic P: Cooled radiofrequency of L5 dorsal ramus for RF denervation of the sacroiliac joint: technical report. *Pain Med* 11:53-57, 2010.
7. Cohen SP, Strassels SA, Kurihara C, et al: Outcome predictors for sacroiliac joint (lateral branch) radiofrequency denervation. *Reg Anesth Pain Med* 34(3):206-214, 2009.
8. Dreyfuss P, Henning T, Malladi N, et al: The ability of multi-depth sacral lateral branch blocks to Anesthetize the sacroiliac joint complex. *Pain Med* 10(4):679-688, 2009.
9. Vallejo R, Benyamin RM, Kramer J, et al: Pulsed radiofrequency denervation for the treatment of sacroiliac joint syndrome. *Pain Med* 7(5):429-434, 2006.
10. Manchikanti L, Singh V, Pampati V, et al: Evaluation of the relative contributions of various structures in chronic low back pain. *Pain Physician* 4:308-316, 2001.
11. Vanelderen P, Szadek K, Cohen SP, et al: Evidence based medicine 13. Sacroiliac joint pain. *Pain Pract* 5:470-478, 2010.
12. Moghadam A, Talebi-Taher M, Dehghan A: Sacroiliitis as an initial presentation of acute lymphoblastic leukemia. *Acta Clin Belg* 65(3): 197-199, 2010.
13. Hwangbo Y, Kim, HJ, Ryu KN, et al: Sacroiliitis is common in Crohn's disease patients with perianal or upper gastrointestinal involvement. *Gut Liver* 3(4):338-344, 2010.
14. Dussault RG, Kaplan PA, Anderson MW: Fluoroscopically guided sacroiliac joint injection. *Radiology* 214:273-277, 2000.
15. Bogduk N: Practice guidelines. In *Spinal diagnostic and treatment procedures*, San Francisco, 2004, ISIS, pp 66-86.
16. Ebraheim NA, Xu R, et al: Sacroiliac joint injection: a cadaver study. *Am J Orthop* 1997;26:338-341.
17. Fortin JD, et al: Sacroiliac joint injection: pain referral maps upon applying a new injection/arthrography technique. Part 1: asymptomatic volunteers. *Spine* 19(13):1475-1482, 1994.
18. Centeno C: How to obtain an SIJ arthrogram 90% of the time in 30 seconds or less. *Pain Physician* 9:159, 2006.
19. Daitch J, Frey M, Snyder K. Modified SIJ injection technique. *Pain Physician* 9:367-368, 2006.
20. Schwarzer AC, Aprill CN, Bognuk N: The sacroiliac joint in chronic back pain. *Spine* 20(1):31-37, 1995.
21. Fortin JD, Tolchin RB: Sacroiliac arthrograms and post-arthrography computerized tomography. *Pain Physician* 6:287-290, 2003.
22. Kim MW, Lee HG, Wo JC, et al: A randomized controlled trial of intraarticular prolotherapy versus steroid injection for sacroiliac joint pain. *J Altern Complement Med* 16(12):1285-1290, 2010.
23. Maigne JY, Aivakiklis A, Pfefer F: Results of sacroiliac joint double block and value of sacroiliac pain provocation test in 54 patients with low back pain. *Spine* 21:1889-1892, 1996.
24. Irwin RW, Watson T, Minick RP, Ambrosius WT: Age, body mass index, and gender differences in sacroiliac joint pathology. *Am J Phys Med Rehabil* 86:37-44, 2007.
25. Cohen SP, Abdi S: Lateral branch blocks as a treatment for sacroiliac joint pain: a pilot study. *Reg Anesth Pain Med* 28(2):113-119, 2003.
26. McKenzie-Brown AM, Shah RV, Sehgal N, Everett CR: A systematic review of sacroiliac interventions. *Pain Physician* 8:115-125, 2005.
27. Schwarzer AC, Aprill CN, Bogduk N: The sacroiliac joint in chronic low back pain. *Spine* 20: 31-37, 1995.
28. Horlocker TT, Rowlingson JC, Enneking FK, et al: Regional anesthesia in the patient receiving antithrombotic or thrombolytic therapy: American Society of Regional Anesthesia and Pain Medicine Evidence-Based Guidelines (Third Edition). *Reg Anesth Pain Med* 35(1):64-101, 2010.
29. Vandermeulen EP, Van Aken H, Vermylen J: Anticoagulants and spinal-epidural anesthesia. *Anesth Analg* 79:1165-1177, 1994.
30. Cohen SP, Hurley RW, Buckenmaier CC, et al: Randomized placebo controlled study evaluating lateral branch radiofrequency denervation for sacroiliac joint pain. *Anesthesiology* 109:279-288, 2008.
31. Cohen SP, Strassels SA, Kurihara C, et al: Outcome predictors for sacroiliac joint (lateral branch) radiofrequency denervation. *Reg Anesth Pain Med* 34(3):206-214, 2009.
32. Dobrogowski J, Wrzosek A, Wordliczek J: Radiofrequency denervation with or without addition of pentoxifylline or methylprednisolone for chronic lumbar zygapophysial joint pain. *Pharmacol Rep* 57:475-480, 2005.
33. Ma K, Yiqun M, Wang W, et al: Efficacy of diclofenac sodium in pain relief after conventional radiofrequency denervation for chronic facet

joint pain: a double blind randomized controlled trial. *Pain Med* 12(1):27-35, 2010.

34. Cohen SP, Hurley RW, Buckenmaier CC 3rd, et al: Randomized placebo-controlled study evaluating lateral branch radiofrequency denervation for sacroiliac joint pain. *Anesthesiology* 109(2):279-288, 2008.

35. Dreyfuss P, Snyder BD, Park K, et al: The ability of single site, single depth sacral lateral branch blocks to anesthetize the sacroiliac joint complex. *Pain Med* 9:844-850, 2008.

36. Ferrante FM, King LF, Roche EA, et al: Radiofrequency sacroiliac joint denervation for sacroiliac syndrome. *Reg Anesth Pain Med* 26:137-142, 2001.

37. Kapural L, Nageeb F, Kapural M, et al: Cooled radiofrequency system for the treatment of chronic pain from sacroiliitis: the first case-series. *Pain Pract* 8(5):348-354, 2008.

38. Hansen HC, McKenzie-Brown AM, Cohen SP, et al: Sacroiliac joint interventions: a systematic review. *Pain Physician* 10:165-184, 2007.

39. Stone JA, Bartynski WS: Treatment of facet and sacroiliac joint arthropathy: steroid injections and radiofrequency ablation. *Tech Vasc Interventional Radiol* 12:22-32, 2009.

40. Cosman ER Jr, Gonzalez CD: Bipolar radiofrequency lesion geometry: implications for palisade treatment of sacroiliac joint pain. *Pain Pract* 11(1):3-22, 2011.

41. Meydani A, Schwartz A, Foye PM, Patel AD: Herpes simplex following intra-articular sacroiliac corticosteroid injection. *Acta Dermatoven APA* 16(3):135-137, 2009.

42. Wong MR, Del Rosso P, Heine L, et al: An outbreak of *Klebsiella pneumoniae* and *Enterobacter aerogenes* bacteremia after interventional pain management procedures, New York City 2008. *Reg Anesth Pain Med* 35(6):496-499, 2010.

43. Mancaarella L, De Santis M, Magarelli N, Ierardi AM, Bonomo L, Ferraccioli G. Septic Arthritis: an uncommon septic arthritis. *Clin Exp Rheuatologu* 27(6):1004-1008, 2009 Nov-Dec.

44. Shealy CN: Percutaneous radiofrequency denervation for spinal facets: treatment for chronic back pain and sciatica. *J Neurosurg* 43:448-451, 1975.

45. Katz SS, Savitz MH: Percutaneous radiofrequency rhizotomy of the lumbar facets. *Mount Sinai J Med* 53:523-525, 1986.

46. Ogsbury JS, Simon RH, Lehman RAW: Facet "denervation" in the treatment of low back pain. *Pain* 3:257-263, 1977.

47. Gevargez A, Groenemeyer D, Schirp S, Braun M: CT-guided percutaneous radiofrequency denervation of the sacroiliac joint. *Eur Radiol* 12:1360-1365, 2002.

48. Habib GS: Systemic effects of intra-articular corticosteroids. *Clin Rheumatol* 28:749-756, 2009.

49. Ward A, Watson J, Wood P, et al: Glucocorticoid epidural for sciatica: metabolic and endocrine sequelae. *Rheumatology (Oxford)* 41:68-71, 2002.

50. Cook DM, Meikle AW, Bowman R: Systemic absorption of triamcinolone after a single intraarticular injections suppresses the pituitary-adrenal axis [abstract]. *Clin Res* 36(suppl A):121A, 1988.

51. Kay J, Findling JW, Raff H: Epidural triamcinolone suppresses the pituitary-adrenal axis in human subjects. *Anesth Analg* 79:501-505, 1994.

52. Knight CL, Burnell JC: Systemic side effects of extradural steroids. *Anaesthesia* 35:593-594, 1980.

53. Boonen S, Van Distel G, Westhovens R, et al: Steroid myopathy induced by epidural triamcinolone injection. *Br J Rheumatol* 34:385-386, 1995.

54. Nesbit LT: Minimizing complications from systemic glucocorticosteroid use. *Dermatol Clin* 13:925-939, 1995.

55. Kapural L, Mekhail N, Hick D, et al: Histological changes and temperature distribution studies of a novel bipolar radiofrequency heating system in degenerated and nondegenerated human cadaver lumbar discs. *Pain Med* 9:68-75, 2008.

56. Burnham RS, Yasui Y: An alternate method of radiofrequency neurotomy of the sacroiliac joint: a pilot study of the effect of pain, function, and satisfaction. *Reg Anesth Pain Med* 32:12-19, 2007.

57. Yin W, Willard F, Carreiro J, Dreyfuss P: Sensory stimulation-guided sacroiliac joint radiofrequency neurotomy: technique based on neuroanatomy of the dorsal sacral plexus. *Spine* 28(20):2419-2425, 2003.

58. Fortin JD, Washington WJ, Falco JE: Three pathways between the sacroiliac joint and neural structures. *Am J Neuroradiol* 20:1429-1434, 1999.

59. Maugars Y, Mathis C, Berthelot JM, et al: Assessment of the efficacy of sacroiliac corticosteroid injections in spondyloarthropathies: a double-blind study. *Br J Rheumatol* 35:767-770, 1996.

17 Complications of Percutaneous Vertebral Augmentation: Vertebroplasty and Kyphoplasty

Paul J. Lynch, Tory L. McJunkin, and Elizabeth Srejic

CHAPTER OVERVIEW

Chapter Synopsis: Vertebral compression fractures (VCFs) can result in debilitating downstream consequences (including spinal deformity and increased mortality) that can be avoided with timely treatment. Percutaneous vertebral augmentation (PVA) techniques consist of vertebroplasty, in which orthopedic cement is injected into painful vertebral bodies, and kyphoplasty, in which a balloon is used to relieve pressure before injection. Although minimally invasive, the techniques carry risks of complications, including needle misplacement, cement extravasation, damage to adjacent vertebrae, and infection.

Important Points:

- Painful VCFs caused by osteoporosis and malignancy are seen more frequently as the U.S. population ages and life expectancies increase.
- Because VCFs can cause debilitating problems, including spinal deformity, impairment of locomotion, decreased lung function, heightened risk of subsequent fracture, and increased mortality, treatment is essential to inhibit the development of deleterious sequelae.
- PVA collectively refers to vertebroplasty and kyphoplasty, two minimally invasive procedures used to treat VCFs.
- Vertebroplasty and kyphoplasty involve injection of medical-grade orthopedic cement into damaged, painful vertebral bodies. Whereas kyphoplasty incorporates the use of a balloon to expand the injection site before introduction of the orthopedic cement, vertebroplasty involves injection of cement directly into the collapsed vertebrae without balloon pretreatment.
- The primary goal of PVA is to reduce the pain associated with VCFs. Secondary goals may include stabilization of crumbling vertebrae and prevention of further vertebral collapse, reversal of height loss (height restoration), and correction of kyphotic deformities that result from VCFs.
- Because of their minimally invasive nature, PVA procedures carry a lower risk of complications than more invasive interventions such as open surgery. However, PVA procedures are associated with serious risks, including errant needle placement, cement extravasation, side effects related to the procedure (e.g., adjacent level fractures), infection, and risks from anesthesia.
- Complications in vertebroplasty and kyphoplasty may be minimized by careful patient selection and by obtaining adequate training and using meticulous technique.
- Good technique in PVA includes safe needle placement, which requires advanced understanding of vertebral anatomy and the ability to skillfully interpret fluoroscopic images, and mastery of bone cement preparation and injection.

Introduction

Worldwide approximately 1.4 million persons currently have vertebral compression fractures (VCFs),[1] which are caused predominantly by osteoporosis and malignancy. The incidence of painful VCFs is increasing as age and life expectancy increase.

Osteoporosis, the leading cause of VCFs, is the most common metabolic bone disorder in the United States, affecting 25 million people and leading to approximately 750,000 new osteoporotic vertebral fractures each year.[2,3] Of these, only one-third receive treatment,[4] and more than one-third become chronically painful.[2] Annualized direct care expenditures for osteoporotic fractures in

the United States were estimated to range from $12 billion to $18 billion in 2002.[5]

Bone malignancy, another leading cause of VCFs, is a consequence of cancer, the second leading cause of death in the United States. Roughly two-thirds of cancer patients develop metastases,[6,7] and vertebral body metastases occur frequently in systemic malignancy. In fact, the skeletal system is the third most common site of metastasis, and metastases favor the spine.[8]

Vertebral compression fractures can cause debilitating spinal deformity with possible impairments in locomotion,[9,10] decreased lung function,[11] a heightened risk of subsequent fracture,[12] and increased mortality.[13,14] Therefore many believe expert and efficacious treatment of VCFs is essential to inhibit the development of deleterious sequelae.

Percutaneous vertebral augmentation (PVA) consists of two minimally invasive procedures used to treat VCFs, vertebroplasty and kyphoplasty. Both PVA interventions involve injection of medical-grade orthopedic cement into collapsed and painful vertebral bodies. This chapter focuses on using PVA for lumbar and thoracic VCFs, although the authors recognize that the treatment can also be used for cervical and sacral fractures. The primary goal of PVA is to reduce the pain associated with VCFs. Secondary goals may include stabilization of crumbling vertebrae and prevention of further vertebral collapse. Other goals might include reversing loss of height (height restoration) and correcting kyphotic deformities that result from VCFs.

Although vertebroplasty and kyphoplasty are similar procedures with largely analogous methodologies and objectives, the chief distinction between them is that kyphoplasty incorporates a balloon to expand the injection site before introduction of orthopedic cement, while vertebroplasty involves injection of cement directly into the collapsed vertebrae without balloon pretreatment. The addition of balloon pretreatment may permit greater gains in vertebral height and kyphosis correction than are achievable with vertebroplasty.[15] Because of the publication of numerous studies that suggest kyphoplasty may have greater efficacy than vertebroplasty, some practitioners consider kyphoplasty to be superior to vertebroplasty for the correction of painful VCFs.[16] However, there exists a comparable number of studies that suggest vertebroplasty is as efficacious as kyphoplasty in stabilizing vertebral fractures and correcting attendant pain and other related consequences. Furthermore, the higher cost associated with kyphoplasty and the outpatient nature of vertebroplasty have made vertebroplasty a more attractive treatment option in many cases.[17]

The exact mechanism(s) of pain relief from vertebroplasty and kyphoplasty remain indefinite, although there are two commonly held theories. The first theory is that the procedures produce an analgesic effect by fixating chronically mobile bone fragments within the vertebral body with an internal cast. This theory is easy to understand because one can see how casting a fracture reduces pain by limiting movement of the fractured site. The second theory is that PVA reduces pain by thermal neurolysis. As the bone cement begins to harden within the body, there occurs an exothermic process capable of producing temperatures as high as 70°C, which could damage (cauterize) nerve endings sufficiently to negate pain.

Vertebroplasty

Originally developed in France in 1986, the practice of vertebroplasty has steadily improved and gained recognition in the United States since the early 1990s. Vertebroplasty is a minimally invasive, nonsurgical procedure that involves fluoroscopically guided placement of needles and injection of biocompatible, orthopedic bone cement (usually polymethylmethacrylate [PMMA] or calcium phosphate) directly into the vertebral body. The procedure has also been performed with computed tomography (CT) guidance by those who have access to that imaging tool. Overall, vertebroplasty is performed to reduce pain. Some have also discussed vertebroplasty as a preventive measure to bolster weakened vertebral bodies destined for fracture, although its use for this purpose has been discouraged by many and has not been supported by prospective studies.

Bone cement may be mixed with antibiotic and barium or tantalum to reduce the risk of infection and facilitate fluoroscopic visibility. Normally, a transpedicular approach is used to access the central portion of the vertebral body in the thoracic and lumbar spine because this spares the spinal canal or segmental arteries flanking the vertebral body. The procedure can be done with an extrapedicular approach as well but may not have as robust of a safety profile. Vertebroplasty can be done unilaterally or bilaterally as desired by the performing surgeon (**Figs. 17-1** and **17-2**). Some experts do recommend a bilateral approach because they believe that this provides increased safety through redundancy and ensures central placement of cement. No current prospective studies have clearly defined the most efficacious method of these two approaches.

Most patients are able to return home the same day as undergoing vertebroplasty and resume normal activities of daily living relatively quickly. This makes the procedure an attractive option compared with more invasive treatments for VCFs.

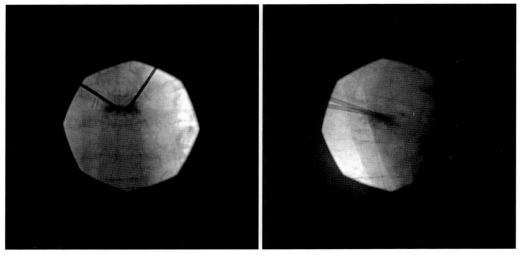

Fig. 17-1 Anteroposterior (**A**) and lateral (**B**) bipedicular vertebroplasty for moderate to severe vertebral compression fracture at T5.

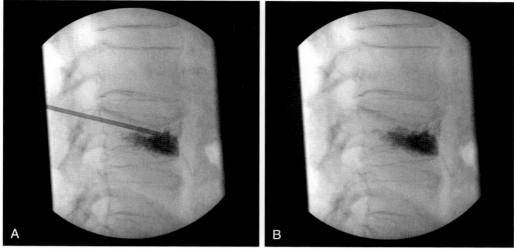

Fig. 17-2   Anteroposterior (AP) (**A**) and postvertebroplasty AP (**B**) views for L3 vertebral compression fracture unipedicular approach.

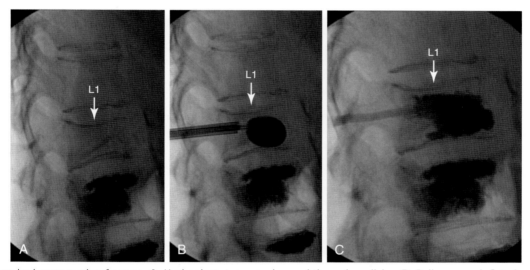

Fig. 17-3   L1 vertebral compression fracture. **A,** Kyphoplasty trocars advanced through pedicles. **B,** Balloons are inflated and then removed. **C,** Bone cement is injected into the cavity created by the balloons. (© 2011 Regents of the University of Michigan.)

Kyphoplasty

Kyphoplasty is a newer therapy indicated for the treatment of painful VCFs. Kyphoplasty parallels vertebroplasty in that it is highly effective in relieving pain associated with VCFs. However, several studies suggest that kyphoplasty can also restore height and reduce deformity compared with vertebroplasty.[18] The data are not completely clear, however, because one study found that kyphoplasty and vertebroplasty produce the same degree of height restoration,[19] although a later cadaver study by the same group[20] found the increase in vertebral height was greater with kyphoplasty than with vertebroplasty (5.1 mm vs. 2.3 mm, respectively).

Normally, kyphoplasty is performed under intravenous (IV) sedation or monitored anesthesia care, but some practitioners prefer to do the procedure with general anesthesia. As in vertebroplasty, fluoroscopy (or CT scan) is used to guide the procedure. Typically, a small incision is made, and the trocars are advanced bilaterally into the vertebral body using a transpedicular approach (**Fig. 17-3**). Kyphoplasty can also be done via an extrapedicular approach, and some systems advocate a unilateral approach (**Fig. 17-4**). When the trocars are in the correct position, a cannulated drill is placed through the trocar, and the bone is drilled by hand creating space within the vertebral bodies for the balloons. The drill is then removed, and the balloons (inflatable bone tamps) are inserted through the trocars. The balloons are filled with contrast medium and carefully inflated under live radiography for easy visualization. Subsequently, the balloons are inflated until they expand to the desired height and then removed, leaving prearranged cavities for the cement within the fractured vertebral body. This process is what is thought to provide the height restoration for the procedure. The cavities are then filled with the same type of orthopedic cement used in vertebroplasty, and the trocars removed. Because of its widely promoted height-restoration effects, many physicians recommend kyphoplasty over vertebroplasty. It should be noted, however, that kyphoplasty is far more expensive a procedure, potentially costing significantly more than vertebroplasty. Clinicians are in need of prospective comparative studies that match these two modalities of treatment to specific types of fractures.

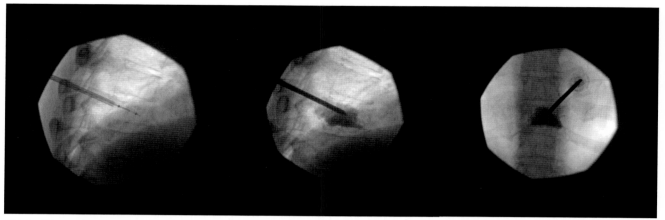

Fig. 17-4   T8 vertebral compression fracture. Unilateral kyphoplasty. Balloons are inflated and then removed. Bone cement is injected into the cavity created by the balloons.

Indications and Contraindications

Percutaneous vertebral augmentation procedures are minimally invasive and designed to treat benign or malignant painful VCFs. Historically, VCFs arising from osteoporosis or malignancy were treated with bed rest and pharmacologic interventions. These measures aimed to decrease the patient's pain but had significant risk. Aside from severe pain, risks for not treating a patient with a painful VCF might include worsening spinal deformity, deep venous thrombosis, pulmonary embolism, and pneumonia, to name a few. In recent times, the development and refinement of minimally invasive interventional techniques have led to an increase in the use of PVA procedures to treat patients with severe pain. PVA can also often help to diagnose the source of the VCF and may lead to treatment of pathologic processes such as osteoporosis and metastatic cancer. Vertebroplasty and kyphoplasty are advantageous in that they provide significant pain reduction as opposed to bed rest and pharmacologic therapy. PVA procedures may also spare patients from more invasive open spinal procedures.

The vertebral compression associated with osteoporosis results from lowered bone strength, a consequence of accelerated loss of bone minerals. Furthermore, kyphosis secondary to osteoporotic VCF shifts the center of gravity anteriorly, increasing the risk of falls and additional fractures. In conjunction with physiologic decreases in lung capacity and appetite, a significant increase in 1-year mortality is associated with a patient's first VCF.[14]

Vertebral compression fractures are most commonly a result of decreased bone strength but can also be a hallmark of malignancy in the spine. It is well known that malignant disease can have a primary bone source or can metastasize to bones with frequent spread to vertebral bodies. Because the length of time a patient lives with cancer is increasing with better treatments, malignancy in the spine will likely become more prevalent among patients.

Absolute contraindications to vertebroplasty and kyphoplasty are rarely seen but include:

- Active infection
  - Spine-related conditions (e.g., osteomyelitis, discitis)
  - Localized infection at the surgical site
  - Systemic infection (e.g., sepsis)
- New neurologic insult related to fracture that is amenable to surgery
  - Spinal cord injury related to fracture: retropulsed vertebral fragments contacting the spinal cord

- Nerve root injury related to fracture
- Spinal bleeding (e.g., epidural hematoma)
- Systemic infection (e.g., sepsis)
- Irreversible coagulopathy

Relative contraindications for PVA treatments include:

- Nonpainful VCF
- Posterior wall of vertebral body is violated (allowing for cement leakage into spinal canal)
- Pedicle instability
- Ineligibility for conscious sedation
- Severe central spinal stenosis (>30%)
- Coagulopathy or thrombocytopenia
- Pregnancy
- Hypersensitivity to cement
- Hypersensitivity to implanted devices
- Neoplastic disease (epidural or intradural) that compresses or encases the thecal sac or nerve roots
- Severe medical conditions in which risks of the procedure outweigh the benefits

Open surgery is another treatment option for patients with painful VCFs. However, unlike more conservative interventions, open surgery addresses deformity but carries a higher risk of complications. In addition, many patients with VCFs are precluded from surgery because they have multilevel disease. As a result, surgery is typically reserved as a last resort for patients who demonstrate neurologic abnormalities on physical examination. Neurologic compromise often results from physical compression of the spinal cord or nerve roots and is often associated with vertebral body bone retropulsion.

Benefits

In the literature, vertebroplasty and kyphoplasty have been described as bringing significant pain relief to patients with vertebral fractures secondary to osteoporosis and solid or marrow-based malignancy (80% to 89% in most reports). For most, relief is usually immediate after treatment, with maximal effect obtained as soon as 2 weeks after treatment. According to one systematic review of the literature, there is fair evidence (level II to III) that 2 years after the intervention, vertebroplasty provides a similar degree of pain control and physical function as optimal medical management. There is also fair evidence (level II to III) that kyphoplasty results in greater improvement in daily activity, physical function, and pain relief compared with optimal medical management for osteoporotic VCFs 6 months after the intervention.[21] Furthermore, a meta-analysis of the literature examining pain relief and complications in vertebroplasty and kyphoplasty patients in 1036 studies found that both vertebroplasty and kyphoplasty provided significant pain improvement as measured by visual analog scores (VAS); vertebroplasty produced greater improvement in VAS scores than kyphoplasty but also carried a statistically greater risk of cement leakage and new fracture.[22]

In addition, the pain relief from both procedures has been noted as long lasting as demonstrated in studies with multiyear follow-ups.[23,24] One such multiyear study, a retrospective single-center consecutive case series with 2-year follow-up, found kyphoplasty markedly improved clinical outcome and produced significant vertebral height restoration and normalization of morphologic shape indices that remained stable for at least 2 years after treatment.[25] Pain scores, patient ability to ambulate independently and without difficulty, and need for prescription pain medications improved significantly after kyphoplasty and remained unchanged or improved at 2 years; furthermore, vertebral heights significantly increased at all postoperative intervals, with greater than or equal to 10% height increases in 84% of fractures. Asymptomatic cement extravasation occurred in 11.3% of fractures, and during the follow-up period, additional fractures occurred in previously untreated levels at a rate of 4.5% per year. There were no kyphoplasty-related complications.

Additional benefits of vertebroplasty and kyphoplasty include the use of IV sedation for the procedure with patients usually able to avoid general anesthesia. Both procedures can usually be conducted on an outpatient basis. In addition, patients can quickly return to the normal activities of daily living, and bracing is not required.

Numerous studies have examined the specific benefits of kyphoplasty. For example, a randomized, controlled trial of 300 patients at 21 sites in eight countries noted significant improvement in quality of life in kyphoplasty patients over the control group as assessed by short form physical component summary.[26] Additionally, a study in 314 kyphoplasty recipients with VCFs as a result of osteoporosis or multiple myeloma found that all patients tolerated the kyphoplasty procedure well, the average Owestry Disability Index score decreased by 12.6 points, and there was no statistically significant difference with regard to functional outcome in the osteoporosis and multiple myeloma subgroups.[27] And a study in 555 patients with a total of 1150 vertebral fractures treated with kyphoplasty noted no cement-related complications as described in the literature and concluded by careful interdisciplinary indication setting and a standardized treatment model that kyphoplasty presented a safe and effective procedure for the treatment of various vertebral fractures.[28]

Despite numerous studies in the literature that support the efficacy of PVA, two controversial original articles questioning the worth of vertebroplasty were published in the August 6, 2009, issue of the *New England Journal of Medicine*. These included reports by Kallmes et al[29] on the Investigational Vertebroplasty Safety and Efficacy Trial (ClinicalTrials.gov number, NCT00068822) and Buchbinder et al[30] on a randomized trial of vertebroplasty for painful osteoporotic vertebral fractures (Australian New Zealand Clinical Trials Registry number, ACTRN012605000079640). In both studies, the authors concluded that vertebroplasty has no greater benefit than placebo in the treatment of painful osteoporotic compression fractures.

Kallmes et al[29] reported, "Improvements in pain and pain-related disability associated with osteoporotic compression fractures in patients treated with vertebroplasty were similar to the improvements in a control group." In this multicenter trial, 131 patients with one to three painful osteoporotic VCFs underwent either vertebroplasty or a simulated procedure without cement (control group). The primary outcomes were scores on the modified Roland–Morris Disability Questionnaire (RDQ) (on a scale of 0 to 23, with higher scores indicating greater disability), and patients' ratings of average pain intensity during the preceding 24 hours at 1 month (on a scale of 0 to 10, with higher scores indicating more severe pain). Patients were permitted to cross over to the other study group after 1 month. All patients underwent the assigned intervention (68 vertebroplasties and 63 simulated procedures). The baseline characteristics were similar in the two groups. At 1 month, it was reported that there was no significant difference between the vertebroplasty group and the control group in either the RDQ score or the pain rating. Both groups had immediate improvement in disability and pain scores after the intervention. Although the two groups did not differ significantly on any secondary outcome measure at 1 month, there was a trend toward a higher rate of clinically meaningful improvement in pain (a 30% decrease from baseline) in the vertebroplasty group (64% vs. 48%; $P = .06$). At 3 months, there was a higher crossover rate in the control group than in the vertebroplasty group (43% vs. 12%; $P < .001$), according to the report.

The Buchbinder et al[30] report described a randomized, double-blind, placebo-controlled trial in which participants ($n = 78$) had one or two painful osteoporotic vertebral fractures that were of less than 12 months' duration and unhealed, as confirmed by magnetic resonance imaging (MRI), and randomly assigned to undergo vertebroplasty or a sham procedure. Participants were stratified according to treatment center, sex, and duration of symptoms (<6 weeks or ≥6 weeks). Outcomes were assessed at 1 week and at 1, 3, and 6 months. The primary outcome was overall pain (on a scale of 0 to 10, with 10 being the maximum imaginable pain) at 3 months. Buchbinder et al[30] reported they found no beneficial effect of vertebroplasty compared with a sham procedure in patients with painful osteoporotic vertebral fractures at 1 week or at 1, 3, or 6 months after treatment. They noted that vertebroplasty did not result in a significant advantage in any measured outcome at any time point, although there were significant reductions in overall pain in both study groups at each follow-up assessment. Similar improvements were seen in both groups with respect to pain at night and at rest, physical functioning, quality of life, and perceived improvement.

In response to these original articles, proponents of vertebroplasty submitted correspondence that critiqued the studies. One group of respondents[31] expressed "serious concerns" over both trials, noting that the study by Kallmes et al[29] involved outpatients exclusively and excluded inpatients hospitalized with acute fracture pain. The same group of commentators noted that the study protocol mandated 4 weeks of medical therapy before enrollment, which they maintained resulted in a study on healed rather than subacute fractures, and noted a more appropriate selection criterion would have been uncontrolled pain for fewer than 6 weeks. They also noted that the Buchbinder et al[30] trial included an inadequate number of patients for a subgroup analysis, substantially limiting statistical power, and that although the study is described as a multicenter trial, two of the four hospitals withdrew early from the study after enrolling five patients each. The authors of the correspondence also argued that 68% of the procedures were performed in one hospital by one radiologist, and the rates of eligible patients who declined to participate were 64% in the Buchbinder trial[30] and 70% in the Kallmes trial[29] (85% in the United States), raising further concerns regarding patient selection.

Another group of correspondents[32] noted that patients with maximal back pain, who tend to have the greatest improvement in pain score after vertebroplasty, would also be the least likely to participate in such studies because they would risk being randomly assigned to the placebo group, as evidenced by the preprocedural pain scores among patients who were enrolled. The correspondents also commented that neither study was sufficiently powered to perform subanalyses, particularly on patients with certain types of fractures that would be more likely to have improved pain scores after vertebroplasty (e.g., those with gas-filled clefts and pathologic fractures).

Also, a singleton respondent[33] questioned whether a group of patients who receive an injection of an anesthetic should be considered a true control because delivery of a local anesthetic can have beneficial effects for a period exceeding the activity of the drug. He also suggested that there may be a significant difference in cross-over rates between the treatment and control groups (12% vs. 43%) in the study by Kallmes et al,[29] which could suggest patient dissatisfaction with the sham procedure that was not fully captured by pain scales.

Certainly, these criticisms provide compelling reasons to question the results of the controversial Kallmes et al[29] and Buchbinder et al[30] studies. Furthermore, it should be noted that these two studies compete with a vast pool of published evidence that supports the therapeutic legitimacy of PVA.

Complications

Because of their minimally invasive nature, PVA procedures carry a lower risk of complications than more invasive interventions such as open surgery. For example, a level III therapeutic study found that kyphoplasty had a complication rate equivalent to nonoperative treatment (1.7% vs. 1.0%), and a lower rate of in-hospital mortality (0.3% vs. 1.6%).[34]

Percutaneous vertebral augmentation procedures are not without significant risk, and care must be taken to avoid the most common and serious risks associated with these procedures. These risks include errant needle placement, cement leakage and its associated problems, side effects related to the procedure, and risks from anesthesia.

Errant Needle Placement

A potentially devastating error in PVA is errant needle placement, which can lead to adverse sequelae such as spinal cord injury; damage to nerves, vessels and organs; and excessive bleeding and pneumothorax.[35]

To preclude errant needle placement, practitioners must develop excellent familiarity with relevant anatomic landmarks, become expert with fluoroscopy, and use modern imaging equipment. Good pathways to achieving the necessary expertise include supervision and mentorship during physician training, cadaver laboratories, and guidance during initial utilization of the modality in professional practice.

Cement Extravasation

The chief complication reported in the literature for both procedures is cement leakage, or extravasation (**Figs. 17-5** and **17-6**). Normally, this complication is asymptomatic. However, patients with symptomatic cement leakage along the spinal nerve roots may experience dysesthesia, culminating in radicular pain or paraplegia (**Fig. 17-7**). Furthermore, cement leakage into vessels can lead to embolism into any vessels, including the pulmonary arteries, depending on the amount leaked (**Fig. 17-8**). Leakage into the spinal canal can lead to tremendous neurologic complications; a study documenting a series of cases of neurologic deficit after vertebroplasty and kyphoplasty found that catastrophic neurologic injury required open surgical intervention in 12 of 14 patients who developed neurologic deficit after undergoing vertebroplasty or kyphoplasty (**Fig. 17-9**).[36]

Despite cement leakage, however, vertebroplasty and kyphoplasty have proven to be safe and effective in many studies in the literature. For example, a 4-year study of 28 patients who underwent either of the two procedures found the only complication was cement extravasation, but no clinical symptom occurred[23] (**Fig. 17-10**). Furthermore, there was no significant difference between the incidences of cement leakage between the two procedures. In addition, there was significant change in

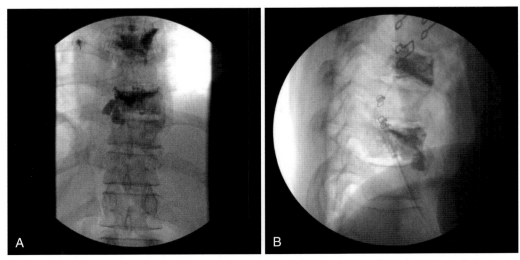

Fig. 17-5 Anteroposterior (AP) (**A**) and lateral views (**B**). The upper fracture shows extravasation of cement inferior and superior to endplate margins. The lower fracture shows lateral and inferior extravasation outside of the vertebral body. The patient had no complications from the previous percutaneous vertebral augmentation procedure and admitted to pain relief.

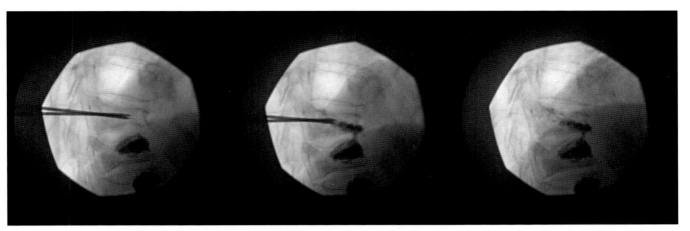

Fig. 17-6   Cement is shown to exit needles and travel toward the inferior endplate fracture and migrate into the inferior disc space, connecting with the previous fracture and inferior level. The procedure is abandoned after minimal cement is placed into the fractured vertebral body. The patient received significant pain relief with no complications.

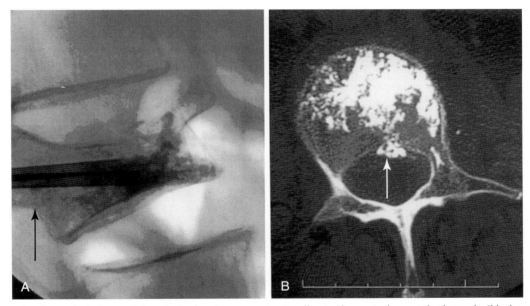

Fig. 17-7   A, Lateral radiograph during vertebroplasty showing cement extending to the posterior vertebral margin (*black arrow*).
B, Computed tomography scan done after percutaneous vertebral augmentation demonstrating a small leak into the epidural venous plexus (*white arrow*). This leak was asymptomatic. (From Mathis JM: Percutaneous vertebroplasty: complication avoidance and technique optimization, *AJNR Am J Neuroradiol* 24(8):1697-1706, 2003.)

preoperative and postoperative VAS and Oswestry scores in both groups.

Because bone cement is a relatively low-viscosity medium when first injected, it carries a relatively high risk of extravasation (**Fig. 17-11**). According to one study,[37] in almost all cases, cement leakage occurs because of premature application of cement before it reaches its optimum thickness. Furthermore, according to the authors of this study, the literature shows a percentage rate of about 9% for cement leakage from balloon kyphoplasty versus leakage rates of up to 41% for vertebroplasty, with some studies reporting cement leakage ratios of 4% to 10% for kyphoplasty versus 20% to 70% for vertebroplasty. Cement extravasation in vertebroplasty, which can result in spinal cord and nerve root compression, cardiac tamponade, and pulmonary and other emboli,[38-40] has been shown to be a direct consequence of the amount of cement injected; this complication is mitigated by the fact that pain relief is not related

to the volume of injection and appears to occur with relatively small amounts of injected cement.[41]

Side Effects from the Procedure

One side effect of PVA often reported in the literature is adjacent level fractures. Independent studies have demonstrated a recurrent fracture rate of 12.4% to 21%, with the majority of these new fracture levels occurring adjacent to the PV level.[42,43] However, the evidence for increased risk of adjacent level fracture after PVA compared with conservative treatment remains inconclusive.[40] A widely posed reason to reject this correlation is that new adjacent level fractures occur in patients with a natural history of osteoporosis regardless of whether they undergo PVA.[44]

One study[45] showed an incidence of 6.16% (18 of 292) of adjacent level fractures after kyphoplasty in patients with a mean age

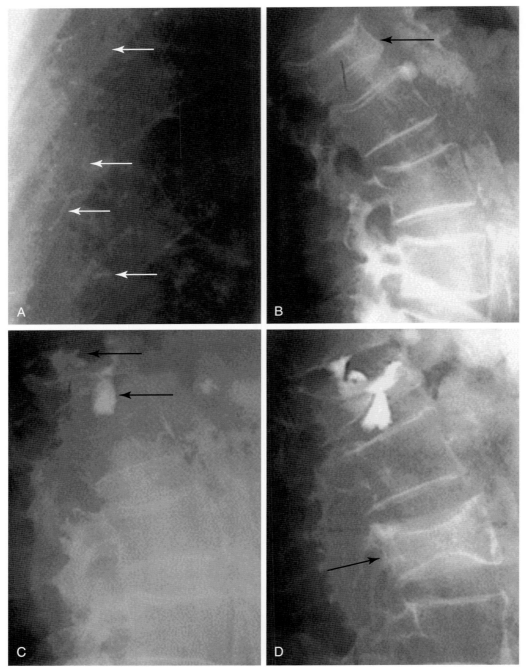

Fig. 17-8 **A,** Portion of a chest radiograph after percutaneous vertebral augmentation showing a small radiopaque cement emboli (*arrows*) in peripheral pulmonary vessels. This patient had no pulmonary symptoms. **B,** Lateral radiograph of the spine showing a moderately compressed vertebra (*arrow*). **C,** After vertebroplasty, there are large leaks of cement (*arrows*) into the adjacent disc spaces. **D,** Six months later, the patient returned with a second fracture (*arrow*). This fracture is not an adjacent level. Adjacent levels did not fracture despite the large disc leaks. (From Mathis JM: Percutaneous vertebroplasty: complication avoidance and technique optimization, *AJNR Am J Neuroradiol* 24(8):1697-1706, 2003.)

of 72.7 years over a mean follow-up interval of 25.6 months, although predictors for new vertebral fracture failed to identify statistically significant risk factors despite a large sample size. Another retrospective study correlating PVA with a subsequent heightened adjacent fracture risk reported that of 38 patients, 10 patients sustained 17 subsequent fractures over the follow-up period, with nine at adjacent-above levels, four at adjacent-below levels, and four at remote levels.[46] Most of those fractures at

adjacent levels occurred within 2 months of the procedure. The authors concluded that the data indicated a higher rate of subsequent fracture after kyphoplasty compared with natural history data for untreated fractures and speculated that because there were only occasional subsequent fractures at remote levels after the 2-month postprocedural period, it confirmed biomechanical studies showing that cement augmentation places additional stress on adjacent levels.

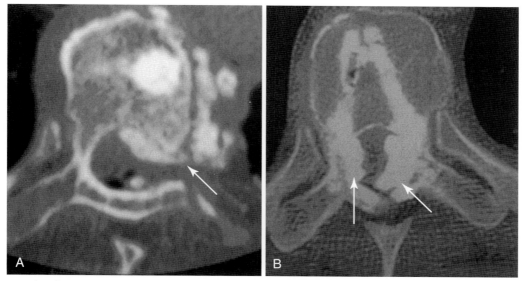

Fig. 17-9 A, Postvertebroplasty computed tomography (CT) scan demonstrating large cement leaks into the spinal canal, neural foramen (*arrow*), and perispinous region. This patient had paresis and radiculopathy. **B,** Postkyphoplasty CT scan showing large leaks into the spinal canal (*arrows*), which created paraplegia. (From Mathis JM: Percutaneous vertebroplasty: complication avoidance and technique optimization, *AJNR Am J Neuroradiol* 24(8):1697-1706, 2003.)

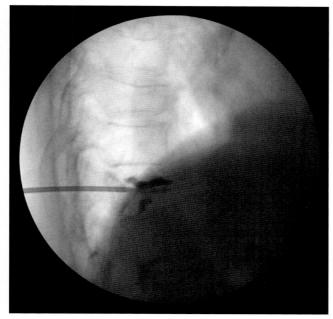

Fig. 17-10 Unipedicular vertebroplasty. Lateral radiograph of an extremely collapsed lower thoracic vertebra. Superior and inferior endplates are identified with bone cement seen to fill the fracture line superiorly and track through the inferior endplate fracture into the adjacent disc space.

One possible cause of new adjacent VCFs noted in the literature is cement leakage into the intervertebral disc, which may necessitate further PVA for pain relief. A retrospective study assessing new adjacent level VCFs after percutaneous vertebroplasty found VCFs occurred in 20 (18.9%) of 106 patients at 22 adjacent vertebral bodies after vertebroplasty during at least 24 months of follow-up, with the difference in number of new adjacent fractures between patients with cement leakage into the disc and those without leakage statistically significant and the risk of adjacent vertebral fracture higher if cement leaked into the disc.[47]

It is important to note that although numerous studies find an association between PVA and adjacent fracture, a relatively equivalent number of reports do not propose a correlation between these events. One study with this viewpoint, involving 188 patients (163 women, 25 men; mean age, 70.9 years; range, 42 to 92 years) who underwent 214 PVA sessions at 351 levels for osteoporotic VCFs, evaluated the effect of intradiscal cement leakage on new adjacent vertebral fracture formation after PVA and concluded that intradiscal cement leakage does not seem to be related to subsequent adjacent VCF in patients who underwent PVA for treatment of an osteoporotic compression fracture.[48] The validity of the study is strengthened because additional risk factors were also analyzed using univariate and multivariate methods, including age, gender, mean bone mineral density (BMD), the vertebral level treated, the presence of an intravertebral cleft or cyst before treatment, the kyphosis angle, the wedge angle, and the injected cement volumes. The authors noted that the only factor correlated with an adjacent vertebral fracture after PVA was thoracolumbar location of the initial compression fracture. In addition, a prospective observational cohort study of consecutive osteoporotic VCFs in patients who were 90 years old and older evaluated at a multidisciplinary, university spine center found vertebroplasty for VCFs in the very elderly appears effective and safe without increased risk of adjacent level fracture.[45] The patient sample, which included consecutive osteoporotic patients with symptomatic VCFs electing to enter the study, were evaluated on a baseline VAS rating, analgesic usage, and duration of symptoms. Subsequent VAS ratings, analgesic utilization, and new fractures were assessed at planned intervals. The mean VAS score was 7.6 at baseline, 3.1 at 30 minutes after the procedure, and 2.3, 1.2, 1.1, 0.9, 0.8, and 0.5 at 2 weeks, 1 month, 3 months, 6 months, 1 year, and 2 years, respectively. Improvement over time was statistically significant, and no complications were encountered during the follow-up intervals. Thirteen new fractures were observed (10.6%) at a mean 20.8 weeks (1 to 52 weeks) after PVA with six new fractures (4.9%) involving an adjacent level in five patients (4.1%). Another study comparing the strength of polymethylmethacrylate and calcium phosphate cement in 24 spinal columns (T10–L2) from human cadavers found that the

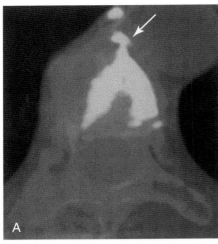
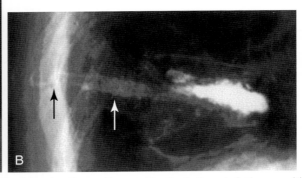

Fig. 17-11 **A,** Postkyphoplasty computed tomography scan. The lateral wall was disrupted by the balloon inflation, resulting in a large cement leak into the mediastinum (*arrow*). For weeks after the procedure, this patient had severe, persistent pain. **B,** Lateral radiograph after vertebroplasty with a slow-set polymethylmethacrylate. The needles were withdrawn, and the cement was still liquid enough to flow into the needle tracts and into the soft tissue (*arrows*). This created local discomfort to pressure. (From Mathis JM: Percutaneous vertebroplasty: complication avoidance and technique optimization, *AJNR Am J Neuroradiol* 24(8):1697-1706, 2003.)

strength of bone filler materials (not cement leakage or other factors) is considered a risk factor in developing adjacent vertebral body fractures after PVA.[49]

A key argument is that subsequent fractures after PVA may be a natural consequence of osteoporosis. A study in 73 consecutive patients with painful VCFs found that more patients with a BMD higher or equal to 3.0 experienced a new fracture than those with a BMD less than 3.0 (odds ratio [OR], 13.00; 95% confidence interval [CI], 1.35 to 124.81), and the risk for adjacent level fractures decreased significantly when the postoperative kyphotic angle was less than 9 degrees compared with that of higher or equal to 9 degrees (OR, 12.00; 95% CI, 1.25 to 114.88).[50] The authors concluded that balloon kyphoplasty and vertebroplasty are methods with a low risk of adjacent level fractures, and the most important factors for new VCFs after a PVA procedure are the degree of osteoporosis and altered biomechanics in the treated area of the spine caused by resistant kyphosis. They also noted that the results suggest that the adjacent vertebrae would fracture eventually even without the procedure and that PVA offers a comparable rate of pain relief.

Low body mass index (BMI) may be another risk factor for VCF in patients with osteoporosis, irrespective of whether PVA is performed. A study found that new VCFs were common in patients with low BMIs, suggesting osteoporosis as a mechanism of fracture, although it should be noted that the new fractures were also associated with proximity to the treated vertebra and greater kyphosis correction.[51] Another study found that lower baseline BMD, older age, and more preexisting VCFs were demonstrated in patients who experienced VCFs two or more times, although it is noteworthy that in 852 patients (1131 vertebrae), 58.8% to 63.8% of new compression fractures after vertebroplasty were adjacent compression fractures, and these occurred much sooner than nonadjacent fractures (71.9 ± 71.8 days vs. 286.8 ± 232.8 days; $P < .001$).[52] Given the risk of subsequent fracture in patients with osteoporosis, postoperative use of anti-osteoporotic medication seems to be an excellent measure for the prevention of new VCFs.[53]

As with any surgical procedure, infection represents a probable adverse outcome of PVA, although the incidence is rare.[54] Signs and

symptoms post-PVA infection may include pain, swelling, rubor, purulent drainage, fever, nausea, vomiting, and chills. Of particular concern are signs of advanced infection, including elevated white blood cell, C-reactive protein, and sedimentation rate counts. Because infection is a definite risk of PVA, practitioners should endeavor to lower the incidence of topical and systemic infection in their patients. Prophylactic antibiotics are given IV (e.g., 1 g cefazolin) because PVA involves injection of foreign material into the body.[55] Beyond administration of antibiotics, screening patients for topical infections, immunocompromised status, and systemic conditions, the most important measure against infection is meticulous surgical technique. To achieve this, iodine or chlorhexidine should be used as a surgical preparation, with a wide area of the back prepared because a variety of angles of approach may be used. Sterile drapes are placed over the patient, and measures such as a surgical scrub and use of masks and gloves should be incorporated.

Percutaneous vertebral augmentation can be performed under mild sedation with local or general anesthesia, but the operation must be convertible in a short time frame to an open emergency operation in cases of severe bone-cement leakage into the spinal canal.[55] Sedative analgesics in the form of fentanyl, midazolam, or propofol can be administered.[56]

Particularly in elderly osteoporosis patients, a notable side effect of surgery is rib fracture from prone positioning on the operating table. Physicians should remain mindful of this possibility and may opt to pad the voids between the patient and the table to achieve maximum extension of the spine, protect pressure points covered by thin skin, avoid rib fracture, and promote patient comfort; it should also be noted that in this largely elderly patient population, rib fracture can occur simply from mobilizing the patient.[57]

Other general side effects of PVA reported in the literature have included cerebrospinal fluid leakage,[58] bleeding,[59] new fracture,[51] nerve damage,[60] and epidural and subdural hematoma.[61] Additional complications have included recurrent back pain,[62] vena cava syndrome,[63] osteitis,[64] epidural abscess,[65] and aseptic osteonecrosis.[66] Development of local metastases along the tract of the needle (needle tract seeding) in a lung cancer patient has also been reported.[67] Additionally, a recent report describes a rare case of anterior spinal cord syndrome caused by a cement embolism in the anterior spinal artery after vertebroplasty.[68] And one group of authors postulates that local infiltration anesthesia is not sufficient for "a substantial proportion of patients" based on the results of a study in 44 vertebroplasty patients.[69]

Bleeding complications also represent a possible adverse effect in PVA. In general, the cement seals most of the bony needle tract from the vertebral body to the pedicle, which should alleviate most of the problem. Still, fracture of a pedicle or tearing of a vein proximal to the spinal canal could lead to a large hematoma in a patient with bleeding diathesis. This can be avoided by verifying that coagulation studies and platelet levels are normal before the procedure.[35]

Reducing Complications

One of the most crucial ways to reduce complications in PVA is to seek adequate training. The best route to achieving this is to obtain adequate supervision initially while performing the procedure. Guidance, repetition, and mentorship may be gained through residency and fellowship experience, cadaver courses, and "real-world" supervision during professional practice. In addition, better results may be expected when there is limited compression of the vertebral body, the fracture is less than 12 months old, or the radionuclide bone scan or T2-weighted MRI indicates the fracture contains active marrow edema.[70]

One of the fundamentals in complication avoidance in PVA is safe needle placement. Beyond practice and skill, mastering this technique requires advanced understanding of vertebral anatomy and the ability to skillfully interpret both normal and abnormal fluoroscopic images. This also requires a fully functional procedure suite with biplane or single-plane high-quality fluoroscopy capabilities. Poor visualization is associated with migration of cement. One study recommended over conventional CT and biplane fluoroscopy the use of isocentric C-arm fluoroscopic cone beam CT (CBCT), a new technique for near real time 3-dimensional volume imaging guidance of percutaneous interventional procedures of the spine. The CBCT has the capability to produce near real time high-resolution image reconstructions in any plane and may be superior to conventional fluoroscopy, but it is not widely used.[71] Failure to master anatomic landmarks, interpret fluoroscopic images, and use high-quality fluoroscopic equipment could result in adverse outcomes such as leakage of cement into the epidural canal, which could result in partial or complete paralysis, neuritis, or embolism. Clearly, development of expertise with fluoroscopy is important in precluding disastrous consequences.

To ensure optimal needle placement, the site of entry should be carefully identified. In the thoracic and lumbar regions, a transpedicular approach is ideal. In contrast, in the cervical spine an anteromedial approach is optimal because the pedicles are too small to accommodate the needles, and a posterolateral approach threatens the vertebral artery.[35] Initially, the fractured vertebral body should be identified with proper counting and visualized in both anteroposterior (AP) and lateral projections. There are many techniques to access the vertebral body in the transpedicular fashion, and most courses teach a systematic way to perform the procedure. Syed and Shaikh[72] also have a technique review that many physicians find helpful. In general after the fractured vertebral body is identified, the endplates are then squared in an AP projection. Through craniocaudad tilting of the fluoroscopic image under live fluoroscopy, the pedicles are then placed in the center of the target area so that the needle traverses the pedicles into the correct portion of the vertebral body. The skin and subcutaneous

tissue are then anesthetized (the authors of this chapter prefer lidocaine 1% with epinephrine) and the tracts are anesthetized down to the pedicles and the pedicles themselves are anesthetized. With the anesthetic needles left in place, one can then visualize the angles of needle trajectory on both AP and lateral views to ensure correct trocar placement in similar fashion. Some will then make a small incision with a scalpel, and the large-bore trocars (typically between 10 and 13 gauge) are inserted through the anesthetized tissue. The trocars are then advanced toward the upper outer quadrant of the pedicles and seated into the bone. The trocars are then advanced with frequent fluoroscopic images monitoring the needle trajectory and position. The trocar should follow a path that is parallel to the superior and inferior edges of the pedicle. In fractured vertebral bodies with endplate depression, a different angle may be required to avoid traversing the endplate. Care must be taken to visualize the medial cortex of the pedicle at all times, and the trocars *must not* violate this boundary as they traverse the vertebral body. Typically, frequent AP and lateral images are monitored as the trocars are being advanced through the pedicles. When the trocars are seen on lateral view to pass the posterior margin of the vertebral body, the spinal canal has been cleared safely. Up to this point, the medial cortex of the pedicle should not have been violated. The trocars can then be advanced to their correct depth within the vertebral body for either the vertebroplasty or kyphoplasty procedure. With vertebroplasty in a lateral fluoroscopic projection, at the posterior vertebral body, the trocars are advanced into the anterior third portion of the vertebral body because this area is mostly devoid of venous plexuses. In kyphoplasty, the trocars are advanced into the posterior third of the vertebral body, and the bone drills are then advanced through the trocars to make room for the inflatable balloons.

Although not commonly performed, some advocate that venography may be performed before cement injection to facilitate accuracy.[73] This is achieved by highlighting the anastomosis of the epidural canal, central veins, and inferior vena cava, which may illustrate an outline of the venous drainage, vertebral cortex fractures, and possible leakage sites. Furthermore, accurate needle placement within the bony trabeculae may be confirmed. Corrections in needle placement should be made early in the procedure when the needle is still in the pedicle.[74] It should be noted there is a risk of fracturing the pedicle because of the large size of the biopsy needle, and CT scan before the procedure can help assess the degree of this risk.[75] Although this technique may highlight the venous anatomy, most practitioners do not use this technique and instead choose to inject thickened contrast-enhanced bone cement into the fractured vertebral body with live fluoroscopy.

Safe cement placement techniques are also important in evading complications in PVA. These techniques include adequate barium radio-opacification of cement; viscous low-pressure delivery of cement; lower volumes of cement; and cement delivery under high-quality, direct fluoroscopic visualization.[76]

Cement should be mixed sufficiently to achieve the optimal, "toothpaste-like" consistency important in precluding extravasation; however, superfluous mixing can result in excessive emulsification of the barium, which lowers fluoroscopic efficacy. Cement must be viscous enough to avoid excessive pressure during placement because this is associated with extravasation. In kyphoplasty, cavities are created before cement is injected. Care must still be taken when injecting the cement into the fractured vertebral body because extravasation can still occur. In vertebroplasty, a small amount of cement should be placed into the anterior two-thirds of the vertebral body. After 30 seconds, the spread of cement may be visualized in AP and lateral views. Pausing during injection to allow curing of the cement can sometimes halt extravasation and allow further filling of the vertebral body.[77] This initial "test dose" of cement should be performed in both vertebroplasty and kyphoplasty to prevent extravasation of cement.

To lower the likelihood of cement extravasation, it is important to observe the spread of cement under live fluoroscopy. This is achieved optimally in the lateral view.[56] Cement extravasation can be promoted by high cement volume because use of excessive amounts of cement invites migration into unwanted areas. In fact, one study finds that the rate of complications in PVA is directly related to the volume of cement injected,[76] but another study asserts that pain relief is not related to volume of cement injected and appears to occur with relatively low amounts of injected cement.[78] High viscosity of cement is another way to mitigate migration; some experts recommend the use of a new high-viscosity cement (Confidence Spinal Cement System) to inhibit cement leakage.[78] This is based on published results of vertebroplasties performed with Confidence cement; the author concluded that highly viscous cements may increase the safety of vertebral augmentation techniques when compared with less viscous cements.

Another tip for successful cement placement includes use of sterile technique to preclude infection which can arise from the injection of foreign material into the body. Less experienced providers should also remain mindful of their personal limitations. For example, performing PVA in more complicated regions, as in the case of high thoracic fractures, is a task best undertaken after obtaining extra instruction and practice.

Tips for Avoidance of Complications from Percutaneous Vertebral Augmentation

- Proper didactic training and understanding of crucial vertebral anatomy
- Hands-on experience performing the procedure on cadavers
- Experienced supervision of initial performance of the procedure
- Correct patient selection for skill level
  - Avoid cervical and high thoracic fractures
  - Avoid severely collapsed fractures with distortion of anatomy
- Ensure that patient does not have preoperative infection or bleeding diathesis
- Know when to stop or abandon the procedure
- Use quality imaging equipment
- Consider preoperative antibiotics
- Meticulous sterile technique and patient scrubbing
- Light sedation if possible to facilitate communication with the patient
- An organized systematic approach to access fractured vertebral body
- Safe needle placement: do not violate the medial cortex of the pedicle until the posterior aspect of the vertebral body has been entered as per the lateral view
- Take a lateral view of the fractured vertebral body and surrounding anatomy before cement is injected as a reference point
- Only inject thickened radiopaque bone cement at the consistency of toothpaste
- Inject cement under live radiography
- Test dose: after the cement is visualized exiting the trocar and entering the vertebral body stop, watch and wait for 30 to 60 seconds
- Take AP and lateral radiographs to view the initial spread of the cement

- If the cement seems to be spreading as expected, proceed slowly with continued cement placed under live radiography in the lateral view
- Stop injecting cement when the cement has reached the posterior third of the vertebral body
- Use lower volumes of cement (e.g., 2 to 4 mL instead of 4 to 8 mL)
- Replace stylet in trocars and slowly remove trocars under radiographic guidance with a twisting motion
- Hold deep pressure over needle entry locations for approximately 5 minutes
- Have a "disaster plan" in place if you suspect any complications (e.g., advanced airway management, transfer to triage center, emergent imaging, emergent surgical decompression)

Conclusion

Despite the limited number of randomized, controlled trials in the literature, vertebroplasty and kyphoplasty are believed to significantly improve quality of life for patients with compression fractures, and evidence of their safety and efficacy is increasing, suggesting that both are more effective than conservative management and carry a low risk of complications.[79] The majority of available evidence supports kyphoplasty and vertebroplasty as effective therapies in the management of patients with symptomatic VCFs refractory to conventional medical therapy.

Complications in vertebroplasty and kyphoplasty may be minimized by careful patient selection and meticulous technique. High-quality fluoroscopic imaging and expertise with operative techniques are necessities. When performed optimally, vertebroplasty and kyphoplasty bring significant, rapid, long-lasting pain relief with few complications.

References

1. HoiKee N: Kyphoplasty for osteoporotic vertebral compression fractures. *JAAPA* 21(7):28-31, 2008.
2. Riggs BL, Melton LJ III: The worldwide problem of osteoporosis: insights afforded by epidemiology. *Bone* 17(suppl 5):S505-S511, 1995.
3. Watts NB, Harris ST, Genant HK: Treatment of painful osteoporotic vertebral fractures with percutaneous vertebroplasty or kyphoplasty. *Osteoporos Int* 12:429-437, 2001.
4. Carmona RH: *Office of the Surgeon General. Bone health and osteoporosis: a report of the Surgeon General*, Rockville, MD, 2004, Department of Health and Human Services.
5. Carmona RH: *Office of the Surgeon General. Bone health and osteoporosis: a report of the Surgeon General*, Rockville, MD, 1984, Department of Health and Human Services.
6. Silverberg E: Cancer statistics. *J Clin Cancer* 34:7-23, 1984.
7. Jaffe W: *Tumors and tumorous conditions of the bones and joints*, Philadelphia, 1958, Lea & Febiger.
8. Gokaslan Z: Spine surgery for cancer. *Curr Opin Oncol* 8:178-181, 1996.
9. Gold DT: The clinical impact of vertebral fractures: quality of life in women with osteoporosis. *Bone* 18(suppl 3):S185-S189, 1996.
10. Sinaki M: Falls, fractures, and hip pads. *Curr Osteoporos Rep* 2:131-137, 2004.
11. Leech JA, Dulberg C, Kellie S, et al: Relationship of lung function to severity of oseteoporosis in women. *Am Rev Respir Dis* 14:68-71, 1990.
12. Kado DM, Duong T, Stone KL, et al: Incident vertebral fractures and mortality in older women: a prospective study. *Osteoporos Int* 14:589-594, 2003.
13. Kado DM, Huan MH, Karlamangla AS, et al: Hyperkyphotic posture predicts mortality in older community-dwelling men and women: a prospective study. *J Am Geriatr Soc* 52:1662-1667, 2004.

14. Kado DM, Browner WS, Palermo L: Vertebral fractures and mortality in older women: a prospective study. Study of Osteoporotic Fractures Research Group. *Arch Intern Med* 159:1215-1220, 1999.

15. Theodorou DJ, Theodorou SJ, Duncan TD, et al: Percutaneous balloon kyphoplasty for the correction of spinal deformity in painful vertebral body compression fractures. *Clin Imaging* 26(1):1-5, 2002.

16. Garfin S, Reilley MA: Minimally invasive treatment of osteoporotic vertebral body compression fractures. *Spine J* 2(1):76-80, 2002.

17. Cloft HJ, Jensen ME: Kyphoplasty: an assessment of a new technology. *AJNR Am J Neuroradiol* 28(2):200-203, 2007.

18. Gan M, Yang H, Zhou F, et al: Kyphoplasty for the treatment of painful osteoporotic thoracolumbar burst fractures. *Orthopedics* 33(2):88, 2010.

19. Hiwatashi A, Westesson PL, Yoshiura T, et al: Kyphoplasty and vertebroplasty produce the same degree of height restoration. *AJNR Am J Neuroradiol* 30(4):669-673, 2009.

20. Hiwatashi A, Sidhu R, Lee RK, et al: Kyphoplasty versus vertebroplasty to increase vertebral body height: a cadaveric study. *Radiology* 237(3):1115-1119, 2005.

21. Hulme PA, Krebs J, Ferguson SJ, Berlemann U: Vertebroplasty and kyphoplasty: a systematic review of 69 clinical studies. *Spine (Phila Pa 1976)* 31(17):1983-2001, 2006.

22. Eck JC, Nachtigall D, Humphreys SC, Hodges SD: Comparison of vertebroplasty and balloon kyphoplasty for treatment of vertebral compression fractures: a meta-analysis of the literature. *Spine J* 8(3):488-497, 2008.

23. Sun ZG, Miao XG, Yuan H, et al: [Assessment of percutaneous vertebroplasty and percutaneous kyphoplasty for treatment of senile osteoporotic vertebral compression fractures]. *Zhongguo Gu Shang* 23(10):734-738, 2010.

24. Dong Y, Wang DY: [Treatment of osteoporotic vertebral compression fractures by balloon kyphoplasty]. *Zhongguo Gu Shang* 23(6):466-467, 2010.

25. Ledlie J, Renfro M: Kyphoplasty treatment of vertebral fractures: 2-year outcomes show sustained benefits. *Spine (Phila Pa 1976)* 31(1):57-64, 2006.

26. Wardlaw D, Cummings SR, Van Meirhaeghe J, et al: Efficacy and safety of balloon kyphoplasty compared with non-surgical care for vertebral compression fracture (FREE): a randomised controlled trial. *Lancet* 373(9668):1016-1024, 2009.

27. Khanna AJ, Reinhardt MK, Togawa D, Lieberman IH: Functional outcomes of kyphoplasty for the treatment of osteoporotic and osteolytic vertebral compression fractures. *Osteoporos Int* 17(6):817-826, 2006.

28. McArthur N, Kasperk C, Baier M, et al: 1,150 kyphoplasties over 7 years: indications, techniques, and intraoperative complications. *Orthopedics* 32(2):90, 2009.

29. Kallmes DF, Comstock BA, Heagerty PJ, et al: A randomized trial of vertebroplasty for osteoporotic spinal fractures. *N Engl J Med* 361(6):569-579. 2009.

30. Buchbinder R, Osborne RH, Ebeling PR, et al: A randomized trial of vertebroplasty for painful osteoporotic vertebral fractures. *N Engl J Med* 361(6):557-568, 2009.

31. Clark W, Lyon S, Burnes J: Trials of vertebroplasty for vertebral fractures. *N Engl J Med* 361:2097-2100, 2009.

32. Baerlocher M, Munk PL, Liu DM: Trials of vertebroplasty for vertebral fractures. *N Engl J Med* 361:2098, 2009.

33. Lotz J: Trials of vertebroplasty for vertebral fractures. *N Engl J Med* 361:2098, 2009.

34. Zampini JM, White AP, McGuire KJ: Comparison of 5766 vertebral compression fractures treated with or without kyphoplasty. *Clin Orthop Relat Res* 468(7):1773-1780, 2010.

35. Miller D, Fenton D, Dion J: Vertebroplasty. In *Image-guided spine intervention*, Philadelphia, 2003, Saunders, p 190.

36. Patel AA, Vaccaro AR, Martyak GG, et al: Neurologic deficit following percutaneous vertebral stabilization. *Spine (Phila Pa 1976)* 32(16):1728-1734, 2007.

37. Bula P, Lein T, Strassberger C, Bonnaire F: [Balloon kyphoplasty in the treatment of osteoporotic vertebral fractures: indications—treatment strategy—complications]. *Z Orthop Unfall* 148(6):646-656, 2010.

38. Cohen J, Lane T: Right intra-atrial and ventricular polymethylmethacrylate embolus after balloon kyphoplasty. *Am J Med* 123(10):e5-e6, 2010.

39. Caynak B, Onan B, Sagbas E, et al: Cardiac tamponade and pulmonary embolism as a complication of percutaneous vertebroplasty. *Ann Thorac Surg* 87(1):299-301, 2009.

40. Röllinghoff M, Zarghooni K, Dargel J, et al: The present role of vertebroplasty and kyphoplasty in the treatment of fresh vertebral compression fractures. *Minerva Chir* 65(4):429-437, 2010.

41. Fourney DR, Schomer DF, Nader R, et al: Percutaneous vertebroplasty and kyphoplasty for painful vertebral body fractures in cancer patients. *J Neurosurg* 98(1 suppl):21-30, 2003.

42. Syed M, Jan S, Patel NA, et al: Vertebroplasty: the alternative treatment of osteoporotic vertebral compression fractures in the elderly. *Clin Geriatr* 14:20-23, 2006.

43. Uppin AA, Hirsch JA, Centenera LV, et al: Occurrence of new vertebral body fracture after percutaneous vertebroplasty in patients with osteoporosis. *Radiology* 226:119-124, 2003.

44. DePalma MJ, Ketchum JM, Frankel BM, Frey ME: Percutaneous vertebroplasty for osteoporotic vertebral compression fractures in the nonagenarians: a prospective study evaluating pain reduction and new symptomatic fracture rate. *Spine (Phila Pa 1976)* 36(4):277-282, 2011.

45. Chen WJ, Kao YH, Yang SC, et al: Impact of cement leakage into disks on the development of adjacent vertebral compression fractures. *J Spinal Disord Tech* 23(1):35-39, 2010.

46. Fribourg D, Tang C, Sra P, et al: Incidence of subsequent vertebral fracture after kyphoplasty. *Spine (Phila Pa 1976)* 29(20):2270-2277, 2004.

47. Lo YP, Chen WJ, Chen LH, Lai PL: New vertebral fracture after vertebroplasty. *J Trauma* 65(6):1439-1445, 2008.

48. Lee KA, Hong SJ, Lee S, et al: Analysis of adjacent fracture after percutaneous vertebroplasty: does intradiscal cement leakage really increase the risk of adjacent vertebral fracture? *Skeletal Radiol* 2011, in press.

49. Nouda S, Tomita S, Kin A, et al: Adjacent vertebral body fracture following vertebroplasty with polymethylmethacrylate or calcium phosphate cement: biomechanical evaluation of the cadaveric spine. *Spine (Phila Pa 1976)* 34(24):2613-2618, 2009.

50. Movrin I, Vengust R, Komadina R: Adjacent vertebral fractures after percutaneous vertebral augmentation of osteoporotic vertebral compression fracture: a comparison of balloon kyphoplasty and vertebroplasty. *Arch Orthop Trauma Surg* 130(9):1157-1166, 2010.

51. Lin WC, Cheng TT, Lee YC, et al: New vertebral osteoporotic compression fractures after percutaneous vertebroplasty: retrospective analysis of risk factors. *J Vasc Interv Radiol* 19(2 Pt 1):225-231, 2008.

52. Tseng YY, Yang TC, Tu PH, et al: Repeated and multiple new vertebral compression fractures after percutaneous transpedicular vertebroplasty. *Spine (Phila Pa 1976)* 34(18):1917-1922, 2009.

53. Moon ES, Kim HS, Park JO, et al: The incidence of new vertebral compression fractures in women after kyphoplasty and factors involved. *Yonsei Med J* 48(4):645-652, 2007.

54. Waldman D: Vertebroplasty. In Fenton D, Czervionke L, editors: *Image-guided spine intervention*, Philadelphia, 2003, Saunders.

55. Ruiz-Lopez R, Pichot C: Vertebroplasty. In *Interventional pain management*, ed 2, Philadelphia, 2008, Saunders, p 560.

56. Raj P, Lou L, Erdine S & Staats P: *Radiographic imaging for regional anesthesia and pain management*, Philadelphia, 2003, Churchill Livingstone, p 216.

57. Ruiz-Lopez R, Pichot C: Vertebroplasty. In *Interventional pain management*, ed 2, Philadelphia, 2008, Saunders, p 561.

58. Jankowitz BT, Atteberry DS, Gerszten PC, et al: Effect of fibrin glue on the prevention of persistent cerebral spinal fluid leakage after incidental durotomy during lumbar spinal surgery. *Eur Spine J* 18(8):1169-1174, 2009.

59. Kwak HJ, Lee JK, Kim YS, et al: Aortic aneurysm complicated with pyogenic spondylitis following vertebroplasty. *J Clin Neurosci* 15(1):89-93, 2008.

60. Stoffel M, Wolf I, Ringel F, et al: Treatment of painful osteoporotic compression and burst fractures using kyphoplasty: a prospective observational design. *J Neurosurg Spine* 6(4):313-319, 2007.

61. Cosar M, Sasani M, Oktenoglu T, et al: The major complications of transpedicular vertebroplasty. *J Neurosurg Spine* 11(5):607-613, 2009.

62. Lin CC, Shen WC, Lo YC, et al: Recurrent pain after percutaneous vertebroplasty. *AJR Am J Roentgenol* 194(5):1323-1329, 2010.

63. Kao FC, Tu YK, Lai PL, et al: Inferior vena cava syndrome following percutaneous vertebroplasty with polymethylmethacrylate. *Spine (Phila Pa 1976)* 33(10):E329-E333, 2008.

64. Wendling D, Runge M, Toussirot E, et al: Vertebral osteitis adjacent to kyphoplasty. *Joint Bone Spine* 77(1):67-69, 2010.

65. Söyüncü Y, Ozdemir H, Söyüncü S, et al: Posterior spinal epidural abscess: an unusual complication of vertebroplasty. *Joint Bone Spine* 73(6):753-755, 2006.

66. Mueller M, Daniels-Wredenhagen M, Besch L, et al: Postoperative aseptic osteonecrosis in a case of kyphoplasty. *Eur Spine J* 18(suppl 2):213-216, 2009.

67. Chen YJ, Chang GC, Chen WH, et al: Local metastases along the tract of needle: a rare complication of vertebroplasty in treating spinal metastases. *Spine (Phila Pa 1976)* 32(21):E615-E618, 2007.

68. Tsai YD, Liliang PC, Chen HJ, et al: Anterior spinal artery syndrome following vertebroplasty: a case report. *Spine (Phila Pa 1976)* 35(4):E134-E136, 2010.

69. Venmans A, Klazen CA, Lohle PN, van Rooij WJ: Percutaneous vertebroplasty and procedural pain. *AJNR Am J Neuroradiol.* 31(5):830-831, 2010.

70. Waldman S: *Atlas of interventional pain management*, ed 2, Philadelphia, 2004, Saunders (Elsevier), pp 587-590.

71. Powell MF, DiNobile D, Reddy AS: C-arm fluoroscopic cone beam CT for guidance of minimally invasive spine interventions. *Pain Physician* 13(1):51-59, 2010.

72. Syed MI, Shaikh A: Vertebroplasty: a systematic approach. *Pain Physician* 10(2):367-380, 2007.

73. Liu J, Bendok B: Osteoporosis and percutaneous vertebroplasty. In *Essentials of pain medicine and regional anesthesia*, Philadelphia, 2005, Elsevier, p 506.

74. Miller D, Fenton D, Dion J: Vertebroplasty. In *Image-guided spine intervention*, Philadelphia, 2003, Saunders, p 202.

75. Ruiz-Lopez R, Pichot C: Vertebroplasty. In *Interventional pain management*, ed 2, Philadelphia, 2008, Saunders, pp 561-562.

76. Moreland DB, Landi MK, Grand W: Vertebroplasty: techniques to avoid complications. *Spine J* 1(1):66-71, 2001.

77. Miller D, Fenton D, Dion J: Vertebroplasty. In *Image-guided spine intervention*, Philadelphia, 2003, Saunders, p 208.

78. Georgy B: Clinical experience with high-viscosity cements for percutaneous vertebral body augmentation: occurrence, degree, and location of cement leakage compared with kyphoplasty. *AJNR Am J Neuroradiol* 31(3):504-508, 2010.

79. Hamady M, Sheard S: Role of cementoplasty in the management of compression vertebral body fractures. *Postgrad Med J* 85(1004):293-298, 2009.

18 Complications of Intraarticular Joint Injections and Musculoskeletal Injections

Eric G. Cornidez

CHAPTER OVERVIEW

Chapter Synopsis: Intraarticular joint and musculoskeletal injections are considered among the least invasive interventional therapies for chronic pain; nevertheless, the procedures carry inherent risks. Complications associated with intraarticular injection can arise from needle misplacement, causing bleeding, infection, or nerve injury, or from interactions with the injectate itself. Injected air can result in air embolism, and hyaluronic acid injection can produce synovitis. The risks of trigger point injection are usually limited to pain at the injection site, but infection and damage to surrounding structures can uncommonly arise.

Important Points:
- There should be a constant awareness of potential complications from interventional pain procedures, and efforts to minimize these complications should be implemented.
- Although uncommon, complications from intraarticular injections arise from needle placement or the injectate itself.
- Trigger points are arguably considered among the safest interventions in a pain practice; however, they are not without risk. This risk includes tenderness at injection site, bleeding, infection, and injury to nearby structures.

Introduction

Over recent years, interventional pain management has grown steadily. Consequently, the prevention of complications from interventional pain procedures should be a very important aspect of pain management. Although the true incidence is difficult to assess, it is extremely important to note and understand the potential risks and consequences. Appendicular intraarticular joint (hip, knee, shoulder, hand) and musculoskeletal injections are deemed some of the safest procedures performed in interventional pain management. The most common complications are infection, although septic arthritis, osteomyelitis, peripheral nerve injuries, pneumothorax, and skeletal muscle toxicity have all been reported (**Table 18-1**). The use of ultrasonography or fluoroscopy can assist in the visualization of nearby structures, thus decreasing the incidence of damage of these structures.

Hip Joint Injections

Hip injection is a common procedure to alleviate hip pain because this is a location commonly affected by osteoarthritis (**Fig. 18-1**). Complications are rare with hip joint injections with proper patient selection, proper sterile technique, and appropriate injection technique. As with other injections, potential complications include bleeding or bruising, infection, allergic reaction to injectate, and increased pain. Injury to the femoral neurovascular bundle is a theoretical complication using an anterior approach to the hip joint, although it has yet to be described. The use of ultrasonography would allow visualization of this neurovascular bundle and would decrease the possibility of injury. Cheng and Abdil[1] (2007) describe air embolism in three pediatric patients undergoing hip injections. During arthrography, injections of a small amount of air can be used to outline the joint for correct needle placement. These injections were done with even small amounts of air (<5 mL). This has not been described in the adult population.

Greater trochanteric bursal injections are commonly given for bursitis-related hip pain. Necrotizing fasciitis has been reported in a case report in 2001 by Hofmeister and Engelhardt.[2] Although this is an isolated incident, this soft tissue infection is limb and life threatening and ultimately resulted in death in this patient.

Glenohumeral Joint Injections

Subacromial and intraarticular injections (**Fig. 18-2**) are commonly provided for shoulder pain when other conservative therapies such as physical therapy, heat and ice, and over-the-counter

Table 18-1: Potential Complications and Avoidance at Each Site

Joint	Problem	Avoidance
Hip joint	Infection Neurovascular (femoral) injury Air embolism Synovitis	Meticulous sterile technique Ultrasonography for visualization Minimal air for injectate Reasonable concentration of corticosteroid
Shoulder joint	Infection Neurovascular (axillary or brachial plexus) injury	Meticulous sterile technique Ultrasonography
Knee joint	Infection Neurovascular injury	Meticulous sterile technique Ultrasonography
Intramuscular or trigger point	Bleeding Infection Myositis Injury to nearby structures	Use smaller gauge needle Meticulous sterile technique Avoid myotoxic local anesthetic (i.e., bupivacaine) Ultrasonography for visualization

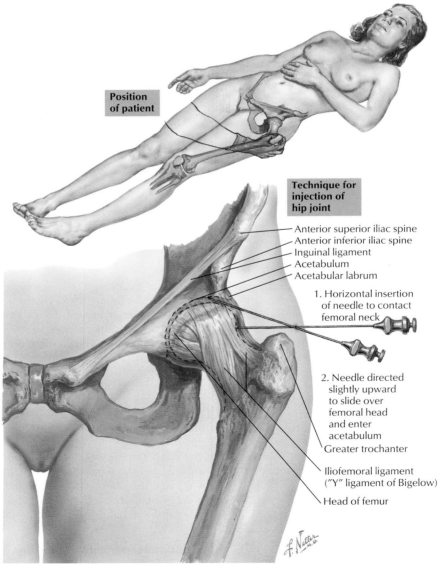

Position of patient

Technique for injection of hip joint

Anterior superior iliac spine
Anterior inferior iliac spine
Inguinal ligament
Acetabulum
Acetabular labrum

1. Horizontal insertion of needle to contact femoral neck

2. Needle directed slightly upward to slide over femoral head and enter acetabulum

Greater trochanter

Iliofemoral ligament ("Y" ligament of Bigelow)

Head of femur

Fig. 18-1 Articulation of the femoral head and the acetabulum of the pelvis. Intraarticular injections would be within this space (as shown). This image also shows the greater trochanter of the femur, the site of greater trochanteric bursal injections. (Netter illustration from www.netterimages.com. © Elsevier, Inc. All rights reserved.)

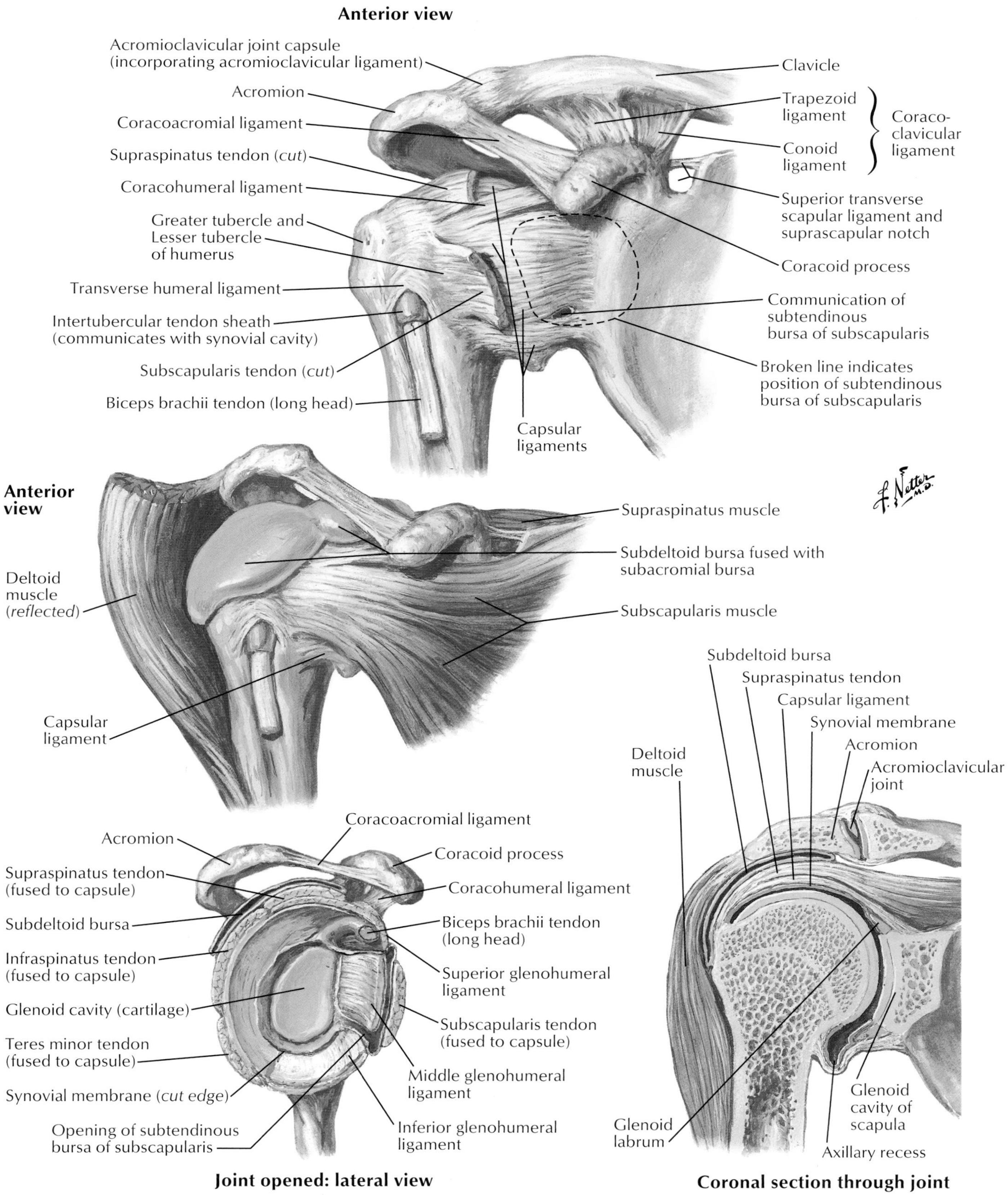

Anterior view

Acromioclavicular joint capsule
(incorporating acromioclavicular ligament)

Acromion

Coracoacromial ligament

Supraspinatus tendon (*cut*)

Coracohumeral ligament

Greater tubercle and
Lesser tubercle
of humerus

Transverse humeral ligament

Intertubercular tendon sheath
(communicates with synovial cavity)

Subscapularis tendon (*cut*)

Biceps brachii tendon (long head)

Capsular
ligaments

Clavicle

Trapezoid
ligament

Conoid
ligament

Coraco-
clavicular
ligament

Superior transverse
scapular ligament and
suprascapular notch

Coracoid process

Communication of
subtendinous
bursa of subscapularis

Broken line indicates
position of subtendinous
bursa of subscapularis

**Anterior
view**

Deltoid
muscle
(*reflected*)

Capsular
ligament

Supraspinatus muscle

Subdeltoid bursa fused with
subacromial bursa

Subscapularis muscle

F. Netter M.D.

Subdeltoid bursa

Supraspinatus tendon

Capsular ligament

Synovial membrane

Acromion

Acromioclavicular
joint

Deltoid
muscle

Glenoid
labrum

Glenoid
cavity of
scapula

Axillary recess

Acromion

Supraspinatus tendon
(fused to capsule)

Subdeltoid bursa

Infraspinatus tendon
(fused to capsule)

Glenoid cavity (cartilage)

Teres minor tendon
(fused to capsule)

Synovial membrane (*cut edge*)

Opening of subtendinous
bursa of subscapularis

Coracoacromial ligament

Coracoid process

Coracohumeral ligament

Biceps brachii tendon
(long head)

Superior glenohumeral
ligament

Subscapularis tendon
(fused to capsule)

Middle glenohumeral
ligament

Inferior glenohumeral
ligament

Joint opened: lateral view

Coronal section through joint

Fig. 18-2 Joint of the shoulder. One can visualize the articulation between the humerus and the glenoid cavity. (Netter illustration from www.netterimages.com. © Elsevier, Inc. All rights reserved.)

antiinflammatory medications are not effective. With proper patients being selected (i.e., no active infection, no bleeding diathesis), using sterile technique, and performing proper injection technique, complications are extremely rare with glenohumeral joint injections. Injury to a neurovascular structure is a potential complication as well, but it should be minimized with proper preprocedure planning and proper technique. In addition, the use of ultrasonography may further minimize this complication.

Infection, although uncommon, is a significant complication. Meticulous adherence to sterile technique is emphasized for performing both subacromial and intraarticular shoulder injections. As in greater trochanteric bursal injection described earlier, necrotizing fasciitis has also been reported during an intraarticular shoulder injection.[3] This patient recovered after extensive surgical debridement, aggressive resuscitative efforts, and intravenous antibiotics. A case of scapular osteomyelitis after subacromial corticosteroid injection has also been reported. Again, meticulous attention to sterile technique has been suggested.[4]

Knee Joint Injections

Knee osteoarthritis is a common disease among the adult population. Knee joint corticosteroid injection is commonly performed for pain management. In addition, intraarticular viscosupplementation with hyaluronic acid–based products has also gained popularity as a potential treatment of knee pain caused by degenerative changes. Complications of knee injections have been noted to be pain at the site of injection, damage to nerves (i.e., saphenous neuropathy), septic arthritis, and granulomatous inflammation of the synovium.

Pain at the site of injection has been noted to have the highest prevalence; it may occur in 20% of patients.[5] However, severe local inflammation and development of joint effusion are rare.[5] Granulomatous inflammation of the synovium was reported in six cases of hyaluronic acid–based injections in 2002.[5]

Although there is a theoretical risk of damage to neurovascular structures, there has been only one case of saphenous neuropathy after a medial approach to an intraarticular knee injection (**Fig. 18-3**).[6]

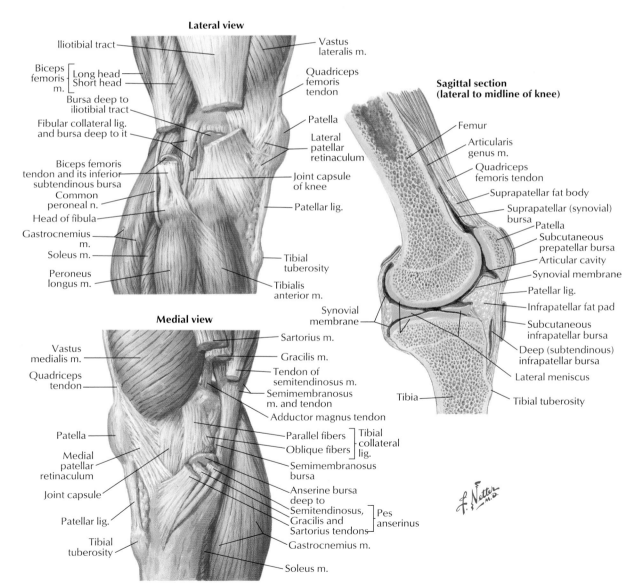

Fig. 18-3 Articulation between the femur and the tibia. Intraarticular injections are commonly achieved by entering just medial or lateral to the patellar ligament. (Netter illustration from www.netterimages.com. © Elsevier, Inc. All rights reserved.)

Septic arthritis has been reported in a few cases with different organisms, including *Actinomyces naeslundii* and *Candida albicans*.[7-9] Aseptic acute arthritis has also been described in two cases.[10]

Trigger Point Injections

Trigger point injections are generally considered very safe. They are common procedures performed by many practitioners, including pain, primary care, and emergency department physicians. Even though they are considered very safe, serious complications can result. Some of these complications include pneumothorax, intrathecal injection, epidural abscess, and skeletal muscle toxicity.[11-14] Of the 276 claims reported in the American Society of Anesthesiologists Closed Claims Project, 17 cases involved trigger point injections in which pneumothorax (15 of 17 cases) was the most common.[15]

Skeletal muscle toxicity is a rare and uncommon side effect of local anesthetics. In fact, intramuscular injections with any local anesthetic can result in reversible myonecrosis. Bupivacaine seems to be the most myotoxic, and procaine appears to be the least.[14] In most cases, there is no sequela and muscle regeneration, and healing usually take 3 to 4 weeks.[14]

Regarding trigger point injections of the quadratus and iliopsoas muscles, there are particular points to mention given the proximity of vital nearby structures. As described before, the quadratus has its origin at the iliac crest and iliolumbar ligament and inserts around the 12th rib and the transverse processes of the lumbar vertebrae (**Fig. 18-4**). It is posterior to the kidney; thus injection should be done with this in mind because renal damage is a potential risk, although it has yet to be described. The iliopsoas muscle is lateral to the vertebral foramen and posterior to the lumbar sympathetic chain and the great vessels of the abdomen, so caution with needle depth is important.

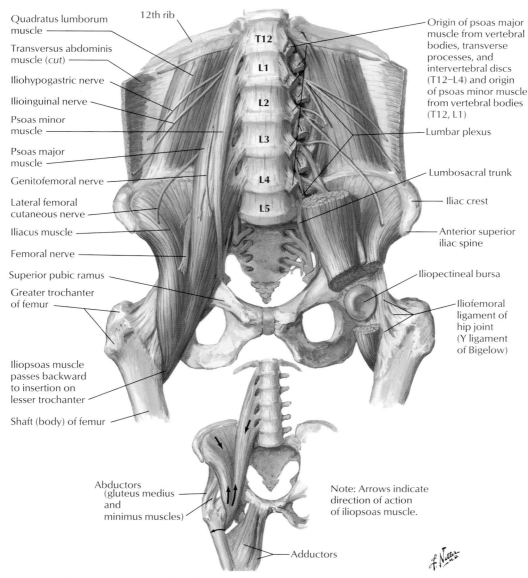

Fig. 18-4 Representation of the deep muscles of the lumbar spine and pelvis. (Netter illustration from www.netterimages.com. © Elsevier, Inc. All rights reserved.)

Conclusion

Intraarticular and musculoskeletal injections are very common in pain management and deemed very safe. The majority of complications are bleeding, infection, increased pain, and damage to nearby structures. Nonetheless, these complications can be minimal with careful patient selection, meticulous attention to sterility, and appropriate technique. The use of ultrasonography or fluoroscopy can aid in further decreasing the risk of injury.

References

1. Cheng J, Abdi S: Complications of joint, tendon, and muscle injections. *Tech Reg Anesth Pain Manag* 11(3):141-147, 2007.

2. Hofmeister E, Engelhardt S: Necrotizing fasciitis as complication of injection into greater trochanteric bursa. *Am J Orthop* 30:426-427, 2001.

3. Birkinshaw R, O'Donnell J, Sammy I: Necrotising fasciitis as a complication of steroid injection. *J Accid Emerg Med* 14:52-54, 1997.

4. Buckley SL, Alexander AH, Barrack RL: Scapular osteomyelitis. An unusual complication following subacromial corticosteroid injection. *Orthop Rev* 18: 321-324, 1989.

5. Chen AL, Desai P, Adler EM, et al: Granulomatous inflammation after Hylan G-F 20 viscosupplementation of the knee: a report of six cases. *J Bone Joint Surg* 84-A(7):1142-1147, 2002.

6. Iizuka M, Yao R, Wainapel S: Saphenous nerve injury following medial knee joint injection: a case report. *Arch Phys Med Rehabil* 86:2062-2065, 2005.

7. Lequerre T, Nouvellon M, Kraznowska K, et al: Septic arthritis due to *Actinomyces naeslundii*: report of a case. *Joint Bone Spine* 69:499-501, 2002.

8. Evanich JD, Evanich CJ, Wright MB, et al: Efficacy of intraarticular hyaluronic acid injections in knee osteoarthritis. *Clin Orthop Relat Res* 390:173-181, 2001.

9. Christensson B, Ryd L, Dahlberg L, et al: *Candida albicans arthritis* in a nonimmunocompromised patient. Complication of placebo intra-articular injections. *Acta Orthop Scand* 64:695-698, 1993.

10. Charalambous CP, Tryfonidis M, Sadiq S, et al: Septic arthritis following intra-articular steroid injection of the knee—a survey of current practice regarding antiseptic technique used during intraarticular steroid injection of the knee. *Clin Rheumatol* 22:386-390, 2003.

11. Shafer N: Pneumothorax following "trigger point" injection. *JAMA* 213:1193, 1970.

12. Nelson LS, Hoffman RS: Intrathecal injection: unusual complication of trigger-point injection therapy. *Ann Emerg Med* 32:506-508, 1998.

13. Elias M: Cervical epidural abscess following trigger point injection. *J Pain Sympt Manage* 9:71-72, 1994.

14. Zink W, Graf BM: Local anesthetic myotoxicity. *Reg Anesth Pain Med* 29:333-340, 2004.

15. Fitzgibbon DR, Posner KL, Domino KB, et al: American Society of Anesthesiologists. Chronic pain management: American Society of Anesthesiologists Closed Claims Project. *Anesthesiology* 100:98-105, 2004.

Index